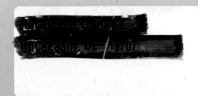

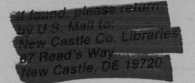

The Complete Guide to Mental Health for Women

The Complete Guide to

MENTAL HEALTH

for

WOMEN

Edited by Lauren Slater, Ed.D.,

Jessica Henderson Daniel, Ph.D., ABPP

and Amy Elizabeth Banks, M.D.

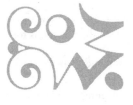

BEACON PRESS

BOSTON

Beacon Press
25 Beacon Street
Boston, Massachusetts 02108-2892
www.beacon.org

Beacon Press books
are published under the auspices of
the Unitarian Universalist Association of Congregations.

This book is meant to educate, but it should not be used as a substitute for personal medical advice. The reader should consult her clinician for specific information concerning her individual medical condition. The authors have done their best to ensure that the information presented here is accurate up to the time of publication. However, as research and development are ongoing, it is possible that new findings may supersede some of the data presented here. The names of organizations, products, or alternative therapies appearing in the book are given for informational purposes only.

Many of the designations used by manufacturers and sellers to distinguish their products are claimed as trademarks. Where those designations appear in this book and Beacon Press was aware of a trademark claim, the designations have been printed in initial capital letters (for example, Prozac).

Excerpt from "A New View of Women's Sexual Problems" by The Working Group for a New View of Women's Sexual Problems, from *Women & Therapy*, Volume 24 (1/2), reprinted by permission of The Haworth Press, Inc.

Illustration on page 222 from A. J. Stunkard, T. Sorenson, and F. Schulsinger, "Use of the Danish Adoption Register for the Study of Obesity and Thinness," in *The Genetics of Neurological and Psychiatric Disorders*, ed. S. S. Kety, L. P. Rowland, R. L. Sidman, and S. W. Matthysse (New York: Raven Press, 1983), 115–120.

Printed in the United States of America

07 06 05 04 03 8 7 6 5 4 3 2 1

This book is printed on acid-free paper that meets the uncoated paper ANSI/NISO specifications for permanence as revised in 1992.

Text design and composition by Wilsted & Taylor Publishing Services

Library of Congress Cataloging-in-Publication Data
The complete guide to mental health for women / edited by Lauren Slater, Jessica Henderson Daniel, and Amy Banks.—1st ed.
   p. cm.
  ISBN 0-8070-2924-6 (hardcover : alk. paper)—ISBN 0-8070-2925-4 (pbk. : alk. paper)
   1. Women—Mental health—United States. 2. Women—Mental health—Social aspects. 3. Feminist psychology. 4. Life cycle, Human.
I. Slater, Lauren. II. Daniel, Jessica Henderson. III. Banks, Amy.

  RC451.4.W6C65 2003
  616.89'0082—dc21   2003010436

Contents

PART TWO: MENTAL DISORDERS

PART THREE: GETTING HELP

PART FOUR: LIFE ENHANCEMENTS

Why *women's* mental health? Why not just *general* mental health? Here's why:

At Ohio State University a researcher by the name of Janice Kiecolt-Glaser has spent the last decade inquiring into the different ways men and women experience stress in marriage. One of her recent experimental designs involves asking couples into her lab, giving them minor skin wounds, and then observing the rate at which healing happens. Kiecolt-Glaser is especially interested in how couples in good marriages fare versus couples in "bad" marriages, marriages in which conflict is expressed negatively, even violently. What she has found: Women in the stress of a difficult relationship exhibit higher levels of immunosuppressing stress hormones and heal from puncture wounds more slowly than their male counterparts. Women in good marital relationships heal well, suggesting that marriage does have health benefits as well as risks. The most surprising finding here, however, is that the men, in neither scenario—the good or bad relationship—exhibit the same intense physiological responses to relational conflict as do women. Men's wounds heal at pretty much the same rate, regardless of what their loved ones are doing or saying. Kiecolt-Glaser wonders why this is. So do we. What we suspect is that men's ability to compartmentalize their experiences offers them a certain amount of protective gloss when it comes to the domestic front, or the warfront, for that matter. In any case, studies like Kiecolt-Glaser's only underscore what common sense tells so many of us: Men and women are different, in mind and body, in soma and psyche. They are different from the first ten weeks of life, when that initial pulse of testosterone does or does not wash its way over the fetal brain. They are different in hormonal development, in brain development, in physiological development, and in social development. More important, even with the rise in the 1970s of women's studies programs, the challenges and strengths of the female gender are still too often ignored in science. Our models of female psychological development are still largely male. Our models in medicine are still almost exclusively male.

Therefore, that's why: *women's mental health.*

Our brains and bodies and the lives that flow from these are women's lives, with problems and challenges unique to our gender.

And we have been overlooked.

Some groups of women, however, have been more overlooked than others. Historically, the voices of middle- and upper-class women have mistakenly been heard as representative of all women. We have taken special care to provide for you a book that includes diverse authors, whose perspectives address the issue of invisibility and silence for a range of women. In here you will find writing by women of color; you will also find writing from and about other marginalized women: women who are childless by choice, women who are victims of terrorism, women who live in poverty. The book is prismatic in that it attempts to capture and refract the full spectrum of female experience with the hope of shedding some kind of light on the topics at hand. We have deliberately chosen to allow the essays in this book their own personal hues; there are many shadings here, many styles, many voices, many women. There is, therefore, no need to read straight through. You can come at this curved and curving, finding the chapters or sections that speak to you most.

However you approach this volume, though, you will find throughout it an attempt to understand women's lives not only by the sicknesses we sometimes suffer, but also by the life stages we all move through, in whichever way we choose to define them. Too often books about mental health focus not on health at all, but on the pathologies. However, while acknowledging the pathologies, we begin our book by talking about ourselves from a position of strength, of growth. All women, all beings, in fact, complete a life cycle while here on this earth, a life cycle with some predictable stages, despite race or class or color. From the smallest, single-celled organism that begins its existence as a nucleus and ends in the much discussed cell atrophy, or cell death, to the human being, who begins her headlong descent in a rush of oxytosin and ends with the inevitable atrophy of billions of neurons, organisms share the fact that we are prompted by and fashioned from the stages that preceded us. For a woman, the first mature stage begins when she exits adolescence. Thus, we have chosen to begin our life cycle section with young adulthood, the point at which the neophyte is poised on the cusp of college or career, about to make a second entry, this time not from the womb but from the walls of her childhood home. From there we move into motherhood as a life stage, with an essay that considers the ups and downs of this sometimes serrated, sometimes smooth journey, and then into a consideration of childlessness by choice. Our life stages section cycles through middle age and old age in an attempt to locate the facets of these experiences that are unique to women.

In this country, women are more likely to be prescribed antidepressants than men. The majority of primary care physician appointments are made by women. Jonathan Metzl, a psychiatrist and scholar at the University Of Michigan, has done a full-scale study of pharmaceutical ads from their first inception in the 1960s through to the Effexor-laced era of our day. He has found, not surprisingly, that the vast majority of these ads picture the (white) female as patient and the doctor as a bald-headed, boxy-looking man in the mythic white coat. Whether women are patients more than men because of cultural forces or whether they are somehow more physiologically vulnerable to certain phenomena in life than men is not a point we want to, or even can, debate here. What is clear is that women, for whatever reasons, do suffer from psychiatric syndromes, some germane only to our gender, such as postpartum depression, others shared fully by both genders, such as depression. The second part of this book deals with these psychiatric syndromes with an eye toward getting as much information across to you, the reader, as possible. We assume that many of our readers who turn to this section will do so because they, or one of their loved ones, are suffering. We hope to be of some help in such a situation, to proffer hope where we can, and to give sound statistics and research in all cases.

Of course, no book on mental health would be complete without a guide to the psychopharmacological components that contribute to our well-being and much of our cultural angst as well. Unlike the other sections of this book, which are written by a wide variety of women with many different professional and personal experiences, the psychopharmacology section is written exclusively by people with a license to dispense the medications they are describing. We have also included a section on medications and pregnancy, as this is an issue millions upon millions of women confront.

In this day and age, much treatment for mental health issues is, in fact, limited to psychopharmacology. We believe this is, in many instances, a mistake. Recent research points to a combination of psychopharmacology and therapy as being the most effective agent of "cure." Even without this research, however, we would still feel as we do: Even an illness that is purely biological in scope affects one's outlook, one's sense of competency, one's sense of security. Psychotherapies are the means by which we make sense of our experiences, and they are always appropriate for anyone with a mental health issue. However, the field of therapy has a range of subsets within it, and women have many options from which to choose. We have tried to provide you with essays by practitioners that describe the current offerings, from cognitive behavioral treatments to dialectic behavior therapy to more controversial interventions like EMDR. Because this is a book about mental health, written by mental health practitioners, we have not included in our therapy/treatment section other possible means of accessing help. We do believe in the efficacy of other means, however. In addition to therapists, there are ministers, rabbis, spiritual guides, best friends; even mothers can do a lot. You take your help where you can find it. Here we are offering finds only within our fields of expertise.

We end the book by talking not about life cycles but lifestyles, the ways in which women can accentuate their own positive experiences through spirituality, exercise, and play. Because, when all is said and done, we are really playing our way through the troughs and peaks of our gendered existence. We played as children, and we continue to play as adults. If this book has any message embedded in it, it may be this: Despite the rising range of cultural and racial diversity in this country, despite the ever-changing demographics of our country and our world, which we have tried to represent here—we are still united by some central human qualities, some central human experiences, deep inexplicable sadnesses, the specter of our own deaths, the growing pains of youth, and the human animal's propensity for joy, that feeling we still get, against all odds. It's there.

PART ONE

Psychology and the Life Cycle

Late Adolescence and Early Adulthood

Imagine that you are standing before a bridge. You had heard about others' travels over the bridge and were told one day you, too, would have to cross it. As a child, hearing about the bridge that will appear before you when you are approximately eighteen years old seemed eons away. It was hard to imagine what it would look like, not to mention what *you* would look like then. Hard to imagine the bridge also because all of the stories you heard from different women about their journey over the bridge were both similar and totally different. The bridge represents the transition from being an adolescent to an adult. One travels the bridge of young adulthood during this time, reaching the other side when you become approximately twenty-two years old.

So there you are, eighteen years old, standing at the foot of the bridge. Imagine that it is wide. Imagine now, for the purposes of this chapter, that there are three paths that run alongside each other for the entire length of the bridge. One path represents work, another represents higher education, and the third represents partnership/marriage and/or family. You cannot see the other side. You cannot tell what the end of each path looks like, and you feel that you do not know where you are going even though you have already chosen which path you will use to cross. These paths are not separated by any barrier and you have been told that you may change your path or walk along multiple paths as you go.

Think of me as your tour guide. I will be pointing out different signposts that may help you identify what you might encounter depending on which path you have chosen as you travel over the bridge. As your tour guide, I will attempt to give you a way to understand the general emotional landscape. Why might you want to identify signposts that you may encounter along the way? The bridge looks straight and simple, right?

Human experience is rarely simple. Experience is made even more complicated when there is change. Change can be perceived as good or as bad, but in either case, usually it is hard. Growth is always paired with loss. In young adulthood, change is paramount, transition is the heart of experience. No matter what path you have chosen to take, you can expect it to be rocky and somewhat unfamiliar. Knowing that may lessen the normal experience of anxiety. In the history of psychology, many theorists have attempted to study the course of development across the life span. Many of the theorists have been men, until recently when female psychologists have begun to study and write about girls' development. The main critique of the male developmental theories is that they are based on examining male development and then applying that to women. Some of the thinking is useful and applicable and some of it falls short.

Psychologist and writer Carol Gilligan has been a pioneer in this area. Gilligan states again and again in her writings that we must pay attention to the fact that women develop in relationship. Gilligan has theorized that when girls move into adolescence they oftentimes "lose their voice." Many women find that the move into young adulthood is a time when they begin to reclaim their voice as they develop a firmer sense of themselves in the world. Erik Erikson, a developmental theorist, conceptualized the life span in terms of conflicts that arise at different stages. He believed that when the environment makes new demands on an individual, conflict arises. The "environment" is a phase of life. He determined the primary task of young adulthood to be centered around the resolution of "intimacy versus isolation." In other words, the primary work in young adulthood focuses on developing intimate relationships or suffering feelings of isolation. If one adds a feminist perspective to Erikson's theory, one could say that for women, the conflict is not only to develop intimacy with others, but primarily to begin to develop intimacy with one's self.

> Human experience is rarely simple. Experience is made even more complicated when there is change. Change can be perceived as good or as bad, but in either case, usually it is hard.

Before we move into what you might expect as you go over the bridge, it is important to consider the cultural landscape the bridge spans. What are the "American" cultural expectations of women during young adulthood? Young women pick up all kinds of messages out there, such as "You can do anything you want," "You should be a mom and raise a family," "You can have it all—a career and children," "You are as valuable as you look," "The thinner, the better," "The nicer, the better," "Put others before yourself," "Men have all of the power," "Women are powerful," "Your work must be meaningful," and so forth. Bear in mind that not only do young women pick up on the many mixed messages regarding expectations, power, and value from the larger culture, each woman's experience is informed by her personal cultural landscape, which is particular to her unique familial experiences/expectations and heritage.

I will be describing experiences that are common during young adulthood that arise on different paths. Of course, it is impossible to adequately describe all the possibilities and variations of experience. In addition, imagine the various emotional responses/struggles I describe as being on a continuum. For example, feelings of sadness can range from feeling blue to mild depression to major depression. Another example would be a continuum ranging from worried feelings to panic. Now, imagine you are back at the foot of the bridge and you take your first step onto the higher education path. You may have traveled far away from home to reach the start of this path, or perhaps home was close by. Imagine now that you are surrounded by all of the other people who are waiting to step onto the path at the same time with you. Maybe you know someone from home. Maybe you do not see a familiar face. You've got plenty of company, but perhaps you still feel alone and scared.

The first year of college has been described by countless women as both intensely scary and exciting. Everything is new. New people, places, classes, and expectations. You may have a new roommate, new cafeteria food, new schedule, and new responsibilities. Sound overwhelming? Usually it is.

Many women find themselves excited and nervous about their newfound freedom and responsibilities. This time of transition allows students to be on their own, but live in a contained environment; this allows for some feelings of security, but is not without its stresses. In college, depression can surface, as can issues of sexuality, competence, and comparison with peers, intellectual exploration, and the stress of competition. In addition, alcohol and drug use is prevalent. Many women have to work to help support themselves during this time in addition to going to school. Economic status has an effect on stress level as does the amount of familial support one has.

As you already know, the longer you are on a path, the more familiar it becomes. This is true in general, but it also shifts as the path bends or winds. So, while the first year is marked by primarily trying to get oriented, the second year is marked more by focusing inward. Friendships tend to deepen and solidify, and relationships are explored further. This, of course, is again both exciting and fear inducing.

In my work in a college counseling center, many women describe feeling a major difference in the second year not while at school but more so when they returned home. I heard many stories about women returning home to find that their families had adjusted to their absence—really well. This often stirs up both feelings of loss and relief. Loss of one's position in the way the family works, but relief that things haven't fallen apart. It can feel confusing when your role in your family shifts and is compensated for.

The third year is often described as the most comfortable. The path feels known and is more easily navigated. Anxiety about graduation begins to seep in, but it still feels far enough away that the anxious feelings usually do not become overwhelming. The final year, however, is marked by intense anxiety and excitement regarding graduation and going out into the "real world." Both the worry of what it will be like to navigate a whole new path and the anticipated loss of friends are paramount. There you are, finally feeling comfortable and competent, moving toward accomplishment, and in front of you, you see yet another bridge, and you recall what it was like when you began school and feel those feelings again. Now you see yourself moving into your role as part of the freshman class of the world.

So, as you travel along this path, you will find many gains and losses and experience a wide array of feelings. Some feelings may seem contradictory but be happening at the same time, like feeling excited to graduate and sad to leave friends and your community. How you respond to those feelings and where you fall on the continuum I spoke about earlier helps you determine which supports might be useful to you. A measure of depressed and anxious feelings along the way is expected; however, if you find yourself feeling overwhelmed, the rest of this book may help you find yourself and aid you in understanding and/or making a plan. Many universities and colleges have mental health centers that are accessible to students, usually for a nominal fee, which makes them a convenient and affordable resource.

Next, let's step onto the path of committed relationship and/or family in young adulthood. If the main task of young adulthood is to develop intimacy with others and oneself, it would make sense that entering into a committed relationship with a partner, and/or a baby for that matter, would present both obstacles and opportunities.

I recently spoke with a nineteen-year-old young woman who has found herself traveling over the bridge with her three-month-old baby girl. I will call this young woman Linda. When I asked Linda what the hardest thing was about being such a young mom, she said that the loss of her friends and social life was the most difficult for her. Although she still maintained connections with her friends, she found her friendships changed due to the lack of freedom she felt. Linda could not identify anything "easy" about being on the path of motherhood at her age, but she did state that she found herself surprised. Linda said that the greatest opportunity for her was the discovery of wisdom that she had no idea she possessed. She said, "It is amazing how much you think you have no idea what you are doing, but then you figure it out. . . . You figure out that you do know what to do . . . you are smarter than you thought you were." Linda's statement is a great example of how feelings of competence are discovered or uncovered during young adulthood. Linda is both surprised and proud of her self-discovery, and she said that this helped to sustain her through the rough spots, like when she feels overwhelmed, exhausted, and frustrated. Or when she might wonder what her life would be like without her baby, but then she can't imagine that either sometimes.

If you decide to cross the bridge with a husband or a partner and/or a child, you might bump into difficulties locating your own needs in the face of others'. Research has shown that women focus outward more often toward significant relationships. It is not to say, though, that women do not or cannot direct care toward themselves, but there is a tendency to focus "out" rather than "in." Because your task is not only to develop intimacy, but also to begin to deepen your sense of who you are in the world, especially during this stage of your life, it will be a greater challenge to continually try to redefine yourself and your place. The demands of a partner and/or child make the task more difficult for young adults because developmentally young adults are called to figure out "who I am" and "what I am going to do now that I am a grown-up."

> You may take side roads, or your path may be straight and narrow.

Most of us remember being asked the question, "What do you what to be when you grow up?" When you step on the path of work, it may or may not be what you had ever imagined you would be doing. Also, you might not feel that you are "grown up" yet either. But there you are, in any case, going to work. Now, when we talk about work, let's remember that often women are not just "working" at a job. Oftentimes, women are working simultaneously at school or on their families, so you might imagine one foot stepping on the path of work while the other falls onto one of the other paths on the bridge. But, for the sake of this particular discussion, "work" will equal "employment."

Like anything else, there will be aspects that feel positive about going to work and aspects that feel more negative. If you find yourself not doing what you had imagined you would be doing at your age, it can feel disheartening and discouraging. One twenty-year-old woman I spoke with expressed dismay at the notion of having to work for the rest of her life in a retail store. She felt scared because she could not imagine how she would be able to shift into a new career and worried that her life would be the same day after day. On the other hand, another young eighteen-year-old woman said that she found work to be "organizing" in that it gave shape to her days and gave her a sense of accomplishment. Much of young adulthood concerns building competence and confidence. One of the ways that happens is in the daily activity of work.

Let me introduce you to Hannah, who has just graduated from college and is starting her first job out of school in a field she did not study and for a lot less money than she had expected. She comes into my office, flops herself down onto the couch, and lets out an enormous sigh. She says, "Okay, let me get this straight, my time in college was supposed to be the best time of my life, right? It's supposed to have prepared me to go out into the world? So, why is it that I felt miserable for the first half of college—you know how depressed I was—and just when I was feeling like I got the hang of school and my life there I had to leave, and now I feel like I am a freshman again, except there is no orientation to the work world. Am I supposed to know what to do here?" I then try help Hannah hold what feel like contradictory ideas, but which are both true. I remind Hannah that the truth is that she does know on some level what to do (she did struggle and learn how to manage her depression, she did secure a job and an apartment with roommates). The truth, also, is that she feels completely disoriented and it is very difficult to stay connected to the part of her that has a sense of her wisdom and competence.

The example of Hannah is a good one because it also points to the fact that change and stress occur *throughout* young adulthood, not just when you stand and face the entrance to the bridge for the first time. It is common to move in and out of feeling competent, connected, and in control. At the same time, it is important to note that young women oftentimes struggle with depression, low self-esteem, distorted body image, procrastination, bouts of sadness, disorientation, and other difficulties. Depression and other mental disorders such as Bipolar Disorder can surface in late adolescence and young adulthood. A biosocial perspective accounts for genetic predispositions toward certain disorders or illnesses in addition to the effects of the environment and then looks at how these two factors interact. For example, if an individual is predisposed to depression, moving into the adult world with the added stressors and the usual lessening of familiar support systems may tip this person into a depressive episode.

Oftentimes, eating disorders such as anorexia and bulimia manifest in adolescence and/or young adulthood. This may be accounted for in the cultural expectations of thinness and its perceived value. Young women frequently report high levels of self-loathing of their bodies even if they do not meet the criteria for a particular disorder. Betty, a young woman twenty years old, has struggled with bulimia since she was fourteen. Betty describes feeling as though she is split—that the emotional/intellectual part of her (neck up) is of value and that she is "a good person inside," but "then there is my body" (the neck down), which she believes is bad and disgusting.

When stressed, Betty has coped by eating enormous amounts of food that she then throws up. She has described the effect as "numbing" and that she feels "more in control afterwards." Betty reports that she had managed to cope in other ways for many years, but that when she moved into young adulthood, the old behaviors became more compelling again and that she found herself "going backwards." She is currently working hard on re-developing other coping mechanisms that are less harmful to herself but finds the constant media bombardment of super-thin women hard to ignore and hard not to internalize. Betty's experience points to the fact that not only can new stressors and difficulties arise, but also issues that had lain dormant for some time can reemerge when there is a developmental shift.

Remember that as you travel over the bridge, you will find that you both know and do not have a clue as to what to do or how to feel in different situations you encounter. It is all practice for tomorrow. Once on the bridge, you can choose to change whichever path you began your journey on, and you may even walk on more than one path at once. You may take side roads, or your path may be straight and narrow.

In any case, whatever you encounter, your job will be to build stronger relationships with those you care for and with yourself, to develop a stronger sense of self, growing areas of confidence and competence and giving voice to whatever choices you make. If you are able to bear in mind that two seemingly opposing emotions often do happen simultaneously, it may enable you to navigate the path with a bit less trepidation.

—Jennifer Coon-Wallman, Psy.D.

RELATED ENTRIES

Anxiety Disorders

Body Image

Depressive Disorders

Eating Disorders and Disconnections

How Do We Define Sexual Health for Women?

Pregnancy as a Life Passage

It's easy to forget that for much of history, a woman's life was taken up with pregnancy and birth. She grew round and large so many times that dress fashion eventually dictated full bodices and hoop skirts voluminous with bustles, as if an adult woman's shape was synonymous with pregnancy.

Like it or not, a woman's body was made to bear fruit and multiply. Crops needed to be harvested. Businesses needed to be managed. Men and women came together to populate the world. A mid-nineteenth-century English working-class woman wrote: "I was my mother's seventh child, and seven more were born after me—fourteen in all—which made my mother a perfect slave. Generally speaking, she was either expecting a baby to be born or had one at the breast" (quoted in *Of Woman Born* by Adrienne Rich).

Middle-class Victorian women, too, lived primarily as reproductive vessels. Although she might average "only" five children, pregnancy and motherhood were seen as her highest and most noble calling. A newly married woman was usually ignorant about sex, pregnancy, or birth and often learned by experience. Custom dictated that a bourgeois woman retreat to the sanctity of her home during the last months of what was called her "confinement." Confinement both protected her famous Victorian modesty and allowed her to focus inward, preparing her nest for the imminent child. Typically, she would prepare a lying-in room, a place she could, ideally, wait out pregnancy's end, give birth, and then, postpartum, literally "lie in"—cared for by her household and caring for the newborn. Pregnancy was seen as a time when a woman should pay special attention to her health. One 1896 manual, *The Glory of Woman or Love, Marriage and Maternity* by Monfort Allen, M.D., and Amelia McGregor, M.D., quoted in *Women at Home in Victorian America* by Ellen M. Plante, advised: "A pregnant lady must retire early to rest. She ought to be in bed every night by ten o'clock, and should make a point of being up and in good time in the morning, that she may have a thorough ablution, a stroll in the garden . . ."

But the fact of life that Victorian women knew too well was the terror of childbirth. Labor pains might be frightening—chloroform anesthesia was not introduced until the late 1840s—but most terrifying to expectant mothers was death by the dreaded "childbed" or puerperal fever. Every Victorian woman knew a woman who died from giving birth. Puerperal fever killed one in four women who gave birth in a Parisian hospital in February 1866. Puerperal fever killed Mary Wollstonecraft when she birthed Mary Shelley. For almost two centuries—until Viennese physician Ignaz Phillip Semmelweis, in 1861, noted the link between physician hand washing and childbed deaths, and then in 1881, when Louis Pasteur demonstrated bacterial infection—puerperal fever killed thousands upon thousands of women. It was thought to be a mysterious epidemic, part of women's curse, and a tragedy for the "weaker sex" to endure.

These high childbirth mortality risks allowed Victorian society to view women as delicate, perishable creatures. How could a woman's life be seen as significant if by fulfilling her highest calling—bringing children into the world—she must be willing to sacrifice her own life?

No wonder, then, that the history of feminism is so closely linked to the history of women's reproductive lives. It is only very recently, in the last forty or so years since the advent of the birth control pill, widespread contraceptive use, and legal abortion, that women have seen pregnancy as a choice, as a part of biology that they can control. Even today, in many Third World countries, family planning is an anomaly. But reproductive choice was a powerful tool for first-wave feminism. Limiting one's childbearing efforts was a necessary prerequisite to women's rise in the workplace, to women's ability to bargain for more equal rights, and to women's economic independence. "Without the full capacity to limit her own reproduction, a woman's other 'freedoms' are tantalizing mockeries that cannotbe exercised," writes Lucinda Cisler in the widely read women's liberation anthology of the 1970s, *Sisterhood Is Powerful*. In 1969, the National Organization for Women (NOW) demanded, as item eight in its Bill of Rights, the following, as quoted in *Sisterhood Is Powerful*: "The right of women to control their own reproductive lives by removing from the penal code laws limiting access to contraceptive information and devices, and by repealing penal laws governing abortion." Today, in

Puerperal fever killed one in four women who gave birth in a Parisian hospital in February 1866.

the twenty-first-century United States of America, the pendulum has swung almost entirely. The U.S. Centers for Disease Control and Prevention report that from 1988 to the near present, women of childbearing age averaged just 1.2 births. As of 1995, almost half of all women who graduated from college were childless, and about 9 percent, or 5.4 million women, had no children and expected none in their lives. In the 1920s, contraception crusader Margaret Sanger endorsed women as free and separate individuals rather than mothers. Her vision appears to have been realized. Never before in the eons of history have women of privilege believed so wholeheartedly and with full entitlement to their childbearing choices.

But has pregnancy become, for women, that much less problematic than it was for our sisters in centuries past? Abortion rights are still being challenged, and today, in the age of technological pregnancies—sonogram, amniocentesis, prenatal tests—the fetal rights movement would again control a woman's pregnant body. Today, the belief that women can control pregnancy extends to the highly lucrative infertility industry. Hormone shots, artificial insemination, in vitro fertilization—the standard repertoire of reproductive therapy—have not only become more widespread, but have received a great deal of media coverage, so much so that not only are women who have difficulty conceiving turning to specialists, but even women who suspect they *might* have difficulty are getting specialists' help with pregnancy.

Ironically, we who have access to more reproductive research and resources than any previous generation of women, and who believe we can have our children when and how we choose, are often as stumped by our biology as women from earlier times. "Once again

I am not pregnant," writes Barbara Shulgold to a newsletter published by RESOLVE, the prominent infertility support organization. "I am trying to be brave through the cramps and, worse, the emotions. I need someone to comfort me, to stop the tears; but I am alone, my husband gone for the week." So begins *Dear Barbara, Dear Lynn,* a series of letters between two women struggling to become mothers, letters that eventually formed a book.

> We who have access to more reproductive resources than any previous generation of women, and who believe we can have our children when and how we choose, are often as stumped by our biology as women from earlier times.

As for pregnancy after infertility, that is a particularly precious life passage indeed, one first known to biblical Sarah, who laughed in disbelief when she conceived in her old age—a fearful, celebratory, treacherous, miraculous passage indeed. Pregnancy after infertility was my own life passage as well, although I was not ninety like Sarah, but thirty-nine years old, when I conceived through a complicated in vitro procedure called intracytoplasmic sperm injection, known as ICSI. My clinic required not one but three consecutive blood tests to verify a viable pregnancy's rising human chorionic gonadotropin (HCG) hormone. At eight weeks gestation, I held my breath when my husband and I saw the fetus's barely decipherable heart beating on a sonogram screen and exhaled only after the physician pronounced everything normal. You might say I was a skeptical newly pregnant woman, having been too often disproved, and the infertility clinic only underscored this belief. For the entire first trimester, my husband continued to inject my buttocks with a nightly intramuscular injection of progesterone because the clinic told us this was a kind of insurance policy on our investment. I became more convinced of my expectant state once the amniocentesis tests revealed that I was carrying a healthy boy, and from then on I relaxed into and enjoyed being pregnant. Technology served me well.

Pregnancy is full of new bonds, both in the sense that a woman feels bound and circumscribed by her becoming-mammoth body, and in the sense that new bonds are forming. First and most importantly, as all the books will tell you, is the bond a woman begins to form with her developing child. For nine months, you are never entirely just yourself alone, but accompanied 24/7 by a tiny human inside whom you cannot see yet know intimately. Whether or not you take drugs or take prenatal vitamins, your actions have an effect on someone other than yourself. And the baby, who you feel kick and turn and lie still and drop down to press upon your cervix and make you constantly run for the bathroom to pee, already has an effect on you. This was one of the revelations pregnancy gave me. For nine months, it is impossible to be a complete narcissist. I have never felt less lonely.

> Successful career women find themselves emotionally challenged by the transition to a new identity that pregnancy and impending motherhood can provoke, an identity for which biology, loss of control, and physical limitation become paramount.

Feminist thinker Naomi Wolf writes in *(Misconceptions): Truth, Lies, and the Unexpected on the Journey to Motherhood:* "Becoming a mother requires a kind of supreme focus, a profound discipline, and even a kind of warrior spirit. Yet our culture prefers to give women doggerel: it often suggests that motherhood is something effortless." In the nearly 300 pages that chronicle her own month-by-month pregnancy in the context of larger societal issues about women and career, women and the obstetrical establishment, women and their bodies, Wolf articulates issues of pregnancy and new motherhood for women of the upper class at the turn of the millennium. Successful career women like herself, accustomed to the rewards of the marketplace—autonomy, freedom, control—find themselves emotionally challenged by the transition to a new identity that pregnancy and impending motherhood can provoke, an identity for which biology, loss of control, and physical limitation become paramount. This is a kind of reversal of the story women have previously told, the story in which women demanded reproductive rights in order to use their minds as well as their wombs. In Naomi Wolf's narrative, pregnancy is a time when a woman, through her own willful agency, prepares for motherhood. That preparation includes a shattering of the myth that pregnancy should happen naturally and blissfully, like a series of scenes through a soft-focus lens—a powerful myth, says Wolf, that blinds women to both their real experience and the pitiful support they receive from society at large.

Wolf and her contemporaries take the story of women and pregnancy full circle—a pregnant woman in the twenty-first century who possesses any historical awareness of how hard won and rare are her self-reliance and independence may have to relearn, in a sense, the very mind-set that made women in earlier generations bound to hearth and home. Virtues like patience, serving others, and dailyness are coming back into vogue. Few contemporary women dare endorse the Victorian practices of the new mother, who, despite her low rung on the patriarchal ladder, was encouraged to rest for a full ten days after delivery and to spend a full postpartum month retired to her "lying-in" room where she could care for her newborn, receive visitors, and recoup her strength. These practices, ones that afford pregnancy and birth a privileged status, and contemporary policies—hospital discharge forty-eight hours after delivery, miserly maternity leaves in most workplaces—make a prolonged postpartum period virtually impossible.

No longer enslaved to near-constant pregnancies, no longer routinely risking our lives in childbirth, no longer bound to home or to hide our pregnant shape, the irony is that our pregnancies may cause us more mental anguish than they did for our choiceless sisters in centuries past. For we have changed; the world has changed. No one wants to return to the oppressive second citizenship women-as-childbearers endured for so many centuries. But our psyches, I think, have not quite caught up. We have not quite accepted the fact that we can exercise choice, but only so much. We can be self-fulfilled, autonomous beings some of the time. We are minds *and* bodies, at work and at home.

—*Karen Propp, Ph.D.*

RELATED ENTRIES

Adoption

Becoming a Mother

Living with Infertility

Living with Infertility

People come to the decision to have children in different ways. Whatever the path to this decision, the wish to have a child is powerful. No one expects to be infertile. It is devastating to realize that the decision to have a child is not within your control. Gone is the assumption that when you are ready, you will conceive.

Approximately 6.1 million people in the United States are having difficulty conceiving or carrying a pregnancy to term. Infertility is a medical condition that results from a problem with either the male or female reproductive tract and prevents either the conception of a child or carrying a pregnancy to term. Living with infertility can mean facing failure month after month. By definition, infertility is a medical problem that has endured for at least twelve months, or six months in women over age thirty-five. By the time a couple is diagnosed with infertility, there have been many months of cycling through hope and disappointment. Many women, up to this point, have experienced a sense of control over life decisions. Infertility often poses the first challenge to their health, their first experience of themselves as a "patient," and often, the first serious crisis in their relationships.

The primary goal of the woman living through infertility is getting pregnant, possibly to the exclusion of many other things. She may wake up in the morning with infertility on her mind (as she takes her basal body temperature), and she may go to sleep thinking about it as well. She may feel that she has lost a sense of balance in her life. Perhaps she feels (or her partner would say) she is obsessed, as she may be living her life in twenty-eight-day cycles of hope, expectation, and despair.

In heterosexual couples, regardless of which partner is diagnosed with infertility, the woman almost always feels some sense of responsibility. It is her body that does not get pregnant or "fails" to maintain a pregnancy. She may be particularly ruthless with herself about the "causes" of infertility. I frequently hear women express the thought that their much-loved partner should leave them and find a more "fertile" woman (even if the infertility is unexplained and could be his body and not hers). Somehow the infertility becomes "hers" rather than "theirs." If you hear yourself in this statement, you might ask, "Why do I take responsibility for something over which I seemingly have no control?" Take a moment to write down a response so that you can refer to it after reading the section entitled "Thinking about Infertility."

Unlike many other chronic medical conditions, infertility carries with it a sense of shame. Women use words like *defective* and *damaged* to describe themselves, saying they feel set apart from the rest of the (i.e., the fertile) world. One woman described this as feeling like she was outside of a snow globe looking in, her face pressed against the glass, watching the (fertile) world from the outside.

The chronic stress of infertility can lead to many feelings, among them, envy, rage, helplessness, despair, and depression. This can overwhelm a woman's usual ability to cope. Many perfectly lovely women struggle with trying to integrate such "negative" emotions into a positive view of themselves. Maria, a woman struggling with infertility, said, "I hate who I have become. I find myself hating pregnant women. I am so angry and jealous. My husband says that he doesn't even recognize me."

Some good news does exist here. There are ways to cope with this stress. Here are some ideas to help cope with living with the emotional impact of infertility.

THE EVALUATION AND TREATMENT OF INFERTILITY

Many women describe the evaluation and treatment of infertility as the most upsetting experience of their lives. In one study, a majority of women rated infertility as being more stressful than divorce when they had experienced both. This is not surprising given that the evaluation and treatment of infertility can involve tremendous physical, social, and financial sacrifices.

The evaluation of infertility can be a long and stressful process. If both partners are generally healthy, specific tests may be recommended. For men, these tests might be a semen analysis examining the number of sperm produced (sperm count), the ability of the sperm to move forward (sperm motility), and the percentage of normal-appearing sperm (sperm morphology). For women, initial tests might include an analysis of body temperature and ovulation, ultrasound of the fallopian tubes and uterus, and laparoscopy (a procedure to view the interior surfaces of the reproductive organs and abdomen). Many women find that becoming a medical "patient" is a difficult transition to make.

> Unlike many other chronic medical conditions, infertility carries with it a sense of shame.

The causes of infertility are varied. Roughly one-third of causes are attributed to male factors, most commonly no sperm cells produced (azoospermia) or few sperm cells produced (oligospermia). Another third of infertility is attributed to factors that affect women, most commonly an ovulation disorder, as well as maternal age, blocked fallopian tubes, endometriosis, structural anomalies of the uterus, and uterine fibroids. The remaining one-third of factors is due to a combination of problems in both partners. For about 20 percent of couples, the cause of infertility is frustratingly "unexplained."

TREATMENT

Most cases of infertility (85–90 percent) can be treated with conventional therapies such as drug treatment and surgical repair of the reproductive organs. The more "high-tech" assisted reproductive technologies (in vitro fertilization [IVF] and similar procedures) account for less than 5 percent of infertility services. The success rate of IVF was 22.5 percent in 1995 (average rate of live delivery). This is about the same chance (20 percent) that a reproductively healthy couple has of conceiving in any given month.

The decision to pursue assisted reproductive technologies may create moral, ethical, or religious dilemmas. Some religions ban in vitro fertilization. It can be very difficult for some couples to resolve the conflict between their religious beliefs and recommended infertility treatment. In addition, there may be disagreement within the couple about whether to pursue treatment, and when. When Deanna and her husband, a couple experiencing infertility, came to the point of making such decisions, her husband was ambivalent about pursuing high-tech treatment, saying that it just didn't seem natural to him, it felt like they were "playing God." Deanna felt desperate and very alone in this decision. Her inability to conceive felt to her like a major disappointment to everyone. Her parents were aging and had no grandchildren. Her husband was opposed to adoption. She didn't feel comfortable with the idea of medical treatment, but felt that it was the only way that she could have a child. She decided to pursue IVF, but she did so with much concern.

> Women living with infertility report twice the rates of depressive symptoms that fertile women do.

The sheer expense of infertility treatment can make the approach prohibitive for many women. The average cost of an IVF cycle in the United States is $7,800. Insurance coverage varies from state to state, with only twelve states currently mandating that insurers offer some coverage for infertility diagnosis and treatment. An excellent information resource on financial coverage is maintained by RESOLVE (www.resolve.org). RESOLVE is a national nonprofit infertility organization with chapters in every state providing public education through brochures, newsletters, support groups, and referral services. It produces a brochure entitled "Infertility Insurance Advisor—An Insurance Counseling Program for Infertile Couples."

DEALING WITH YOUR FEELINGS

What is the emotional impact of infertility? Some women manage infertility relatively well. For others, the onset of menstruation each month, and the "failure" that it signals, can trigger depression and anxiety, two common emotions of women seeking treatment for infertility. Some research shows that women living with infertility report twice the rates of depressive symptoms that fertile women do. Nine to 11 percent of these women would meet the criteria for an episode of major depression, and a majority (75 percent) report negative changes in their mood. Depressive symptoms fluctuate, depending on where a woman is in her cycle. Prior to an IVF cycle, 34 percent of women in one study reported depressive symptoms, and this increased to 64 percent after it was clear that pregnancy did not occur. One large research study found that, following IVF failure, a majority of men and women reported psychological symptoms, such as sleep and appetite disturbance, nightmares, anxiety, and panic. They also found that 13 percent of women were so distressed that they had some suicidal thoughts. Clearly, the experience of infertility treatment can overwhelm even the healthiest woman.

> Despite the fact that infertility is not life threatening, the emotional impact of infertility is comparable to that of serious, sometimes life-threatening medical conditions.

As you would expect, infertility distress increases with time. After two to three years of infertility, depression peaks, returning to normal only after the sixth year. In general, women report greater levels of distress than men do at every point along the way.

The impact of infertility has been compared to other chronic medical conditions. How do women going through infertility feel compared to women with cancer, heart disease, HIV-positive status, or chronic pain? Levels of anxiety and depression are the same across all of these groups with the exception of patients with chronic pain. The conclusion of this interesting study is that despite the fact that infertility is not life threatening, the emotional impact of infertility is comparable to that of serious, sometimes life-threatening medical conditions. Yet, friends, coworkers, and family typically rally around someone when they go through cancer or heart disease. There isn't the same level of societal understanding for infertility or the same knowledge of how to support a loved one going through this experience. This is particularly true for women of color, single women, and lesbian women for which the decision to attempt pregnancy can be a difficult process with many obstacles.

Infertile lesbian women generally report all the same distress symptoms as heterosexual women, but are more likely to be isolated and receive less support because of homophobic reactions to their desire to be parents. Further, when treatment options are exhausted, adoption for single and lesbian women may be hindered by the refusal of some adoption agencies to accept them as potential parents.

Infertility is usually seen as solely affecting affluent, white, heterosexual women. The public image of infertility rarely includes women of color. The stereotypical image is of an African American woman struggling with too many children, not with infertility. Rosario Ceballo interviewed one infertile African American woman who felt like she was "the only black woman walking the face of the earth that cannot have a baby." Most infertility research is based exclusively on samples of white, middle-class women, and this is the group most likely to seek treatment. High-tech, high-cost treatments are often inaccessible to racial and ethnic minorities, gays and lesbians, and single women.

COPING WITH INFERTILITY: THREE SURVIVAL SKILLS

Women can develop skills to gain control over their responses to infertility rather than feeling controlled by them. Three things that a woman can do to improve how she feels are: (1) reduce stress through relaxation exercises, (2) work to change how you think about infertility, and (3) join an infertility group. The following sections describe such techniques.

Relaxation Training Imagine your first day back at work after an intrauterine insemination (IUI). You are trying hard not to obsess about whether you will get pregnant this time. At lunch, a coworker announces that she is pregnant. Groan. She's reaching for the ultrasound pictures. You feel like everyone is looking at you. You notice that your face is flushed, your heart is pounding, your stomach is suddenly sour, and your legs feel wobbly. What is happening?

You have just experienced the "flight-or-fight response." Your body has been flooded with a surge of stress hormones (among them adrenaline). In response, your blood pressure, heart rate, and breathing rate surge upward. You are ready to fight or flee. This is a hard-wired, physiological response that prepares you for danger and, when needed, could be life saving. Think of times when you have used this response to good effect—for example, stepping in front of a moving car and leaping back to safety. The same physiological response occurred as the coworker reached for her ultrasound pictures. In one scenario, the threat is physical, in the other, psychological. Hearing that someone is pregnant is not a life-or-death situation. Your body, however, does not know the difference. Dealing with the chronic stress of infertility can overstimulate this flight-or-fight response. Think of how many situations in a day might lead to activating this response. The result? You may begin to experience stress-related symptoms (e.g., irritability, insomnia, neck and shoulder pain). You may feel "on the edge" or "crazy." You can't avoid the world and the stress of infertility—what can you do?

> Three things that a woman can do to improve how she feels are:
>
> ▶ reduce stress through relaxation exercises
>
> ▶ work to change how you think about infertility
>
> ▶ join an infertility group.

The relaxation response is the antidote to the flight-or-fight response. The relaxation response turns off the stress response, slows down your heart and breathing rates, and decreases blood pressure. *The Relaxation Response*, by Herbert Benson, M.D., describes the importance of eliciting this response and the health benefits of doing so. There is nothing mysterious about relaxation, but it is not the same as watching television or sleeping. Yoga, progressive muscle relaxation, meditation, deep breathing, all are ways to elicit the relaxation response. Some people can achieve this with repetitive prayer. With regular use, all of these techniques can effectively calm the mind and the body and generate significant health benefits. While you may not be able to control your fertility, you can control your breathing.

> ✦
>
> Stop and take a moment to write an answer to the following question. "Why is infertility happening to me?" Your answer will give you information about the beliefs that you bring to understanding your own infertility.

This is a simple technique with powerful results. Take a moment to practice: sit comfortably and close your eyes. Relax your hands and uncross your legs. Take a deep breath, in through your nose. Hold it, allowing your chest to expand fully, and release it slowly. Concentrate your thoughts on the sensation of breathing. If you feel distracted, gently bring your thoughts back to your breathing. Now do this a few times. Notice the feeling of relaxation spreading over you. In the next few breaths, as you breathe in, think of breathing in a sense of calm, and as you exhale, breathe out anxiety, tension, anger, whatever you are feeling. Do this a few times. This is a simple technique that you can use anywhere to manage stress and it is one way that you can take some control over how you feel. You can elicit this relaxation response through breathing at work, when you see a pregnant woman, or while waiting for a return telephone call from your doctor's office.

Thinking about Infertility Infertility can certainly *feel* like a punishment, but just because you feel something doesn't make it true. How you think about something, however, can affect how you feel. Understanding this concept is the easy part. In actuality, it is hard work to change patterns of thinking. Drs. Aaron Beck and David Burns are two pioneers in the field of cognitive therapy. The information in this section is based largely upon their work and applying it to the problem of infertility.

We are in constant dialogue with ourselves, engaging in an internal conversation. Pay attention to what you are saying to yourself. A lot of this dialogue is negative, either about yourself, others, or situations. You see a pregnant woman in the grocery store. What are your thoughts? What do you say to or about yourself? A cognitive therapy approach emphasizes *choices*. We can make choices about how we talk to ourselves. The cognitive approach assumes that stress and suffering can arise from how we perceive situations. Thoughts that yield stress are usually negative, unrealistic, and distorted. This can be especially true around emotionally laden issues like infertility.

Now, as the belly of the pregnant woman at the grocery store rounds the bend, what might your internal dialogue be? "Her life is perfect. She probably has three kids and another on the way. I'll never be happy. I'm a failure as a woman." This chance meeting in the grocery story is an event, a neutral event. When living with infertility, starting your period used to be a neutral event too, but can become a very negative event. In fact, there may have been times, before attempting pregnancy, when starting your period was a relief! Think of

ORGANIZATIONS AND RESOURCES

RESOLVE, Inc.
National Headquarters
1310 Broadway
Somerville, MA
(617) 623-1156
Helpline: (617) 623-0744
www.resolve.org

American Society for Reproductive Medicine
1209 Montgomery Highway
Birmingham, AL 35216-2809
(205) 978-5000
www.asrm.org

The Mind/Body Center for Women's Health at Boston IVF
40 Second Avenue, Suite 300
Waltham, MA 02451
(781) 434-6578
www.conqueringinfertility@BostonIVF.com

Support Groups

RESOLVE is a national nonprofit infertility organization with chapters in every state offering support groups (www.resolve.org). *For information about infertility mind/body groups, contact www.conqueringinfertility@BostonIVF.com.*

an event as similar to an elevator door opening: you can push up or down. There is a choice in response. How you perceive and respond to seeing a pregnant woman in the grocery store can have a significant impact on your mood.

In the midst of an emotionally charged situation, we may be barraged by "automatic thoughts" (a concept introduced by Dr. Burns). These thoughts are knee-jerk responses, usually just below consciousness, so that you might not even be fully aware of what you are thinking. They are negative thoughts, have a flashy quality, and are usually stated in extreme language (e.g., "I'm a failure as a woman"). They also tend to come in rapid fire, clustering together. Whether or not you are fully aware, these thoughts can strongly influence how you feel in your daily life. Your body doesn't know the difference between a true and an untrue thought. In *The Wellness Book*, Benson and Stuart use the example of a scary movie. Even though you know on some level that the movie is not real, your body reacts as if it was: sweaty palms, racing heart, and so on.

These automatic thoughts are like tennis balls flying out of an automatic serving machine. Without a tennis racket, you would be barraged and pummeled by balls. You're defenseless. *Cognitive restructuring* is the process of building a tennis racket to deflect these automatic negative thoughts. One example of an automatic thought might be, "I will never be happy unless I get pregnant." Ask yourself some questions. Is this logical? Is this true? Can this kind of statement affect how I feel? You bet it can. A statement like, "I will never be happy unless I get pregnant," if left unchallenged, can significantly impact your mood. You might feel angry, sad, or hopeless. If this thought was below consciousness, you might not even be aware as to why your mood soured.

Asking yourself questions following an automatic thought is one way to interrupt the cycle. First, you must hear the dialogue and be aware of what you say to yourself in an emotional situation. Then you can "talk back." If you decide the negative thought is inaccurate, restructure it. Whack that tennis ball back. Referring to our example, a restructured thought might be, "I'm doing everything that I can to have a baby. Even though it's hard to imagine now, I do think I will find some happiness in my life no matter what the outcome." The point of cognitive restructuring is not to gloss over difficult or true feelings. Acknowledge what is true in a thought, but state it accurately. It is true that not becoming pregnant causes much unhappiness, but the statement, "I will never be happy" is likely untrue.

JOINING AN INFERTILITY GROUP

Participating in a RESOLVE support group or a mind/body group can be invaluable during the experience of infertility. In addition to the social support provided by a group, there is some interesting recent research by Harvard psychologist Dr. Alice Domar that suggests another potential benefit to joining a group: participation can significantly decrease symptoms of distress (depression, anxiety, and anger) and can also enhance the chances of conception.

The relationship between stress and infertility is complex. In the Domar study, women who completed a ten-week mind/body group had significantly increased viable pregnancy rates when compared to women who did not participate in a group. Recall that depression peaks at two to three years of infertility. Dr. Domar hypothesizes that it is important to intervene *before* that two- to three-year surge in depression to stave off possible harmful psychological and reproductive effects. Her best advice is to join a support group or mind/body group while experiencing infertility. The "Organizations and Resources" section has information about locating infertility support groups and mind/body groups.

MAKING SENSE OF CHILDLESSNESS

Stop and take a moment to write an answer to the following question. "Why is infertility happening to me?" Your answer will give you information about the beliefs that you bring to understanding your own infertility. Some people do not ask "Why?" because they don't believe there is an answer. Others are plagued by the question and search unforgivingly through their past to dredge up a reason. I have found that some people's beliefs follow a rational path, but more superstitious reasons almost always lurk about that people use to explain their infertility. These "reasons" usually include negative or unpleasant distortions about the self: "This is my punishment for my promiscuity in college."

Examine your own beliefs about your infertility. Can you imagine saying such things to someone else you care about? Imagine, for example, telling your sister that perhaps she can't conceive a child because she really doesn't deserve to be a mother? Anger at infertility often becomes anger turned on the self.

FINDING MEANING AND MOVING ON

Given continuing advances in infertility treatment, it has become increasingly difficult for couples to reach a point at which they have exhausted all medical possibilities. There is always one more procedure or one more cycle to hold out hope. Arthur L. Griel notes that couples no longer define themselves as "childless," but as "not yet pregnant." He states that "parenthood for the infertile is a status that can neither be achieved nor abandoned." When is enough, enough? The couple or individual, not the medical team, must draw the line on when to stop treatment.

In my clinical experience, individuals and couples who do best are those who generate a plan that includes an articulated end point. The range of what people can tolerate (and the amount of time that is healthy for them to pursue treatment) is varied. There are no clear-cut answers about when to stop. Some couples endure years of treatment reasonably well, while others are just about undone by brief encounters with infertility treatment. Periodic assessment of how you are doing and how your relationship is doing in the midst of treatment is important.

Make a Plan Plans can always be revised, but having a plan is vital. In their books *Surviving Infertility* and *Missed Conceptions,* Linda Salzer and Anne Mullens pose some helpful questions to use in evaluating when to end treatment. Their basic ideas are (1) How would you feel if your doctor presented you with the news that there was some promising new treatment? (2) Do you feel that your relationship with your partner is at risk because of continued treatment? (3) Are you comfortable with how much you are postponing other life plans because of infertility treatment? (4) Have you given treatment a "reasonable chance" of working? (5) When might you be ready to stop treatment? Is there a logical end point?

Grief over not being able to conceive and deliver one's own child can be tenacious. For most individuals, there is a period of mourning the loss of genetic parenthood, not unlike grief over other losses. However, there is no established ritual mourning process and often no public recognition for these feelings of grief. Some women welcome, with relief, the end to the attempt to conceive. Most women do move on and successfully redefine their life goals without a genetic child.

—*Angel Seibring, Ph.D.*

RELATED ENTRIES

A Guide to Grief and Bereavement

Anger: That Most Unfeminine Emotion

Choosing Childlessness

Becoming a Mother

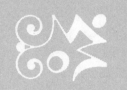

A *Psychobiosocial Transition* in a *Woman's Life*

Although our culture no longer insists that a woman become a mother in order to be considered a fully mature adult, for most of the 3.5 million U.S. women who give birth for the first time each year, becoming a mother is a major developmental milestone. Personal accounts of first-time motherhood leave little doubt that this is a life transition of enormous psychological complexity and richness. The birth of a child marks a process that not only involves establishing a highly distinctive kind of relationship to another human being, but also a reorganization of a woman's sense of herself and her other significant life relationships and commitments. At the end of her remarkable thirty-year study of women's development, psychologist Ruthellen Josselson concluded:

Motherhood is such a powerful framework for identity that the having or not having of children is the single most silent distinction among the adult women I studied. All the mothers, regardless of their occupational success or commitment said that their children were the most important aspect of their lives, their self-realization, and their sense of who they are. Aside from severe trauma and life-threatening illness, becoming a mother seems to be the most potent identity-transforming event in a woman's life.

Our scientific understanding of motherhood, its developmental course, and the attendant psychological processes and consequences is limited. Researchers in the United States have rarely studied motherhood in terms of the woman's development. Instead, most studies focus on the child and narrowly conceptualize a mother as either a "detractor" or "enhancer" of her child's development. Consequently, we know a great deal about "at-risk" mothers: teen mothers, psychiatrically disturbed mothers, low-income mothers, and substance-using mothers.

The study of normal populations of mothers most often proceeds from the same overriding interest in the growth and development of children. Research on maternal personality factors that facilitate or undermine healthy attachment between mother and infant and on the effects of postpartum depression further illustrate this child-centered outlook. Moreover, research in the United States that has explored the normative experience of becoming a mother has focused almost exclusively on first-time mothers and on maternal adjustment only through the first year postpartum. English, Canadian, Australian, and Finnish scientists have similarly tended to study mothers only through the first year after birth.

The absence of systematic and sustained attention to questions of maternal development and, in particular, to questions of the emotional health and well-being of women as they engage in mothering *across the life span* is both intriguing and troubling. It reflects both the cultural notion of mothering as "natural" to women and thus executed "reflexively," and more particularly to our culture's tendency to place concerns deeply relevant to women outside the mainstream of scientific inquiry. Researchers have also disproportionately studied mothers who are white, college educated, middle class, and married. With rare exception, the psychological adaptation and development of mothers who adopt children, are single parents, are lesbian or of ethnically, racially, or culturally distinct backgrounds or socioeconomic classes other than middle class, and have less formal education have not been adequately represented in the study of maternal development and adaptation.

> Personal accounts of first-time motherhood leave little doubt that this is a life transition of enormous psychological complexity and richness.

Keeping these limitations in mind, I surveyed the empirical literature on the transition to motherhood in the United States of the last fifty years. In order to understand a woman's experience of being a mother over time, I focused exclusively on investigations that followed the same group of women either for a minimum of a year postpartum or those that followed the same group of women through their pregnancies and then for at least six months following the birth of their baby.

Is fifty years too lengthy a time span given the numerous social changes that have occurred since the 1950s? Despite the advances in the social and economic status of women and demographic changes such as increased numbers of working mothers under the age of eighteen and the advancing average age at which women give birth to a first child, the experience of becoming a mother has been remarkably consistent in the last half century.

My review has been guided by the following two questions:

- What phases and challenges can be expected in a new mother's life?
- What factors enhance the emotional well-being of women as they mother their children?

First, here is a brief summary of the studies from which I conducted my review.

STUDIES OF ADAPTATION TO FIRST-TIME MOTHERHOOD, 1950 TO 2000

Over the past fifty years, six groups of American researchers have studied women's early psychological adaptation to motherhood: Each has approached its studies with the same general purpose, but with slightly different emphases and research methods. They are as follows:

Louis Sander Beginning in 1954, child psychoanalyst Sander and his research team observed the development of the mother–child relationship from birth to six. This careful examination was based on the premise that a child's personality development is directly related to the quality and characteristics of the mother's personality and the way she interacts with the baby and young child. As a result of his study, Sander proposed five periods of child development from birth to eighteen months, each with its own unique, central challenge to the first-time mother's caregiving skills. These periods were "Initial Adaptation" (birth to two and a half months); "Reciprocal Exchange" (two and a half to five months); "Early Directed Activity of the Infant" (five to nine months); "Focalization on Mother" (nine to fifteen months); and "Self Assertion" (twelve to eighteen months).

Pauline Shereshefsky and Leon Yarrow (1977) This multidisciplinary study of sixty-two couples about to become parents for the first time was conducted during the mid-sixties. The women ranged in age from eighteen to twenty-eight, with most of them between the ages of twenty and twenty-four. Sixty-nine percent were white, 21 percent African American, and all participants were described as "socially upwardly mobile." These investigators looked at whether it was possible to predict a woman's adaptation to her role as mother from aspects of her life history such as her relationship with her mother, personality attributes, marital situation, and external stresses. The researchers interviewed women and their husbands when the women were three to four months pregnant, at month 7 and month 9, and at delivery and evaluated the mothers and their infants at four weeks, six weeks, three months, and six months postpartum.

Myra Leifer (1977) Nineteen white, middle-class first-time mothers, between ages twenty and thirty-five participated in this study, based on the view that pregnancy and parenthood function as an impetus for "change, reorganization, and integration" in a woman's personality. Interviews were conducted a total of five times: at each trimester of pregnancy, the third day after the birth of the baby, and six to eight weeks postpartum. Each new mother completed a follow-up questionnaire at seven months postpartum.

Frances Grossman, Lois Eichler, and Susan Winickoff (1980) This group of psychologists focused on understanding women's experience of pregnancy and the first postpartum year, with the goals of identifying factors early on that predict problems adapting to pregnancy, delivery, and the first year of motherhood. They met with ninety-three women and most of their husbands five times over an eighteen-month period. Women who participated were between twenty-one and thirty-four years old, predominantly Caucasian and middle class. Only about half of the women were first-time mothers. Visits to the couples' home occurred in the first and third trimesters of pregnancy, in the hospital right after the baby was born (at which time the baby was assessed as well), and at two months and one year postpartum.

Ramona Mercer A Ph.D. nurse with a specialty in maternal and child health, Mercer studied the development of maternal identity from the late 1960s through the mid-1990s. She regarded a successful "attainment" of a woman's identity as a mother to have occurred when a woman "integrated the [maternal] role into her self system with a congruence of self and other roles; [is] secure in her identity as a mother, is emotionally committed to her infant, and feels a sense of harmony, satisfaction, and competence in the role" (1995, p. 14). The 294 women in her study of first-time mothers were divided into three age groups (15 to 19; 20 to 29; 30 to 42) and were observed interacting with their babies by the research team at one, four, eight, and twelve months postpartum. Based on the interview data, responses to questionnaires, and observations of the mother–baby pair, Mercer proposed a stage model for the development of maternal identity: stage 1: physical recovery (0–1 month); stage 2: achievement of role (2nd to 5th month); stage 3: disruption of role (6th to 8th month); and stage 4: reorganization of role (8th to 12th month).

Alison Fleming and Colleagues Fleming et al. conducted one of the largest studies on adjustment in mothers with a sample of women about to become, or who had recently become, mothers for the first time between 1981 and 1983. This research had many objectives, among them to clarify the nature of "normal" depressive feelings in the postpartum period and to test whether these feelings interfere with either the mother's capacity to care for her child or the quality of the relationship she has with her baby.

> Whether a woman enjoys the physical changes of pregnancy or not, the changes greatly assist her mental preparation for motherhood.

The researchers met once with 667 women, ages eighteen to forty-two, comprising six groups. The groups of this cross-sectional sample were (1) women who were planning to conceive in two years; (2) women in their first trimester; (3) women in their second trimester; (4) women in their third trimester; (5) women in their first month postpartum; and (6) women in their third month postpartum. Women were predominantly Caucasian, middle income, English speaking and were either married or living with their male partner. Interviews of this sample allowed comparisons of women at different stages of pregnancy or motherhood. A second group of fifty-one women comprised the longitudinal sample. These women completed interviews in their ninth month of pregnancy, on one of the first days after their baby's birth, and at the end of the first, third, and sixteenth postpartum month. Questionnaires were given at each time point, with the exception of the sixteen-month postpartum in-person visit.

MATERNAL PHASES AND MILESTONES OF THE FIRST YEAR POSTPARTUM

Being Pregnant: Physical Changes and Psychological Adaptations The most obvious changes that a woman goes through while carrying a child to term are the physical ones, the ones visible to the outside world. These changes, such as weight gain and loss of figure, are the ones that signify to the world at large that something is about to change in a woman's life, that she is mak- ing a journey to a new identity. In *Birth of a Mother*, Daniel Stern and Nadia Bruschweiler-Stern point out that whether a woman enjoys the physical changes of pregnancy or not, the changes greatly assist her mental preparation for motherhood. The belly grows, breasts swell, the center of gravity shifts. These external, bodily changes are, the authors note, a "constant reminder of the baby-to-be," mirroring the internal process of a woman's psychological preparation for her "birth" as a mother.

R. P. Lederman, author of *Psychosocial Adaptation in Pregnancy*, interviewed pregnant women at several points during their pregnancies and found weight gain and body change to be one of the most consistent concerns spontaneously brought up by women. They worried about being seen as fat, "unsightly," unattractive, and even used the phrase "circus freaks." Moreover, many, if not most, women fear the weight they gain will remain long after the baby is born. There is some truth to this—some studies have found that body weight change after pregnancy is probably not only from weight retention from pregnancy but also lifestyle adjustments when there is a new baby. Evidence suggests that a single birth results in the average woman gaining four to seven pounds of weight over pregnancy and the first

Fetal attachment, or the psychological preparation for motherhood that takes place during pregnancy, is a process that includes:

- Thoughts and feelings about the unborn baby
- Actively preparing for the baby's needs
- Actively preparing for the changes in your lifestyle after the baby's birth
- Envisioning oneself as a mother
- Envisioning a real, live, healthy baby
- Engaging in good health practices—eating better, sleeping more, getting prenatal care

year of motherhood. Retaining the weight one gains with pregnancy is influenced by a variety of factors including the amount of time that has passed between pregnancies and weight prior to pregnancy. Greater weight retention occurs when pregnancies are closer together and when prepregnancy weight is greater.

Grossman, Eichler, and Winickhoff's study illustrates the close association between the physical symptoms of pregnancy and other factors. They found that women who had reported experiencing more marked symptoms of premenstrual syndrome (PMS) prior to their pregnancy reported more symptoms during pregnancy. Pregnant women whose socioeconomic status was less than middle class reported more pregnancy symptoms. And whether pregnant for the first or second time, women with greater marital satisfaction experienced fewer pregnancy symptoms. For first-time mothers-to-be, fewer symptoms were associated with a more equal division of household chores with their husbands.

Perhaps the most important psychological preparation that takes place during pregnancy is becoming attached to the unborn child, a process known as fetal attachment. This bond includes thoughts and feelings about the unborn baby, as well as actively preparing for the baby's needs and the changes in one's adult lifestyle that will accompany the baby's arrival. Becoming attached to one's baby before he or she is born is a gradual process, one that involves envisioning oneself as a mother and envisioning a real, live, healthy baby. Thus, attachment is strengthened by events such as receiving normal results from genetic testing, quickening (feeling the baby move), and the growth and physical movement of the baby in utero. The outward signs of this attachment include selecting names and pet names, debating the pros and cons of breast- versus bottle-feeding, talking to the fetus, and touching and stroking one's expanding belly. Less obviously, research has shown that attachment is strengthened when a pregnant woman engages in good health practices, such as eating better, sleeping more, exercising, and getting prenatal care. Lederman notes that "toward the end of the [last] trimester attachment culminates in a readiness and eagerness to get through the pregnancy and hold the baby."

Psychological Preparation for Labor and Delivery Labor and delivery in most industrialized societies is a female rite of passage associated with great emotional significance and is not uncommonly suffused with fears and anxieties, including fear of losing self-control and self-esteem in labor, fears about anesthesia, and fears of helplessness and pain. A great deal of attention has been devoted to figuring out what helps women cope with this milestone in their transition to motherhood. The role of anxiety in the labor and delivery experience is well documented. The more fearful a woman is about labor, the longer and more problematic labor can be. Women with high anxiety during labor showed slower progress in second-stage labor. Anxiety was also associated with use of forceps, while lower anxiety was associated with spontaneous vaginal delivery. Research demonstrates that the more information one has about labor and delivery, the less anxious and fearful one is. In fact, information seeking is an invaluable coping strategy throughout pregnancy.

An interesting study compared women according to their attitude regarding the use of medication. Group 1 women did not want medication because they wanted to have the "whole" experience. They fared quite well in labor itself. Group 2 women did not want medication because they were afraid of losing control or being unconscious. This group of women had very low confidence in their ability to handle the labor process. Group 3 women insisted on medication because they felt a complete lack of confidence in their ability to handle labor and delivery. The group for whom labor and delivery was most positive was group 4. These women indicated they did not initially want medication, but were open to its use if it was needed.

Thus, it appears that women who are able to face their fears about labor and delivery and try to anticipate what life would be like after the baby arrives fare much better at the time of actual delivery than those who do not prepare themselves in these ways. This may be because the women who were psychologically ready to labor and deliver were also women who were more likely to have actively researched and prepared for birth and motherhood. A finding by Lederman that poor marital relationship was associated with poor preparation for labor raises the question as to whether some women are less prepared because they receive less encouragement and support to do so by their partners.

Birth: Physical Recovery and Moving toward a Maternal Self In the earliest days of motherhood, a woman is in a phase of physical recovery from labor and childbirth that is often masked by the sheer exhilaration, relief, and joy at having delivered a healthy baby. As she copes with the physical discomforts of the postdelivery phase, she faces the process of getting to know the new person that has entered her life. This first-time mother, writing the day after her delivery and as quoted from Leifer's *Psychological Aspects of Motherhood,* discovers that her feelings about this life change are more of a jumble than expected:

I have found it hard to sort out my feelings about her. I have felt exhausted, sore from the stitches, perhaps more focused on myself than on her right now. And that makes me feel guilty. I have the sense that a good mother should feel a lot of love toward her baby, and I really can't say that what I feel is love. I'm a little frightened by her, I'm also delighted by her and find that I would like to just watch her and get to know her, but in all honesty, I can't say that I feel like a mother yet.

Although we know that not all women choose to breastfeed their infants,[1] for those who do, the first postpartum days involve the additional task of learning this complex maternal skill that involves physiological as well as behavioral and psychological facets. Milk pro-

---

1. A 1992 study found that women who are older, are better educated and of a higher socioeconomic status are the most likely to breastfeed their infants. Breastfeeding rates among white mothers are double that of African American mothers (Maternal and Child Health Bureau, 1994). However, according to a 1991 study, regardless of race or ethnicity, better-educated mothers are more likely to breastfeed while the less-educated and poor are less likely to do so. Although a mother's work status makes some difference in the decision whether or not to breastfeed, more specifically, whether work outside the home affords the flexibility necessary to maintain breastfeeding over time, the majority of women who do not work also do not breastfeed.

duction begins halfway through pregnancy. At that time, the hormone prolactin is produced in abundance to prepare the body for breastfeeding, but progesterone stops the process short of actually releasing milk. After birth, progesterone and estrogen levels drop dramatically. While this can trigger depression in some women, it also prepares the cells in the breasts for breastfeeding. Breastfeeding can hold significant emotional advantages for both mother and child as most mothers report the experience of breastfeeding brings about feelings of intimacy and closeness that are incomparable to other experiences they have with their infant. The hormones produced during breastfeeding help shrink the uteruses of women following birth and inhibit ovulation. Breastfeeding also helps mothers react to stress better, as research has shown that the level of stress hormones is lower in mothers who breastfeed their infants than those who bottle feed them. As an example, some researchers have looked at levels of the hormone oxytocin in women who are nursing. Oxytocin is released during breastfeeding; the longer a woman breastfeeds, the more oxytocin is released. Secretion patterns differ among women; some women secrete it in bursts, while others release continuously. The women with "bursts" of oxytocin actually ended up with more oxytocin in their blood. Women who had higher levels of oxytocin in their blood reported feeling calmer, more emotionally accessible, and more attached to their children. As natural as the physiological process of a woman's body preparing for lactation is, breastfeeding itself is a learned behavior and not one that works for every mother. Some mothers have no problems with breastfeeding—they love it, they talk about how good it feels. Even when away from their baby, a woman's milk starts flowing if she thinks about breastfeeding or hears a baby cry. Other women may not ever get the hang of it, often because nature seems to be conspiring against the most determined new mother—stress hormones disrupt milk flow, nipples become dry, cracked, and bleed. Whether breastfeeding is successful or not depends on a variety of factors that have nothing to do with a woman's adequacy as a mother.

Postpartum: Months One to Three As physical healing and recovery proceed through this next phase of a new mother's adjustment, she is faced with a multitude of new emotions and emotional challenges. Despite the image of early motherhood as uniformly happy, it is very clear that women have different feelings about themselves as mothers, about their babies, and about their husbands and that these feelings are simultaneously positive and negative. This is truly a period of complex and intense thought and feeling.

At this point, a typical new mother wonders whether she will ever be able to sleep through the night and feel rested again. She has (but cannot admit to anyone for fear of being seen as a bad mother) fleeting regrets about having had a baby. She worries about the new tensions that have surfaced with her partner. And she wonders a great deal about whether she is taking adequate care of their newborn. But less obvious to the new mother is that her feelings about herself and how she is doing are still closely tied to the process of her physical recovery; in fact, it has been found that the *more tired* a new mother is at the one month postpartum mark, the *less adequate* she feels as a mother.

In trying to capture the challenges of motherhood at four to eight weeks, Shereshefsky and Yarrow comment:

One would have to deal with the impact on the woman of the need for new concepts of time, a different organization of self, and a changed coordination of routine. Women ... have first of all to unlearn the virtues of adherence to time schedules and become attuned to a new kind of demand, one that emanates from the infant or from within the self. Keeping one's self ready for feeding on demand, awakening from sound sleep to determine the basis for an infant's discomfort (or of one's own discomfort, from too-full breasts), trying to take advantage of the infant's hour of sleep either to gain much-needed rest, meet other obligations, or undertake a cherished outing—all this requires a new organization of one's time and energies.

Postpartum: Months Three to Six By three months, in response to the baby's physiological maturation and the increased regularity in his patterns of eating, sleeping, waking, and crying, most women are feeling less anxious about their ability to take care of their babies. The exception to this are mothers who described their three-month-olds as "more difficult"; they tend to question their adequacy as mothers more than women with "less difficult" babies. Women who have more temperamentally demanding infants face a greater challenge developing a sense of themselves as competent caregivers, a critical facet to one's maternal identity. Both Leifer and Mercer note there is a difference between feeling confident about taking care of one's baby and having established a sense of oneself as a mother; the latter development is a milestone that does not occur for most women until sometime after the fourth postpartum month, although there is a small percentage who feel not yet like mothers even at their baby's first birthday.

For the women in Mercer's study, satisfaction with being a mother was at its absolute highest during the second quarter of the first year. She attributed the improvement to the combination of a woman's physical recovery, the infant's physical maturation, and two of the baby's social milestones: the baby begins to recognize and respond to his or her own mother as distinct from, and preferred over, all other caregivers, and, as important, the baby starts to smile. Others similarly attribute the mother's deep emotional satisfactions during this phase to the baby's growing responsiveness and sociability. Sander highlighted the ten-week postpartum mark as ushering in a new and exhilarating aspect of mother's relationship to her baby, the opportunity for mother to interact in a playful and emotionally reciprocal way.

Writer Anne Lamott, in her book *Operating Instructions: A Journal of My Son's First Year*, recorded a milestone in her life as a mother:

[Sam] laughed today for the first time, when Julie from upstairs was dangling her bracelets above his head while I changed his diaper. His laughter was like little bells. Then there was the clearest silence, a hush, before total joyous pandemonium broke out between Julie and me.

Postpartum: Months Six to Twelve During the second half of the first year, the reciprocal nature of the relationship between mother and baby becomes more evident as a powerful influence on a woman's experience of herself as a mother. Sander describes these six months as the time when the baby's focus on his mother as the center of his universe is "intense and unremitting." He goes on to say that this period separates "those with flexibility from those without, those whose sense of identity as mothers is secure from those who are only partially committed." For the mothers Mercer studied, the second six months postpartum were marked by a shift toward a more negative feeling tone. Mercer attributes this change to the "discontinuity" in the care-taking skills that are required of mothers as the infant becomes more mobile and expressive of needs and preferences. The terms "*disrup-*

> Satisfaction with being a mother was at its absolute highest during the second quarter of the first year.

tion" and *"reorganization"* to describe the two stages of this second half of a mother's first year refer to this process of adapting to the baby's changing requirements, as well as to the parallel process of disorganization and reorganization of a mother's personal identity.

In spite of the often overwhelming number of adaptations that pregnancy and the first year of motherhood present, there are predictable phases and milestones that give it shape and coherence. Unlike the popular conception of early motherhood as a period of pure joy, fulfillment, and delight, it appears to be a time of tremendous, although manageable, emotional disequilibrium. Intertwined with the pleasures and satisfactions of being a mother, new mothers also routinely report feeling despondent, overwhelmed, self-doubting, angry, regretful, and simply exhausted by the physical demands of caring for a baby. While certain milestones for a mother are delighted reactions to the progress of her baby's unfolding development—understanding his reactions to environmental stimulation, becoming familiar with the rhythms of his physiological states, his increasing responsiveness and sociability— the research to date suggests that the significant milestone of feeling as though one is a mother and defining oneself as a mother to oneself follows a developmental course less closely linked to her baby's emerging capacities.

FACTORS ASSOCIATED WITH A MOTHER'S EMOTIONAL WELL-BEING

It is easy to imagine a multitude of influences that might either support or diminish a new mother's sense of emotional well-being: aspects of her personality, the functioning of the couple and their extended family, interactions with the work environment and day care providers, and social or governmental policies like family leave. We describe here only the better-studied factors relating to a first-time mother's emotional well-being. These include her prior experience with babies and children, the quality of her relationships to her husband and own mother, the strength of her broader social support system, and the baby's health and temperament. The lack of discussion about broader societal influences such as employment, housing, and day care options reflects only an absence of reliable data that speak to these issues, and most definitely not their lack of importance in determining a woman's postnatal experience.

> ✦
>
> Information from outside "experts" may be of the greatest value to women during pregnancy, and soon after the baby's birth, support that helps new mothers separate their feelings of "doing it right" from their babies' reactions to them and the world may be more useful.

Prior Experience with Babies and Children

Interest in children and experience in caring for babies and children have been found by several researchers to be associated with positive adaptation to motherhood. The Fleming group suggests that mothers with more childcare experience have already learned some of the skills involved in caring for a newborn and therefore more quickly feel that they are doing a good job as mothers. Or it may be that their familiarity with babies and children, even those not their own, makes them less likely to blame themselves if their infant is difficult.

Baby's Temperament

Relatively recently, researchers have begun to consider the "reciprocal influence" of mother and baby upon each other by asking not only how a mother's parenting style affects her infant's development, but also how aspects of the infant's personality influence how mothers respond to them and, as a result, how they adjust to being a mother.

Babies' temperaments, or style of interacting with the world—for example, fussiness, regularity of eating and sleeping schedules, reactions to changes in routine—contribute not only to mothers' enjoyment of mothering, but also to their evaluations of themselves as mothers. Rather than attributing their difficulties to a source outside themselves, mothers of more temperamentally difficult infants often blame themselves and feel less adequate as mothers than mothers of easier babies.

Relationship to Mother The Fleming group found that during pregnancy, women who had positive relationships with their own mothers were more self-confident as they imagined being mothers themselves, and they also believed they would be involved, protective, and knowledgeable as mothers.

Social Support Psychologists Thomas Power and Ross Parke, in their review of research on the transition to motherhood, propose that how easily a woman adapts to becoming a mother is determined in large part by the nature and availability of her social supports. They describe four types of social support. *Relational support* comes from emotionally close relationships and includes emotional support and enjoyment of recreational activities. *Ideological support* refers to support for beliefs about mothering, such as whether to return to work after the baby's birth. *Physical support* is the provision of goods and services, such as money, housecleaning, and babysitting. *Informational support* is defined as factual information about pregnancy and motherhood, for example, about nutrition or day care. Power and Parke hypothesize that women benefit most from these different forms of social support at different times during the transition to motherhood, depending on their physical and emotional needs.

Psychologist Carolyn Cutrona conducted one of the most thorough explorations of the role social support plays in the transition to first-time motherhood. Her study examined relationships among social support, stress, and depressive symptoms in eighty-five women between the ages of eighteen and thirty-five years. As in the other studies described, most participants were married, Caucasian, and middle class. Interviews and questionnaires were given at four times: during the third trimester, two weeks after delivery, eight weeks after delivery, and at one year postpartum.

At two weeks after the baby's birth, women's moods were unrelated to the social support they received, perhaps because the hormonal influences on mood were so strong then. However, what Cutrona called "child-related stress"—poor infant or maternal health, difficulty with feeding or sleeping, tension with other adults related to the baby—did predict women's depressed feelings two weeks following the baby's arrival. For those women with fewer stressors, guidance and advice from others helped offset depressive feelings. But for women experiencing high levels of stress, these forms of informational social support did not buffer depression. Thus, in the early days after the new baby's arrival, informational support is helpful for some women, but when a new mother is coping with higher levels of child-related stress, information alone can't mitigate depressed mood.

The Fleming group similarly found that once a baby was born, obtaining information from books or people did not bolster the confidence of new mothers. What best predicted a woman's self-confidence was personal experience with her own unique infant and, in particular, how temperamentally easy the baby was. However, women they studied actively sought information during their pregnancies, many relying heavily on information from books. Those pregnant women who received the most information on motherhood, pregnancy, or labor and delivery tended to feel more self-confident in anticipating motherhood and to perceive themselves as more likely to possess the personal qualities that allow them to fulfill the responsibilities of being a mother.

Taken together, these findings suggest that information from outside "experts" may be of the greatest value to women during pregnancy, and soon after the baby's birth, support that helps new mothers separate their feelings of "doing it right" from their babies' reactions to them and the world may be more useful.

By the time mothers in Cutrona's sample were eight weeks postpartum, the critical importance of social support was very clear. In the broadest terms, women with the least support felt the most depressed. Several aspects of relational social support emerged as particularly important to a new mother's emotional well-being. Specifically, women who felt themselves part of a group of friends with whom they could share common concerns and recreational activities were less depressed. And women who had others on whom they could rely for help under any circumstances felt better, as did women with colleagues or coworkers who recognized them as competent and skillful.

Power and Parke's review elucidates the importance of having social support networks not simply of other mothers, but of mothers with similar views on motherhood and values and goals for themselves and their families. They cite research that found that career-oriented women without the social support networks of more traditional women were less satisfied with motherhood. Although the study couldn't answer *why* adequate social support is so crucial for new mothers' well-being, it seems likely that having others on whom one can rely for concrete forms of assistance, such as money and babysitting, as well as more intangible forms of help such as advice, would help women keep the demands of new motherhood in a manageable perspective. For example, being able to turn to knowledgeable mothers who can answer questions such as, "Is this normal?" "Am I doing something wrong?" "Am I the crazy to be feeling this way?" could facilitate a woman's own efforts to cope with the early challenges of being a mother. Support from knowledgeable others helps women to see the demands of motherhood as surmountable and may also help women avoid blaming themselves for difficulties.

In addition, women who know other mothers may be less likely to feel that they are unique in their problems and may ease the intensity of women's early doubts and anxieties. Cutrona's study also highlighted a particular irony related to becoming a parent. While strong social support was related to better postpartum mood in her sample of new mothers, a year after the baby's birth women received less social support in certain areas *than they had during pregnancy*. The mothers of one-year-olds were *less likely* to have their skills and abilities acknowledged and less likely to have relationships in which they felt a sense of safety and security. Thus, even though we know that the emotional transition to being a mother can take a full twelve months, the social support that is so vital to a first-time mother does not continue for as long as is necessary for a woman to optimally adjust to the transition.

Relationship to Partner Studies looking at new mothers who are married or in committed relationships find that a woman's partner is her most critical source of support. Power and Parke note that husbands are in a position to provide all four types of social support simultaneously, and research consistently concludes that men's relational and physical support greatly facilitates women's adaptation and satisfaction throughout the pregnancy and post-partum period. However, the postpartum period is also frequently a period of tension between new parents. Many men and women become less satisfied with their marriages in the months following a new baby's arrival. Part of the explanation for women's declining satisfaction is that despite their increased workload following the baby's birth, husbands often offer *less* relational and physical support than they did during pregnancy.

Psychologists (and spouses) Carolyn and Philip Cowan conducted one of the most rigorous and long-term studies of how relationships between partners change when they become parents. The Cowans' research team met with seventy-two expectant couples from their pregnancies in 1979 and 1980 through their children's kindergarten year, as well as with twenty-four couples with no immediate plans to become parents. Ninety-five percent of the couples were married; the others were living together. The couples had a wide range of education and income, and more than three-quarters were Caucasian. The inclusion of a nonparent group allowed the Cowans to better understand which changes in couples' functioning were due to the addition of a baby to the family and which changes were more likely due to normal maturation of the couple.

As in other studies of partners becoming parents, the Cowans found that most, but not all, couples became less satisfied with their relationship following the birth of a baby. In their sample, about one-fifth of the couples studied showed modest increases in marital satisfaction from pregnancy to six months after the baby's birth. Other researchers such as Jay Belsky found for at least half the couples he studied, the arrival of a baby had no or even a slightly positive effect on their relationship.

The Cowans found that postpartum decline in marital satisfaction was particularly true for couples aged thirty and above. Older couples tend to have clear expectations about how their marriage ought to function; perhaps these expectations were not met after baby's arrival. Mothers' marital satisfaction declined steadily from birth to when the baby was eighteen months old, whereas fathers' satisfaction declined more sharply between six and eighteen months after the birth of the baby. When asked about levels of conflict and disagreement between them, 92 percent of the new parents described having more conflict and disagreement after the baby's birth.

Interestingly, the Fleming and Ruble group observed that in their cross-sectional sample, postpartum women did not feel any less close to their husbands than women who were thinking about pregnancy but not yet pregnant. They suggest that women feel *more satisfied than usual* with their partners during pregnancy, and that part of the decline in satisfaction seen in many studies after a baby's birth may simply reflect a return to more typical, or prepregnancy, levels of marital satisfaction.

What, then, accounts for many women's feelings of dissatisfaction with their most im-

---

TYPICAL THOUGHTS IN NEW MOTHERHOOD

- Will I ever sleep through the night and feel rested again?
- Should I really have had a baby?
- Am I taking good care of my child?
- What effect is having a child having on my marriage?

portant supporters? The Cowans found that both men and women overwhelmingly state workload imbalance as the issue most likely to cause conflict in the first two years of parenthood. The importance of "who does what" was found by the Fleming and Ruble group as well. They note that even mothers employed full-time outside the home still have more responsibility for managing the family work and child rearing than husbands typically do. On average, across many different household tasks, men and women in their sample divided household tasks fairly evenly before the baby was born. After the baby's birth, men did more of the cooking, cleaning, and grocery shopping than they had before, but women still did more of those chores overall than men. And men did less of other chores, so although the overall responsibility for managing the household did not shift very much, parents became more specialized, and traditional, in terms of what they did. Although shifting to more traditional arrangements was common, couples expressed dissatisfaction with these changes. Chores like cooking meals and cleaning up after children—unrelenting and repetitive—tend to be more stressful than chores that are flexible and intermittent, such as household repairs and automobile maintenance.

Also related to women's satisfaction with their marriage is how supportive fathers are of their parenting. Belsky found that supportive co-parenting was an important predictor of which marriages continued to function well and which marriages took a downturn after the baby's birth. He defined "unsupportive co-parenting" as when one parent undermined the other parent's goals, such as a mother removing a toddler from his high chair right after his father had asked him to stay in his chair to finish his milk.

Along with the actual division of labor, *expectations* about the division of labor have been consistently found to play a role in women's sense of well-being. During pregnancy, both men and women predict that fathers will be *more involved* in childcare than they actually end up being at three and six months postpartum. In Fleming and Ruble's sample, 40 percent of the pregnant women expected an equal division of childcare, but at three months postpartum, only half of them described that to be the case. Only 17 percent of the pregnant women expected to do *much more* of the child care relative to their husbands, but after the baby was born, 41 percent of these women reported doing "much more." Not surprisingly, women are less satisfied than men with how childcare gets shared between them and experience a corresponding decline in marital satisfaction and describe their baby's birth as having more of a negative influence on their marriage. In contrast, men's violated expectations were not related to their marital satisfaction.

Though difficult to achieve, it may be that more realistic appraisals of how much childcare she will be providing can help a woman's adaptation to motherhood. That said, let us underscore the Cowans' finding that when fathers were more involved in taking care of the baby, mothers *and* fathers of six-month-olds described their marriage as more satisfying, the family as more cohesive, and parenting as less stressful. Even a year later, fathers who are more involved with their children have wives who are happier with the quality of the marriage and family life.

The overall conclusion? Despite the challenges inherent in crossing the great divide from independent adult to mother, women can and do adapt with grace, humor, and joy to their new role.

—*Bonnie Ohye, Ph.D., Cynthia W. Moore, Ph.D., and Ellen Braaten, Ph.D.*

Adoption

Despite the intense emotion, celebration, and ritual surrounding families created by birth, the practice of adoption is a phenomenon that has existed since the beginning of recorded history. According to researchers, "adoption has been a means of securing heirs, satisfying political and religious needs, obtaining labor for families, and building alliances" since ancient times. Today, adoption in the United States has become an increasingly more common way to build a family. However, the issues of birth and adoption continue to be powerful and controversial in the legal, political, religious, and personal realms. Cases of adoption covered by the media have increased the general public's awareness of adoption issues, but have at times increased misunderstanding rather than created a more open environment for adoption. There are some major social, psychological, and developmental issues to consider in adoption, for the adoptees, adoptive parents, and birth parents.

DIFFERENT TYPES OF ADOPTION

There are many ways to create a family through adoption: One can adopt domestically or internationally. Adoption can occur between members of the same race or can take place transracially. Many parents prefer to adopt infants, but some choose older children. Increasingly, there are single parents and lesbian or gay parents adopting, and people may decide to adopt through an open or semiopen process, as opposed to the closed adoption processes of the past, in which the birth parents remain anonymous to the adoptive parents and the adoptee. And many families may grow through more than one of the preceding variations of adoption. Not infrequently, adoptive families may already have one or two birth children and choose to have one or more children through adoption.

Same-race adoption has been the traditional form of adoption in the United States. In the past, the policies of adoption agencies were to match the characteristics and background of the adoptee to that of the adoptive parents whenever possible, including ethnic or religious backgrounds (i.e., Catholic or Jewish families worked with Catholic and Jewish organizations to identify matching children). In the United States, until the 1960s this was the most common form of adoption—usually a childless, white, middle-class couple adopted a child who was matched for similarity according to ethnic, religious, and physical characteristics. With the increased acceptance of birth control, single parenthood, and women pursuing more professional careers, the policies of agencies to match race started to change. This was less a matter of increasing liberalism and more of a "function of the market"—in other words, healthy white babies became increasingly scarce.

Transracial adoption can occur domestically or internationally. Within the United States, transracial adoption was almost always practiced by white, middle-class parents who adopted children of a minority racial background, whether African American, Native American, Latino/Hispanic, or of a multiracial background. However, the policies shifted again in 1972, when the National Association of Black Social Workers and then, similarly, Native American leaders took the position that African American and Native American children should be placed only in same-race families. There was a significant focus on the part of agencies to recruit more African American and Native American families in the 1970s, but the numbers of families fell (and continue to fall) short of the numbers of children needing adoptive homes.

> Adoption has been a means of securing heirs, satisfying political and religious needs, obtaining labor for families, and building alliances since ancient times.

In the United States and in Western nations, adoption has involved both same-race and transracial international adoption. In the first half of the twentieth century, international adoptions usually involved white, middle-class Americans adopting orphaned children and children whose parents could not keep them due to war or economic devastation (for example, adoption from Italy or Greece post–World War II). In the second half of the twentieth century, the first major wave of transracial international adoption occurred between Korea and the West following the Korean War. The vast majority of these Korean children came to the United States, as the United States was actively involved in the Korean conflict and continues to have a significant military presence there. Likewise, Vietnam became a source for adopting children following America's involvement in war there. Later in the twentieth century, international adoptees often came from countries dealing with political and economic instability, such as Romania, Russia, India, and Latin American countries.

Increasingly, gay and lesbian adoption has given gay and lesbian couples a means of creating families. In some cases, a gay couple may know the birth mother of the child they adopt in an informal arrangement that then becomes legal. In the case of some lesbian couples, one of the parents may be the biological parent with a known donor, and the other member of the couple adopts the child legally. In other cases, gay and lesbian couples have adopted children who have, in the past, been considered "hard to place"—children who are often of a different race than the adopting parents, who may have been in foster care systems in the United States, who may be older, or who may possibly have physical limitations.

Single-parent adoption is almost always by a single woman who wants to adopt a child (single men do adopt, but rarely). It is likely that single prospective parents are often treated by adoption agencies similarly to gay and lesbian prospective parents—and are often not afforded the same access to children that married, Caucasian, heterosexual parents of middle- to upper-middle income levels are. However, there are some agencies that are more open to single and gay/lesbian prospective parents than others.

> Single-parent adoption is almost always by a single woman who wants to adopt a child.

Open adoption "is the process in which the birth parents and adoptive parents meet and exchange identifying information. The birth parents relinquish legal and basic child rearing rights to the adoptive parents. Both sets of parents retain the right to continuing contact and access to knowledge on behalf of the child." In an open adoption, the degree of contact and frequency of the communications varies depending upon the desires of the individuals involved, including the adoptee, the birth parents, and adoptive parents. Semiopen adoption is a variation on open adoption in which the birth parent(s) and adoptive parent(s) have agreed to set some limits on contact.

DEVELOPMENTAL, PSYCHOLOGICAL, AND SOCIAL ISSUES

For all members of the adoption triad—adoptee, adoptive parent, and birth parent—the feelings, attitudes, and ways of adjusting to and growing with adoption are as numerous and varied as are the members of the triad. While adoptees and adoptive families tend to seek mental health services at rates higher than the general population, the vast majority of adoptees and adoptive families are very satisfied with their families. As with birth families, the lives of adoptive families span the range of human experience.

Adoptees Loss—concrete loss, in terms of physical separation from birth parents, as well as the more abstract, in terms of adoptees' loss of the idealized or fantasy birth parents—is probably the issue given the most attention by professionals who study the field of adoption. For some adoptees, these losses can relate to a kind of loss of self. Reactions to the separation from birth family change with the adoptee's development and can differ based on the age of the child at adoption.

It is generally thought that the longer a child remains in the birth family, the greater the attachment and therefore the greater the distress when the child is separated from the birth parent. However, even when children are adopted in infancy, the child can experience grief many years later. In this situation, the child is grieving imagined birth parents—a mental representation of what she or he has lost—rather than known birth parents. This loss can be further complicated for children adopted into completely different environments, such as adoptees born in a foreign country or adopted into a racially or ethnically dissimilar family.

Secrecy, perhaps more than the fact of adoption, is the cause of a great deal of difficulty for many adoptees. "Why do adoptees feel so alienated and invisible to themselves and others?" is a question of great debate. The secrecy inherent in the closed adoption system is considered a factor, as is the "cumulative adoption trauma"—separation from the birth mother, learning that one was born to parents other than those one calls mother and father, and then the denial of knowledge of birth parents— which most damages the adoptee's sense of self. Indeed, it is a qualitatively different experience for adoptees who do not have access to information about their birth families because they are denied it (whether actively or passively) than it is for adoptees who choose not to seek information about the origins of their birth.

> Open adoption is the process in which the birth parents and adoptive parents meet and exchange identifying information.

Secrecy can often be a less significant issue for transracially/internationally adopted individuals than for those matched for race and ethnicity, even though most of these adoptions are also closed birth records. However, when there are visible physical differences in race between the adoptee and the adoptive parents, the fact of adoption is usually not secret. There does typically remain the same complications as exist for most adoptees—little or no access to information about the birth family. And, for some internationally adopted children, the possibility of obtaining information about birth families may seem so unlikely as to make their birth country feel unreal.

The family romance fantasy is a notion taken from psychoanalysis that suggests one way in which children cope with conflict with parents in the middle years of childhood. Most children (adopted or not) have the fantasy that their parents are not their "real" parents and imagine they have secretly been adopted. Their "real" parents would never scold or punish them and would always love them and gratify their every wish. During moments of anger, one adoptive mother reported this kind of exchange between her and her ten-year-old:

Child: You're not my *real* mother!
Mother: Oh, yes, I am.
Child: You're ruining my life!
Mother: That proves I'm your *real* mother!

This fantasy usually occurs when the child is upset or angry and feels the conflict of loving and hating a parent simultaneously. Eventually, most children resolve this conflict and are able to integrate the "mean" parent and the "loving" parent they live with. For adoptees, however, the family romance is not just played out at the level of fantasy. One can imagine that resolving this fantasy might be a bit more complex and, for some, may take longer to resolve. For some adoptees, the family romance fantasy gets reversed, with the attribution of all positive qualities bestowed upon the adoptive family and all the negative qualities deposited with the unknown birth family. Sometimes, an adoptee might say, "You're my favorite mother" or "You're my best Mom."

COMMON PSYCHOLOGICAL
AND DEVELOPMENTAL
ISSUES FOR ADOPTEES

Loss

Secrecy

The Family Romance Fantasy

The Search for Birth Parents

The general experience of loss can be expressed in a number of different ways and may vary depending upon the developmental stage at which the loss occurs or the loss is recognized. In an infant or small child, this loss may be expressed as despondency, irritability, or lack of connection. For children who experience this loss a little later (perhaps in the middle years between ages seven and ten), it may express itself as confusion, anger, feelings of rejection, or lowered self-esteem. Teens may act out with defiant behavior and/or depression and sadness. We are all aware that teens, adopted or not, are prone to these kinds of reactions; therefore, it is likely that the experiences of feeling different and confused are intensified for the adopted adolescent. One adult adoptee looks back and believes her mother said some "amazing things" in response to her teenage anger: "When I screamed at her when I was seventeen, she would say 'you're stuck with me . . . you can hate me as much as you want, but we're here.'"

Of course, adoptees don't all experience the loss inherent in the adoption process in the same way. Adoptees who feel very securely attached and well matched to their adoptive families, who experience open communication within the family and the larger community, and in whose families differences (race, nationality, sexual orientation, etc.) are valued have an easier time dealing with being adopted. This does not mean that the teen years for these adoptees are completely smooth, but they may not be significantly different from those of fairly well adjusted nonadoptive teens.

Common sense might tell us that identity development might be more complicated for adoptees than for those who are not adopted. While all children and adolescents struggle to become independent of their parents, adoptees contend with further issues, and transracially and internationally adopted individuals deal with yet another layer of issues. Again, most adoptees manage to navigate these difficult adolescent years in ways not so dissimilar to other adolescents. For others, there may be difficulties that arise that are related to their experience of adoption. Being different is a significant concern for all kids, especially in the preteen and teen years. However, visible differences and invisible differences affect how other people respond to adoptees. Transracially adopted and internationally adopted children who grow up in communities where no one looks like them are likely to face racism and prejudice in their many forms (teasing on the playground, being stereotyped or misunderstood, difficulties dating, and occasionally more blatant and aggressive forms of racism). For example, one transracially adopted woman said:

When I was growing up? There was a lot of self-hatred. . . . I turned on my Mom a lot. I tried to make myself look different. Yeah . . . that was probably until college. . . . I really didn't want to be Asian. At some point, you sort of convince yourself that if you *do* enough things, you won't *be* as Asian. And you're really kind of surprised when people can still tell . . . I wore a lot of makeup and I had a lot of perms. . . . So, I would always have a lot of really bad hair.

On the other hand, children of the same race as their adoptive parents may hear negative or disparaging remarks about adoption by peers unaware of their adoption status. These issues then will naturally complicate the adolescent's questioning of "who am I?" and "where do I belong?" which precede teenagers' natural attempts to separate from their parents. Separation from adoptive parents can be complicated then, as most nonadopted teens usually contrast themselves to their parents—yet have the secure knowledge of being fundamentally linked to their parents, at least genetically. Some adoptees may feel alienated from their parents—feeling they have never really "belonged" to their families. Others, conversely, may struggle to maintain their connections and similarity for fear of losing the only parents they know. For many adoptees, adolescence is a particularly complex and confusing time to navigate between the different poles of connection and disconnection to the adoptive parents.

The search for birth parents or birth family has become a much more common and acceptable practice among adoptees and within adoption communities in the last fifteen to twenty years. There are different ways for adoptees to seek and discover information about their birth families and possibly reunite with them (private investigators, their adoption agency, search organizations).

> Adoptees who feel very securely attached and well matched to their adoptive families, who experience open communication within the family and the larger community, and in whose families differences are valued have an easier time dealing with being adopted.

Adoption professionals now almost insist that adoptees search, implying that adoptees are in denial or cannot be "whole" without going through the search process. As with any intense emotional issue, the search process is a deeply personal one. For some adoptees, searching for their birth parents is a long-held desire they have nurtured since early childhood. For other adoptees, the search is a process they have thought about but have not actively pursued—perhaps because they were preoccupied with other pressing concerns (friends, social life, school, college, marriage, etc.). It may be they were waiting until they felt more stable in their lives and more certain of their own identities.

Other adoptees may have never thought of searching; perhaps they feel very solidly connected to their adoptive families and do not feel the need to meet or know of biological family. Some may be afraid of what they may find when they search. And for yet others, searching for birth family is a very concrete manifestation of their adoption status, and they may fear that this too clearly differentiates them from others. Whatever the reasons for searching or not searching, the important thing is that the opportunity to search exists, although not all adoptees choose to take this path.

> For many adoptees, adolescence is a particularly complex and confusing time to navigate between the different poles of connection and disconnection to the adoptive parents.

A reunion with one's birth family, in contrast to the search, is less common. This, however, is also increasing in frequency. Some adoptees simply want basic medical and factual information about their birth families when they search. Others are very focused on meeting a member or members of their birth family and developing a relationship. Adopted women search in much higher percentages than men and often at significant junctures in their lives (birth of their own child, pregnancy, death of an adoptive parent). Most often, the focus of the search is on the birth mother and somewhat less frequently on the birth father. However, many adoptees wonder whether or imagine that they may have brothers and sisters—and may fantasize they could encounter a member of their birth family without realizing it.

The reunions themselves are rich and often varied in terms of adoptees' satisfaction. For some adoptees, the birth family and the adoptive family become a rich part of their ongoing lives—albeit usually with some adjustment difficulties. I spoke with one adoptee who had both her birth parents and her adoptive parents at her wedding. Other adoptees who establish contact may maintain contact sporadically perhaps because the adoptee and the birth family do not have much in common, or there are language or cultural barriers. Some adoptees have talked about the frustration of feeling that the birth family denies the past and expects the adoptee to fit into the birth family's lives as if the years apart had not existed. Other birth families mostly express relief in knowing their child is safe and well or educated in a way they could not have provided, and these families leave decisions about contact up to the adoptee.

Adoptive Parents Adoptive parents differ from each other as all parents differ from one another. However, in making the decision to adopt, many have one thing in common: The adoption of their child/children was the "most thrilling, exciting thing in [their] lives." The reasons for adopting range from fertility and health issues to a desire to "rescue" orphans or reduce population growth or, most commonly and simply, "to have a family."

Fertility problems have become increasingly common in the postindustrial United States. With more and more women obtaining advanced degrees and couples waiting to start families, the average age of first-time mothers has increased. Today, women from their teens to forties are having children for the first time. Men have also had increasing fertility problems. Some couples choose to adopt because having children by birth might put the mother at some health risk or there is evidence for genetic disorders in the family history.

In the process of dealing with fertility issues or health risks prohibiting pregnancy, many women and men go through a process of loss. For some prospective parents, it is the loss of the child they imagined they would have, who might share physical and genetic similarities to them. In some cases, the woman or man might deal with this concern fairly quickly and consider alternatives. Other couples may work with medical professionals for many years and arrive at the decision to adopt after some significantly painful and exhausting experiences.

Raising an adoptee is a complex topic, and most would agree there is no one correct way to raise any child. However, there are a few points that do promote healthy adjustment in adopted children. One finding, based on a 1995 U.S. study of Korean adopted women, suggests that a "positive and openly communicative relationship with the adoptive parents and family is the best predictor of positive self concept in adoptees."

This finding had some significant implications for "culture camps" that have been growing in number and popularity in recent years. Culture camps are designed to teach internationally adopted children about their heritage and expose them to children of similar backgrounds. This study points to the need to not only teach adoptees about their ethnic and cultural background, but also to talk openly about feelings related to adoption issues, both within larger groups and within the family. Directors of some of these camps and many mental health professionals stress that learning about the adoptees' cultural or ethnic background is not just the task of the adoptee, but of the entire adoptive family. Overall then, talking about adoption issues early on, in developmentally appropriate ways, is very useful. For transracial adoptees, comfort in and knowledge of the adoptee's culture of origin as well as the adopted culture is related to higher self-esteem.

Another significant and related finding is that acknowledgment of differences within the family rather than the denial of differences contributes to healthy self-esteem and adjustment in adoptees. In the 1960s and 1970s, liberal attitudes promoted equal rights and a "color blind" approach. However, that approach sometimes ignored the realities of adopted children when they left the comfort and security of their families and small communities. For example, from the perspective of one adult Korean adoptee:

> Um, I'm actually very thankful that I'm here, you know.... And, I don't have a lot of anger towards my parents because I think they're very wonderful, loving, caring people who cared about my ethnicity. I mean, it wasn't just "OK, now you're a part of our family, and now let's not ever deal with issues...." They were always involved in different groups. I think at one time, they were involved in "friends of Vietnam..." so a lot of Vietnamese families would get together with us, so we could be exposed to other kids who kind of looked like us. So, they were very conscientious about getting us involved.

When and how to share information about the child's past with their son or daughter is a common question most adoptive parents have. Most children, whether adopted or birth

> ✦
>
> Culture camps are designed to teach internationally adopted children about their heritage and expose them to children of similar backgrounds.

children, love to hear about their entry into the family. Again, this is an extremely complex question and may vary a great deal depending upon the child and the circumstances. One adoptive parent, who is herself an adoptee, said this about her approach to the topic with her five-year-old daughter: "I will often say things, just to keep things open. Sometimes, I'll bring up her birth mother . . . mostly so she knows that she can bring it up whenever she wants to."

What is generally useful is to provide ample opportunities for a child to ask questions early on—and when the child does ask, to try to assess what it is he or she is asking. Parents may feel they have to share everything they know about the child's past when their child first asks about his or her birth origins. However, your child may not be asking for much information and is likely not ready for all the details—but he or she may want to know something simple or more basic. It is a balancing act to provide an environment in which children are supported to raise questions, concerns, and show curiosity—and yet it is important that adoptive parents do not take over the issues of adoption for their children. Sometimes, very well meaning parents become so concerned with making sure their child is talking about adoption and knowledgeable about his or her origins that the child may not feel he or she has ownership of the process anymore.

For most families who have openly acknowledged and valued adoption and differences, the adoptee's search for birth family can be a process that is supported when and if the adoptee is interested or ready. What can make this process significantly easier for an adoptee is the knowledge that searching for the birth family is not going to jeopardize or threaten the adoptee's relationship to the adoptive parents. In many cases, the search and reunion with the birth family can be a process that increases closeness between the adoptee and his or her adoptive parents. For many adoptees, the search for birth family is an experience they may need to do on their own, but having the support of their parents facilitates this process immensely. One adoptive mother always expressed to her children an interest in meeting her daughter's birth mother: "I want to thank her for bringing you into this world and for sharing you with me." Adoptees whose parents chose a semiopen or open adoption have a significant advantage in this realm, as they have likely grown up knowing that information and/or a birth parent is accessible, when and if they are interested.

On the other hand, many adoptees do not show any significant interest in searching for their birth families. In recent years, a bias seems to have developed in the adoption field that searching is the only way for adoptees to feel "whole." This may be a response to the past when all adoptions were closed and shrouded in secrecy. While some adoptees may indeed feel more "complete" when they have gone through the process of search, other adoptees may never feel an interest—because they have fears and concerns that prevent them from searching, or because they feel their lives are rich and satisfying and simply have other stronger interests.

> For most families who have openly acknowledged and valued adoption and differences, the adoptee's search for birth family can be a process that is supported when and if the adoptee is interested or ready.

> While some adoptees may indeed feel more "complete" when they have gone through the process of search, other adoptees may never feel an interest—because they have fears and concerns that prevent them from searching, or because they feel their lives are rich and satisfying.

Birth Parents Historically, mothers have held the weight of the decision to place their children for adoption. Birth fathers have rarely been involved, and their rights were not recognized legally in the United States until the 1970s. While there is a multitude of reasons for a birth mother to relinquish a child, always there is some force (individual, group, or society) acting upon her that prevents her from feeling she can take care of the child in the way she wishes. These forces may include one or more of the following: (1) the social or religious stigma of raising a child out of wedlock, (2) disapproval of extended families, (3) birth parent(s)' acknowledgment of their own immaturity and lack of readiness for a child, (4) financial difficulties for the mother/parents, (5) major social or political upheaval or mass poverty in the birth country, (6) death of one or both of the parents, (7) racism or prejudice (e.g., the child is biracial or multiracial), (8) conception resulted from coercion or violence, and numerous other possibilities. Whatever the circumstances, there is physical and psychological loss associated with relinquishment of a child. In many cases, this loss may be felt in varying degrees throughout the life of the birth parent.

Throughout the history of women having children outside of marriage or relinquishing children to adoption, society has placed blame and ascribed moral deviance or psychopathology to the birth mother. Even today in the United States, women who have children outside of marriage continue to be condemned. So, in addition to experiencing the personal grief in the loss of a child, the birth mother also faces shame and secrecy imposed upon her by a society that would rather blame her than address the systemic problems leading to some her choices. In most cases, birth mothers (and fathers) choose adoption in the hope that they are providing an opportunity for a better life for their child. During a reunion between a birth family and an adoptee, one of the birth brothers was able to say, "Our mother, she always worried about your education," and he also talked about how much the birth family worried and thought about the adoptee, especially during holidays and family events.

For birth parents, not knowing about the adoptee's life situation can be very complicated. In some international adoptions, birth families are given misleading information—for example, that the adoptee will return to the birth family once he or she has received his or her education abroad. For many birth parents, there is a simultaneous desire for information about the child as well as a desire not to know because it is too painful.

As an outgrowth of social changes taking place in the 1970s and beyond, birth mothers have come together to speak out about their experiences, to increase awareness of their situations, and to help change agency practices.

—*Kunya S. Desjardins, Ph.D.*

RELATED ENTRIES

A Guide to Grief and Bereavement

Becoming a Mother

Choosing Childlessness

Living with Infertility

Choosing Childlessness

On a clear, bright day last fall, I started to wonder whether something was wrong with My attack of self-doubt began under highly unlikely circumstances. My husband and I were on vacation in a charming medieval hill town in Italy, surrounded by miles of rolling hills, vineyards, and unspoiled countryside. It was lovely and lush; we were having a fine time.

The setting was Felliniesque: an elegant picnic on the site of an archaeological excavation. Fifty guests, all wearing sunglasses, clambered up and down the Roman ruins, dressed formally in suits and ties, gowns and heels. A long table had been set under the cypresses, covered with a white linen tablecloth and laden with a banquet. Just as we started to enjoy the feast, I struck up a conversation with the tall blonde woman to my right. She was an Italian business executive from Rome. After a minute or two, she asked me if we had any children.

"No, we don't," I said.

"But why not?" She looked stunned.

"We . . ." I faltered. "We just don't," I said. I wasn't sure what to tell her. The answer was both simple and complicated. Above all, it was private.

"But you *must* have some!" she said, pressing my arm with her tanned fingers. "My sons are the most wonderful things in my life. You *have* to have children. Quickly. Don't miss it."

I opened my mouth, but didn't say anything. Though many people had raised the topic over the years, few had been quite so blunt or intrusive as this woman. "You know," she said, earnestly, "if you don't have children, you'll regret it. Don't wait until it's too late." She picked up her fork and speared an olive.

I couldn't respond. I had no words with which to defend my choice. Back home in Brooklyn, my relatives had been dropping similar hints. It seemed that in electing not to have children, I'd made a decision that few people, aside from my husband, could support or comprehend. Most of my closest friends were becoming mothers. I excused myself from the party early, and when I got back to the hotel room, I locked myself in and cried.

CHILDLESS BY CHOICE: THE WOMAN OF MYSTERY

I decided to research the topic of women who are childless by choice as soon as we got back. The first thing I did was to contact a sympathetic expert, a woman I considered to be a leading authority on all matters pertaining to the human female. I called Natalie Angier, the author of *Woman: An Intimate Geography*. The book explores how cultural biases about gender have led researchers to draw inaccurate, discriminatory conclusions about "female nature"—like the stereotype that women are born to be monogamous while men are born to philander. I thought Angier might agree with my own suspicion: that not every woman is meant to be a mother, that our biology need not be our destiny, and that "the maternal instinct" is a myth.

I was wrong. Natalie Angier had no such reassurances for me. Women who reject motherhood are few and far between, she said. To the scientific mind, the woman who is childless by choice remains a mystery. "The evolutionary imperative is to reproduce," said Angier, a Pulitzer Prize–winning science writer for the *New York Times*. "It's such a strong drive: to preserve the species, to pass your genes along. In fact, it's fundamental to life. There isn't a satisfactory explanation for why women decide against motherhood. It's a *tiny* minority. Like homosexuality, intentional childlessness presents, for the biologist, an unsolved puzzle."

In the eyes of science, I was a freak. While I didn't relish being thought of as an oddity, I was intrigued by the notion that I belong to a minority group. Perhaps, like homosexuals in the early dawn of the gay rights movement, women like me have been marginalized, made to feel "Other." Left out. Even deviant. Had we been rendered silent and invisible by a boisterous, procreating majority? Maybe my problem—if I had one—had more to do with my sense of shame than with my decision. Instead of "coming out" as childless by choice, I'd stayed in the darkness of the closet.

That winter, I devised my own research project. Over a period of six weeks, I conducted a study of women like myself. My research methods were as follows: I asked everyone I knew to give me the name and phone number of a woman who was childless by choice. Once a week, after dinner, I plunked down in an armchair, poured myself a glass of wine, and made a phone call. I interviewed ten women who I've never met. I don't know their ethnicity, where they live, or what they look like. As we talked, I imagined they were standing behind a screen, out of sight, the way coifed and powdered noblewomen were required to do in tenth-century Japan. In voices that ranged from throaty and gruff to high and girlish, they introduced themselves—jewelry designer, tax accountant, hatmaker, poet. One by one, they confided the most personal elements of their lives, discussing romances, ambitions, miscarriages, desires, dreams, and fears. Portraits emerged of distinct, diverse women—from the brusque and decisive to the sensitive and introspective.

THE WOMAN WHO DOES WHAT SHE WANTS TO DO

Suzanne Ostro, a rare book dealer, is in her seventies. A woman of strong opinions, her attitude is impish. She talks with bravado, a verbal swagger. "Let me tell you right now, I'm going to throw your whole damn study off," she drawls. "Everyone who knows me says that the reason I don't have kids is that I hate them. They say, don't ask Suzanne to baby-sit, whatever you do." She isn't complaining or protesting, but making mischief, teasing, almost bragging. Unlike others I'd speak with later, the accusation of child hating doesn't distress her. Ostro bristles with confidence. She's a cheerful rebel, and always has been.

Ostro grew up in a radically different America, before Madonna or Monica, the Equal Rights Amendment and the sexual revolution, rock and roll and World War II. With few exceptions, the women she knew, as a girl in the 1930s and 1940s, were housewives. Though her middle-class Baltimore home was fairly traditional, her own mind-set was not. "All my friends wanted to do was get *married* and have *kids*," she says, with great scorn and disgust. "They were typical women of that generation. They thought college was a waste of time. If they even bothered to go, it wasn't to get themselves educated. It was just a convenient place to wait. Their primary occupation was looking for a husband."

Ostro was raised to think of herself differently. "I was never aware of any prejudice against me as a female, whatsoever," she says. "I had an aunt who was a doctor. She came to America from Russia at the age of twenty-three. In 1916, she became the first woman to graduate from her medical school. My other aunt was also a career woman. At the time, that was rare. For some reason, I was oblivious to the prevailing attitudes. I grew up thinking I could do anything I wanted to! My father was extremely supportive of me. He told me, Suzanne, you'd better figure out what you're going to do, or you'll wind up washing some man's laundry."

> Had we been rendered silent and invisible by a boisterous, procreating majority? Maybe my problem—if I had one—had more to do with my sense of shame than with my decision. Instead of "coming out" as childless by choice, I'd stayed in the darkness of the closet.

Ostro has had several stimulating careers, many relationships, and two marriages. She's traveled widely. "I've always done exactly what I wanted to do," she states, with her chipper, endearing bluntness. Ostro followed her own impulses. They never included having children. Where did a woman raised in prefeminist America acquire so much irreverent spunk?

"Right from the start," she says, "I was armed to make independent decisions. I never cared about what other people thought. Part of it is my personality. My mother used to call me headstrong. I am. I wanted to be free to move around and do as I pleased."

Asked how she reacted to the social stigma of childlessness, Ostro says, "I didn't care what society thought about it—on any level. Not just about childlessness. About anything. The worst thing, for anyone, is to pay attention to what society tells you to do."

Motherhood isn't interesting to Ostro. "There are people who think their whole role in life is being a mother," she says. "I find that irritating. It's as if they wouldn't know who they are unless they were mothers. If everyone had kids for the right reasons, the population would drop 80 percent. The attitude that nothing else matters—the obsessiveness—is exasperating."

As Ostro notes, "Throughout history, there have always been women who have done just what they've wanted without caring what people think. And I'd be willing to bet they've never been looked at fondly by society."

Looking back on seven decades, Ostro is content. "I'm extremely pleased with how it worked," she says. "If I'd had children, they'd get in my way. I'm a reasonably selfish person. I couldn't have stood all that being tied down. The best thing about not having kids was that I could leave my husbands when I wanted to! I lived in Paris for five years. I've been to Europe, Greece, Morocco, all over the place. I have the freedom." Asked if she had any advice for younger women who were moving toward childlessness, Ostro says, "When I was a kid, my aunts would say: No one can tell you what to do. Men don't go around apologizing for not having children. Why should we? It's that simple."

By the way, does she hate kids? "Well, no. Not really," she confesses, with a sigh. She sounds disappointed, as if it might be more fun to say she did.

THE WILD AUNT OF AMERICA

Lola Ehrlich is a fifty-four-year-old hat designer. She spent her childhood, in the 1950s, in a rural neighborhood outside of Paris. Sprawling and isolated, "It looked just like an impressionist painting," she recalls, in a husky voice with a French accent. Her parents, a journalist and a painter, were bohemian. They were opposed to providing any formal schooling for their two daughters. Neither Ehrlich nor her sister attended elementary school, high school, or college. She learned to read as a small child, and, after that, she educated herself. She disliked the anarchic atmosphere of her household and craved routine normality. "My parents lived the life they chose," she says. "They spent most of the day in bed."

Ehrlich left home while in her teens and, at eighteen, fell in love with a man who was thirty years her senior. They married when she was twenty-one. She embarked on many illicit love affairs. She recognized that the unconventional marriage wasn't a secure enough environment for children. At twenty-six, she became a widow. Ehrlich, a single woman for the first time in her adulthood, now yearned to be a mother. Upon moving to the United States in 1974, she became pregnant while involved with a married man. Her miscarriage four months later was traumatic. She had badly wanted a baby. As she recovered from the loss, she subjected her feelings about motherhood to scrutiny. "I realized I wanted the child because I wasn't happy in the relationship. It became a pattern. For several years, if I felt I wasn't loved or didn't love enough, I got pregnant." Each of her four pregnancies ended in abortion or miscarriage. After a string of disappointing relationships, she met a man whom she married. Once she was secure, happy, and fulfilled, the desire to have a child vanished. "I realized a child was an idea, not a reality, for me," she says. "It represented love." They've been married for over twenty years.

The decision not to have children was difficult, however, because Ehrlich's husband adores children. After much discussion, they agreed that the ultimate choice should be hers. "I gave myself a deadline, set a date on which to decide. On that day, I said 'no.' You have to make up your mind and say it aloud. I have never once regretted it," she says. The marriage hasn't suffered the strains that Ehrlich believes small children inevitably bring. "We're like a young couple," she notes. "We're independent, but also very close. We talk a lot. We enjoy each other's presence."

Having worked on the periphery of the fashion industry since the 1970s, Ehrlich had dreamed of designing hats ever since she was a child. When she turned forty, she began taking night classes in hat design. She opened a one-woman storefront in New York's East Village in 1989. Today, she has two shops and a staff of thirteen. Thousands of her hats are sold each year around the world. Though she's designed hats for the runway shows of such luminaries as Oscar de la Renta, Donna Karan, Michael Kors, and Calvin Klein, the glamour of her profession isn't what she cherishes. "I love what I do," she says, with quiet intensity. "I love the people I work with. It's a small studio, and I only hire people that I like. So I'm surrounded by friends all the time. We're a team. They're so supportive of me."

In addition to the extended family of colleagues, Ehrlich is attached to her nieces, aged sixteen and twenty-one, who frequently visit from France. "To them," she said, bemused, "I'm the wild aunt of America, you know? And yet, for all the craziness of my youth, I'm now a proper *bourgeois,* very reasonable and rational."

THE PRAGMATIST

"I wake up every morning and I *thank God* that I don't have kids," announces Leslie Journet, emphatically. "I don't have a maternal or a motherly bone in my entire body." It's a rather shocking thing to say, the more so because her voice is sweet and low. Journet speaks with a lilting Southern twang. It sounds extremely "feminine." A yoga instructor, age forty-six, she was born in a small town in southern Georgia. Her initial assessment of motherhood was negative, and that impression has endured. "When I was growing up, my father had re-married. They had five kids, and I often took care of my step-brothers and step-sisters. I changed a lot of diapers. I saw how much work it was, firsthand. If I were going to have kids of my own, I intended to be with them full-time for the first few years. I felt they deserved their mother's full attention." She pauses, then delivers her zinger. "But," she says, pleasantly, "if I had to stay home with a kid, I'd lose my mind."

Like many of the women I spoke to, Journet is refreshingly honest. She knows herself and doesn't feel she has to soft-pedal her likes and dislikes, to equivocate, or to minimize unpleasant realities. She's a pragmatist. "On a practical level," Journet says, "quality of life entered into my decision. I wasn't interested in *schlepping.* I was living in New York City, in a walk-up, on no money. Carrying a stroller and groceries and children up and down five flights of stairs didn't beckon to me. I thought it would be nice to have an elevator, at least."

Journet was a professional modern dancer for the better part of a decade. When she married, at thirty-five, she considered becoming a mother. "I didn't want children," she realized. "I saw what had happened to my friends' lives when they had kids. One had moved out to Long Island. She was totally isolated. Another friend seemed beaten down and exhausted by juggling work with motherhood. After a grueling week, she'd spend all weekend planning events for her children. I'm too selfish to spend my whole weekend that way," she says, frankly. "I have a strong ego. I never saw any need to replicate myself, genetically." Reviewing her choices, Journet feels they were the right ones.

THE EXPLORER

"You often hear about women who regret not having children," observes Mary Mackey, novelist and screenwriter. "But there are just as many women who regret having them." Mackey's own mother was a chemist who gave up her career to raise children. The sense of opportunities lost shadowed Mackey's childhood, and she regards women's knowledge of their mothers' frustrated ambitions as a motivating force behind the feminist movement of the 1970s. "It was fueled," she says, "by the awareness of what our mothers had been forced to give up." She came of age at a time when fresh possibilities were just opening to women. Even in childhood, Mackey knew she wanted to be an author. "I was influenced by Sylvia Plath," she says. "She dealt with motherhood and career—not very gracefully. I watched her destroy herself." Children, she surmises, can be a mistake. Leery of sacrifice, Mackey gave a wide berth to the choices made by Plath and other thwarted female talents of that generation.

Mackey, who holds a Ph.D., is the author of thirteen books, including *The Earthsong*

Trilogy, a series that draws on the work of the late feminist archaeologist Marija Gimbutas (who theorized the existence of an ancient goddess-worshipping matriarchy). To research her novels, Mackey has journeyed far and wide. She's been to the Amazon several times, as well as Brazil, Bulgaria, Colombia, Mexico, and Romania. She has traveled to unstable and remote regions, living in the forests of Costa Rica and twice coming under machine-gun fire. In South America, she's stayed in huts with people who were suffering from malaria. She's flown over jungles in small propeller airplanes. "Ran out of gas, more than once," she says, with evident pride. This, in short, is a woman who takes chances. Unwilling to leave rugged explorations to the likes of Hemingway, she's intentionally exposed herself to situations that she believes are typically identified with males. Her adventures have been both exhilarating and frightening, increasing Mackey's confidence while broadening her personal and professional horizons. "People talk about women's writing being 'domestic,'" she says. "That's because women with small children just can't afford to take those kinds of risks."

> "You often hear about women who regret not having children," observes Mary Mackey, novelist and screenwriter. "But there are just as many women who regret having them."

Yet Mackey loves children. In the ideal universe, she would have liked to be able to do it all: to have twelve kids, a successful career, and the ability to travel extensively. She views that combination as an impossible fantasy, one that many women chase after to their detriment. She's dismayed by the current expectation that women balance a high-powered profession with perfect parenting. Men and women are not yet equal partners, at home or in the workplace. "Women are still paid so much less than men," she observes. "Even with a high salary, a woman feels torn—guilty about her job, and guilty about her kids. Women are under pressure from family and friends to have children, while under pressure from employers *not* to have them. Discrimination is illegal, so this is unspoken. But a high-level executive who has children knows the truth: that she's jeopardizing her career by being a mom. No one likes to say it, but it's true. We've got a lot of tired, ragged-out women today."

Mackey feels she has a happy, successful life. Though she has no regrets, she has felt vulnerable to criticism. She's encountered many people who assume that childless women are "cruel and selfish." She's disturbed by the frequent questions she receives about why she doesn't have kids. "People who ask this are insensitive. For all they know, you may have tried desperately to have children. You may have had a baby who died. Men aren't questioned like that."

Becoming a mother is of paramount importance to some women, she says. To others, it is not. "The truer you are to your soul in making choices," she notes, "the happier you'll be with your life."

Like Mackey, acclaimed author Mary Gaitskill is adventurous. Gaitskill's fiction explores circumstances that women have been taught to avoid, and she's shown a similar disregard for convention in her own life. At the age of sixteen, she ran away from home to become a stripper, and later began to pen stories while holding down a series of menial jobs. Gaitskill often wrote through the night in her tiny studio, determined to achieve the mastery of language and emotional complexity that her fiction is celebrated for. "I feel certain that if I'd had a family I would not be a writer," she says. Over the phone, Gaitskill—who recently married—explains that it was key to her artistic development to be both single and childless. She needed time and solitude to hone her skills. "If I'd been a mother," she said, "I would have been embittered."

At the age of eight, Gaitskill alarmed her grandmother by proclaiming that she never wanted to have children. The sentiment remains unsettling. "Women who don't have children are disapproved of," she observes. "Part of it is the need to believe there is something all tender and all nurturing in the world. The world is so violent and so full of cruelty. If no one seems willing to be the nurturer, the gentle one, that's scary."

> Becoming a mother is of paramount importance to some women, she says. To others, it is not. "The truer you are to your soul in making choices," she notes, "the happier you'll be with your life."

For many years, Gaitskill felt her choice not to be a mother was unremarkable. But at the end of the 1990s she sensed a deep prejudice emerging against women who elect not to have children. "A journalist asked me if not being a mother had 'narrowed my palette,'" she recalls. "I agreed that it probably has, but so has not being in a war. I let the question go, but it haunted me." In her fiction and nonfiction, Gaitskill has written incisively on this issue. Though she has tentatively weighed the possibility of adopting, she is bothered by the implication that the only fulfillment a woman can find, artistically or otherwise, is through motherhood.

THE BALLET STAR

Pamela Pribifco's voice exudes power and dignity. Now nearing retirement, she was for many years a principal dancer with the Cleveland Ballet. She began training at the age of six and was dancing professionally at thirteen. Ballet is her passion. Her friends and family recognized her unique aptitude early on. Pribifco was never pressured to marry or have children and has had no second thoughts. She regards dance as a calling. "You won't succeed unless you give it your full effort," she says. "It's just too hard. It requires tremendous determination and discipline, years are required to refine one's technique, hours are spent practicing each and every day, in peak physical condition. If I had had children, I would have regretted it," she says, echoing Mackey. "I wouldn't have done, in my life, what I came here to do."

For a principal ballet dancer, she tells me, childlessness, far from being "freakish," is the norm. "In the ballet world," she explains, "we say that creativity is your child."

A SIGNIFICANT MINORITY

On a chilly December evening, in a state of confusion and doubt, I'd begun a telephone treasure hunt—without quite knowing what I was looking for. I quickly saw that what I'd been missing were role models. In the extraordinary women I spoke to, I found them. While I've only written about a few of the women I interviewed, all those I spoke with had satisfying careers in common. Half of my unscientific study participants were in a long-term partnership. More than half said they didn't perceive childlessness as bearing a social stigma. Five out of ten women were aware, from an early age, that they had no desire to have children. The others came to a gradual decision. Only three of my respondents said they had gone through periods of deep ambivalence. I'd intended to interview gay women as well as heterosexuals, but the three lesbians I contacted, all in their thirties, are undecided about motherhood.

Women who wish to explore this issue for themselves might make their own round of phone calls, or take a stroll to their local library. With childlessness steadily rising since 1975 (a trend that applies to all age groups, according to the Census Bureau's 1998 report "Fertility of American Women") more attention is being paid to the topic. Ten years ago, when Rochelle Ratner first began gathering material for an anthology devoted to childlessness, she found little was available on the subject. "In the last five years," she said, "there's been a surge of interest. The issue has become more visible, and more acceptable. It's gotten easier to talk about. But there continues to be a sense of shame attached to it. The emphasis is on how a woman has 'made up' for being without children. It's important not to frame it negatively."

"It's been called the last taboo," notes Molly Peacock, whose engaging memoir revolves around her choice not to have children. She leads workshops for those who are considering this option. "Women who make this decision do so from a deep level of awareness of their own internal conflicts, and those in the culture," she says. "Instead of accepting the myth that we can have it all, they recognize their own limits, not as a deficiency, but as a part of the human condition. They don't allow the culture to tell them who they are, but follow a powerful intuition about their own natures."

My unscientific telephone study bears this out. And the fact that my study was unscientific points to the biases that still exist regarding this topic. While the ranks of women without children continue to grow, there are still few researchers who have taken the time or have the inclination to study the phenomenon as an acceptable, visible force. Why study something so marginal as to be irrelevant? In a sense, that's what Angier was implying. If your job is to study the natural world, and childlessness by choice is outside the natural world, then of course no one will turn an inquiring eye toward it.

What we need are scientific psychological studies of childlessness, the decision-making processes that women go through, their growth and development throughout the life span, how women without children negotiate the developmental challenges of middle and late age versus their procreative counterparts. We need these scientific studies because they are interesting and because they can shed light on the phenomenon in a way an anecdotal study, like mine, simply cannot. I look forward to the day when I will be able to turn to a body of literature that gives me an organized and cohesive thesis about the whos, whys, and wheres of childless women by choice, because then I will know; we have entered Angier's arena. We are not freaks. We are, perhaps, nature's answer to overpopulation. We are, perhaps, evolutionary imperatives. We are many things, and we are just starting to tell our stories.

—Lisa Dierbeck

RELATED ENTRIES

Play

Women and Spirituality

Issues for Women in Middle Age

Middle age (defined roughly as the time from age forty to age sixty-five) has traditionally been seen as a rotten time for women, who are thought to be afflicted with major issues such empty nest syndrome, retirement, developmental tasks, and health issues, specifically breast cancer, heart disease, and menopause. But does the scientific evidence support these traditional views?

IS THERE AN EMPTY NEST SYNDROME?

The empty nest syndrome refers to the psychological distress that women are believed to experience when their children are grown and have left home, leaving Mother rattling around in an empty nest. We have thought that the empty nest syndrome would strike most at women who were full-time moms and homemakers and should be less difficult for women who have been employed. The idea is that people's identity and meaning in life derive from their major roles, and if a major role is taken away, the result can be psychological distress such as depression. All mothers lose a role when their children become adults, but for full-time moms the loss is thought to be more serious because they do not have the work role to soften the blow.

Sociologist Lillian Rubin challenged many ideas about the empty nest syndrome. She studied 160 women, a cross section of mothers aged thirty-five to fifty-four, from the working, middle, and professional classes, all of them white. To be included in the sample, a woman had to have given up work or her career for at least ten years after the birth of her first child, thus representing the group that should be most vulnerable to the empty nest syndrome. Many of these women said, "My career was my child." Rubin found, in striking contrast to popular thinking, that although some women were momentarily sad, lonely, or frightened, they were not depressed in response to the departure or impending departure of their children. The predominant feeling of every woman except one was a feeling of relief! Rather than experiencing an immobilizing depression, most of the women found new jobs and reorganized their daily lives.

Other studies consistently find that women, on average, are no more depressed in midlife than at other times. The Massachusetts Women's Health Study found that 85 percent of women were never depressed during the menopausal years, 10 percent were depressed occasionally, and just 5 percent were persistently depressed.

Some psychologists go one step further and argue that the early fifties are the prime of life for women. In one study of women college graduates between the ages of twenty-six and eighty, the women in their early fifties were the most likely to describe their lives as "first rate." Health was better and income was higher at this age than others. These women displayed confidence, involvement, security, and depth in their personalities.

In short, the empty nest syndrome does not dominate the lives of middle-aged women, and, in fact, for many women these years are the prime of life.

RETIREMENT

Today in the United States, employment is the norm for adult women; among women between the ages of fifty and fifty-four, 73 percent are employed. Although we once considered retirement to be a men's issue, it has now become an issue for women as well. Unfortunately, most of the research on retirement has been based on all-male samples.

Women are more likely than men to retire because of a spouse's retirement, particularly because women tend to marry men who are somewhat older than they are. The combination of one spouse being retired and the other still employed is associated with strains on the marriage. Women are also more likely than men to retire because of their spouse's ill health. Professional women and self-employed women are less likely to retire early than are women in other occupations.

Income is a concern for retired women. Women are more likely than men to report that their retirement incomes are not adequate. One reason is that retired women, on average, receive considerably smaller Social Security checks than retired men do. This occurs because Social Security payments are based on a person's preretirement earnings, and the wage gender gap continues to ensure that women have smaller earnings and therefore smaller Social Security payments.

DEVELOPMENTAL TASKS

According to the famous developmental theorist Erik Erikson, those in the middle adult years face a particular developmental task, the crisis of generativity versus stagnation. Some exit this crisis with the feeling that their lives are stagnant, going nowhere and have little purpose. Those who resolve the crisis positively have a sense of generativity; they invest time and energy in the next generation and find this satisfying. For women, generativity often derives from parenting one's own biological children and supporting them as they develop into competent young adults.

In an era in which women have had unprecedented opportunities for and successes in careers, women's generativity may also result from mentoring younger people in their own field of work. Just as they raise their own children, so too may they raise the next generation of professionals in their field.

Recent research on generativity has extended the concept to caring for elderly parents. Compared with other women, generative women report feeling less burdened by caring for their aging parents. Generative women also report that they feel embedded in a reciprocal, intergenerational caregiving network in their family in which they, too, receive care.

HEALTH ISSUES

The two leading causes of death for American women are, in order, heart disease and cancers. It may be surprising to learn that heart disease is the leading killer of women, because we tend to think of heart attacks as men's problem. Nothing could be further from the truth.

Unfortunately, the belief that heart disease is a masculine ailment is also held by many physicians, often leaving women's heart disease undiagnosed or misdiagnosed.

Men are more likely to first present with heart disease by having a myocardial infarction (MI, or heart attack), but MIs are more often fatal for women, especially black women. The problem is that women are more likely to have "silent" heart disease that doesn't manifest itself in the dramatic way men's heart disease does, with a collapsing-on-the-ground, painful heart attack that everyone notices. Women are more likely simply to experience angina (chest pain), which is often ignored both by them and their physicians.

Heart disease is influenced by genetics, age, and behavior. High cholesterol levels and high blood pressure are two of the leading risk factors for heart disease, and cholesterol levels are genetically influenced. Estrogen keeps cholesterol levels in check, so estrogen helps protect women from heart disease before menopause. In terms of behavioral factors, cigarette smoking is a major risk, and women are, unfortunately, catching up to men in rates of smoking.

Breast cancer is the second most common form of cancer in women, exceeded only by skin cancer. Breast cancer is rare in women under twenty-five; however, a woman's chances of developing it increase every year after that age. About one out of every nine American women has breast cancer at some time in her life.

Women diagnosed with breast cancer face important but complex decisions regarding the best treatment. Several decades ago, the medical establishment believed that radical mastectomy—removal of the entire breast, the underlying muscles, and the associated lymph nodes—was the only solution. Today physicians choose much more conservative treatments, using only lumpectomy for cases in which the cancer has not spread beyond the lump itself. Further decisions are involved as to whether the surgery should be followed by radiation therapy or chemotherapy.

Many women feel depressed or anxious around the time of diagnosis, although the period immediately following discovery of the lump is rated as the worst psychologically. The great majority of women show good adjustment after lumpectomy or mastectomy. Nonetheless, many experience considerable distress at some point in the process, so it is important for counseling to be available. In many towns, the American Cancer Society organizes support groups for breast cancer patients. Some controversy exists among psychologists as to how effective these support groups are in relieving psychological distress. One study found that educational classes that provided relevant information were more effective than support groups in terms of benefits to quality of life. For women who are more severely distressed, cognitive behavioral therapy with a trained psychologist can be very effective.

Some psychologists argue that there is such a thing as post-traumatic growth, defined as positive life changes following highly stressful experiences. Many breast cancer survivors show evidence of post-traumatic growth, particularly in relationships with others, appreciation of life, and spiritual growth.

While the issues facing middle-aged women are sometimes significant, they are not for the most part insurmountable nor are they cut-and-dry as researchers may have assumed. And the issues change with almost every generation. Women have coped well with aging by taking care of their physical and mental health throughout life, and they seem to continue to do so.

—Janet Shibley Hyde, Ph.D.

The Fires of Menopause

Menopause is a process, a long slow metamorphosis over a range of years, roughly between a woman's mid-forties until her mid-fifties. It is a story marked by fluctuations. We are turning toward a broader view, the second half of life, the down sweep, and a new freedom.

Technically, *menopause* refers to the last menstrual flow of a woman's life. The time near and around menopause is referred to as the *climacteric,* and indeed the body's climate is shifting like the planet's thermals, meltings, sea-changes. Even the terminology we use tends to fluctuate in meaning. Part of the confusion comes from the linear world of medicine that tends to think of menopause as a single event rather than a process. The climacteric can last up to twenty years, some say. Another view is that it is synonymous with the term *perimenopause,* the year before and after the last period. So, you see, from the onset, things are soupy, colliding, overlapping.

The story quite often begins with our sleep being disturbed. Our body temperature seems erratic: we are too hot, bedding is tossed, then we're too cold. We awaken cranky, our bones ache. All of our rhythms seem to be in flux. Emotions, particularly anger, can run hot; weeping may take us by surprise. We feel a vague familiarity with adolescence, or a constant sense of PMS. These symptoms may be slight in the early years. For each woman, it will be different. We scratch our heads. *Is this it?* As soon as you begin to ask, herbalist and author Susan Weed writes, the process has begun.

The central shift, of course, is the menstrual cycle itself. The calendar grid with its predictable twenty-eight-day blocks begins to swim before our eyes. The red marks we made with a felt pen start to run wild or fade pink. Our rational self chatters on, explaining why a period was skipped, why it was lighter or heavier in flow. *Is this it?* This is it. We may bleed heavily two weeks straight, or none at all for an entire year only to have our period return. But, by then, we know.

What is going on in our bodies? The very things that can appear so out of balance for a woman entering menopause are actually overseen by an area of the brain called the hypothalamus, which regulates body temperature, water balance, sleep patterns, metabolic rate. But as the perimenopausal woman's ovarian hormones, estrogen and progesterone, decrease, the brain pumps greater and greater amounts of the hormones follicle-stimulating hormone (FSH) and luteinizing hormone (LH) into the blood. So, the established rhythms we've known for years begin to do a different dance. Nothing is "wrong"; it's supposed to work this way.

Of course, the symptom that confirms the entry point to the process, experienced by 90 percent of American women, is the hot flash, that lightning bolt that moves up the body, flushing the face like a hot red pepper. It may be intense, like the first real contraction in labor when a woman breaks out into a sweat. *Oh my god, this is real,* she thinks. And it may be mild; the range of "normal" is very wide.

Again, fluctuating hormones, those plummeting and soaring estrogen levels, are believed to bring on the hot flash. The skin temperature suddenly elevates, causing the skin to redden and the flushing to spread, then the body breaks out in perspiration to try to cool.

> Of course, the symptom that confirms the entry point to the process, experienced by 90 percent of American women, is the hot flash, that lightning bolt that moves up the body, flushing the face like a hot red pepper.

The sweater you have taken off, the blouse you have unbuttoned is put back on and buttoned again because a chill sets in. There are plenty of things you can do: the age-old advice of dressing in layers. Drinking plenty of fluids helps, as well as herbal and homeopathic remedies.

Once you know this, you can avoid experiences of mega-hot flashes (if you choose) like the one I had after a sweltering hot day at the beach. In an air-conditioned restaurant, I ordered a cold beer and a spicy pizza. Hot and cold, my body didn't know what to make of it. What it did make was a hot flash that lit up the whole restaurant. It gathered force, building and retreating on the horizon like an orgasm. I felt like Meg Ryan in *When Harry Met Sally,* only silent. My friend's face across the table was one of awe. She mouthed "hot flash?" Soon after, a group of high school friends came to town for a reunion. One woman passed out caps for all of us to wear; on the brim she'd painted a gold lightening bolt, like Zorro's, I thought, and the words *Hot Flash* underneath. We laughed together, marking our common state in our mid-forties, the strange wood we'd found ourselves in. For all the joking, we were also trying to say, let's see this differently from our mothers. Let's look at this as a powerful time, rather than the beginning of the end. But what did it mean beyond the little party hats?

Behind the hormone story is the story of our lives. We wake in our mid-forties to discover that our children have left and perhaps we are alone for the first time; or we have no children and the clock has run out. We wake to the pains of divorce or the pains of never having fully said "yes" to a partner. We long to return to a self put aside when we raised a family; or we are exhausted by the work world and long for home. Our creativity has been channeled into others.

Acknowledging our grief is part of the story. For most women, there is the sense of our eggs dwindling. The 400,000 you were born with are almost gone, and those that remain in the ovaries will not mature. We grieve the death of ourselves as fertile women, an important part of the work we need to do. So, where is the power? Where is the creativity?

If we allow ourselves to think metaphorically, to treat this as a personal journey, we will be fed by the depth of our experience. We will allow ourselves to be transformed. Otherwise, the passage of menopause could easily be reduced to supplements and resentment. In mythic terms the way is marked by fire. Fire has always been the elemental symbol for initiation. The fire heralds change, burns away everything inessential, clears dead wood. Fire purifies, holds us steady in our intent, keeps us warm. Even grief, for all its water, contains the fires of betrayal, the rage that accompanies loss. The perimenopausal hot flash can be seen as the outer symbol of the cooking inside.

There is a lot of knowledge in the bevy of books on menopause now available to us, but the wisdom, for me, came through a close association to the Native American tradition. Elders, or Grandmothers, speak a language that rounds out our understanding, elevates our passage to one of "growing into the wisdom years." Quite a different view from the linear culture we live in. The physician Christiane Northrup in her book *The Wisdom of Menopause* calls the menopause process one of switching from AC to DC current. During a woman's twenty-eight-day cycle, the hormones FSH and LH peak or alternate, pulling us inward toward the intuitive self. This process is dramatic and erratic during menopause; however, by postmenopause these hormones have become a constant, steady flow, or direct current. She writes, "The intuitive wisdom that was once available most clearly during only certain parts of the menstrual cycle is now potentially available all the time."

> If we allow ourselves to think metaphorically, to treat this as a personal journey, we will be fed by the depth of our experience.

So, hot flashes are good, to be explored. We are forging a new relationship with the self. Women are used to giving away energy. We are caretakers, harmonizers; we nurture and bend to accommodate, include. But we all know the drained feeling when there is nothing left for oneself. Fire ignites the voice. The initiation is one of finding the authentic howl, whimper, groan, or song that is you.

The first time I heard that new voice, I donned my running shoes and ran out of the house on a spring day. It was after a session with a client that had been an epiphany for both of us. I realized I could leave an unhappy relationship with the man I lived with. I ran around a nearby empty playing field in the thawed earth with the smell of mud, yelling, *I can leave! It's okay to leave!* Why had I thought I couldn't?

Metaphorically, our journey through menopause includes facing our own mortality. It is no mistake that the loss of a parent so often coincides with the menopausal journey of our forties and fifties. As we undergo our own symbolic death, we are turning toward the second half of life during which we not only look at death, we eventually must accept it. I recall a moment noticing my mother at her kitchen sink, her hair thinned, her shoulders rounded, her height shrunk. She seemed to be disappearing, and the stark truth paraded before me: someday *I would too.*

> There is something to be said for not rushing in to "fix" or "do."

What begs for transformation is our own fear. We must look into the darkness, descend into ourselves. *Roget's Thesaurus* tells us *transformation* is a noun, meaning "complete change." Our mothers' generation whispered with an ominous tone, "Oh, she's going through The Change." The Navajo peoples have an archetype they call Changing Woman. She who continually shapeshifts, transforms, renews. Yes, complete change.

Women ask, "What should I do?" when hot flashes, insomnia, fatigue, and other symptoms appear. There are many things we can do to bring more balance into our systems, some of which I've already mentioned. But there is really nothing to "do" overall but trust in your body, have faith in process. Powerful contractions of the uterus push the baby out, our systems follow a course for closing down shop at death—the body is good at passages. Ask yourself, what is being born? What is being let go?

We also don't have to be stoic, enduring extreme discomforts or pain. Our mothers were often silent and enduring, ashamed of their darkness. We baby boomers have brought The Change out of the closet, and that knowledge is power.

But there is something to be said for not rushing in to "fix" or "do." My friend Patricia has frequent, intense flashes throughout the day, making her quite uncomfortable. When she discovered her mother-in-law had experienced a similar pattern, she asked her, "Well, what did you do?" Her mother-in-law replied, "I loosened my collar a bit." We roll our eyes over our mothers' generation that persevered. On the other hand, there is something to be said for a certain healthy acceptance. It's important to remember that menopause is *natural;* it's not a disease or a medical problem. The body is not to be mastered; it has an intelligence and wisdom all its own.

One of the things you *can* do is make time for yourself. Dr. Christiane Northrup says we are biologically programmed at this time in our life to turn inward. Even if a charming cottage in the woods is not available, find a room or a corner of your home where you can meet yourself free of distractions. We want to schedule every moment—these days some women even protest they haven't got *time* to labor at birth. Let go of the linear track. Listen. This is the time.

> Even if a charming cottage in the woods is not available, find a room or a corner of your home where you can meet yourself free of distractions. We want to schedule every moment—some women even protest they haven't got *time* to labor at birth. Let go of the linear track. This is the time.

I followed the overwhelming impulse to part from others, moving to a country farmhouse on a couple of acres. It was fall and the giant sugar maples that lined the dirt driveway were ablaze. In retrospect, I recall wearing mostly orange clothes. I made a kiln in the yard for sawdust firings, the black pots that would cook for days.

I drove into the city a few days a week to see clients; otherwise, I was at home or on the nearby trails of Bare Pond. Any move toward dashing into the city for a bit of culture was thwarted, as if a hand gently pushed me back down on my chair. I nursed old partnership wounds. The driveway filled with snow. It was quiet, unbelievably quiet, as if I could hear for the first time. I began to write my first poems of true intent.

These are spiritual fires. There is so much more going on than we acknowledge or understand. In the ancient mystery schools of Egypt and Greece, women's cycles were seen as part of a great initiation. The fires of menopause announce the way, your own way. If we can hang in there for the duration of its stay, the rewards are rich, the transformation complete; we have passed through the burning gateway of middle life.

What is it like on the other side of the menopausal moment? Well, we are told to wait one year after our last period to officially proclaim ourselves in the land of postmenopause, so we don't really know it's our last flow when it's happening—the moment itself is anticlimactic. The average age is fifty-one, although it can vary widely. As a process, the fluctuations are smoothing out.

Our sexuality is challenged. Just as the eggs have dwindled, so may our desire. Sexual arousal is not the same as at thirty-five, and this is part of the grieving we've done. For many women, natural lubrication of the vagina decreases. There are plenty of synthetic lubricants that can help. But we must engage our imagination, find a different image of ourselves. Perhaps we feel free that we are not driven by our sexual passion. Or maybe we begin to feel sexy and passionately turned on to all of life.

Our bones are thinning, becoming more porous. Again, this is meant to happen to a certain extent. The process even begins in our mid-thirties. But the danger is that bone density loss can lead to a condition of osteoporosis in which the bones turn brittle and can break easily. It is a time to be vigilant about calcium intake and exercise. During the first five years after menopause, the rate of bone loss speeds up. Eat a calcium-rich diet—think leafy greens. And practice weight-bearing exercise—walking, jogging, yoga, bicycling.

Two other areas need our attention. One is keeping our heart healthy. Cardiovascular disease rises postmenopause. Research on hormone replacement therapies, or HRT, has recently added more fear and confusion. But, as Susun Weed writes, 90 percent of all heart disease is preventable with lifestyle changes. Our hearts thrive on low-fat diets, exercise, lowering blood pressure, stopping smoking.

As we move through perimenopause into postmenopause, we mostly notice the winds have died down, the fires have abated, and our feet feel planted on the earth again. Our bodies can feel alive with creative urges; there is the "postmenopausal zest" anthropologist and author Margaret Mead referred to.

Creativity feels different to us. We are reservoirs, holding the full cycle of life that includes dying. We may make art, write books, garden, but there is also an ever-growing acceptance of the way things are.

I was age forty-nine when my last flow took place. Of course, I can't remember, it was just a mark on a calendar. What I do know is that one year later I was living with the man who was to become my husband; two years later we bought our first house. After a decade of turbulent moves, I was finally building a nest, and with a partner. A great love burned as well as a new eroticism. The passage led me into totally new terrain. Deep relief settled in my bones for the end of ambivalence around childbearing. I noted with a smile that it wasn't until postmenopause that I finally opened to home and partnership.

This passing opens a different lens on beauty, too. When the grocery clerk at the checkout counter recently asked me for my senior card, I was horrified. When I arrived home, I stood before the mirror examining the gray hairs at my temples, running my hand over the tiredness that sat on my skin. *How could I look that old?* But a photograph taken of me standing in window light in Maine showed me a different side of my new face. I saw a look of strength, ease, and something like character bleeding through the creases and furrows.

We are new. And we are full of completions. We forgive ourselves for all we are not, for all those we did not please. The approval moves inside. The great grief swell over loss and relationships subsides. We have turned. Holding layers of what went before, we grow into the long view. We see in both directions and in many dimensions.

—Nadine Boughton, M.A.

RELATED ENTRIES

Aging and Its Effects on Mood, Memory, the Brain, and Hormones

Issues for Women in Middle Age

Menopause and Psychiatric Illness

Older Adulthood

What comes to mind when you think of older women? Women over forty? Women in their sixties and older? Women past age eighty? Your answer likely depends on your age. Psychological research indicates that the subjective mark of older adulthood moves up as we get older. Your answer also depends on where you live and how long you expect to live. If you are from a country like Haiti, where women's life expectancy at birth is about fifty years, your view of the age at which older adulthood begins is likely to be different from the view you might have if you are from the United States, where life expectancy at birth for women is about eighty years.

Your cultural background is also going to influence your perception of the threshold of old age. In some cultures, women are defined as "old" once they are past their reproductive years. For example, according to a study by psychologist Mary Gergen, in the United States, women have been assumed to be "finished at forty."

Currently, in the United States older adulthood is typically defined as the time of life beyond age sixty. In this country, like in other industrialized countries, this period of life encompasses not only many years of life, but also a significant range of experiences. This has led social scientists to break down older adulthood into three stages: a young-old stage (the period between age sixty and seventy-five), an old-old stage (the decade between ages seventy-six and eighty-five), and an oldest-old stage (the late eighties onward). These age markers help map the vast territory of older adulthood. However, they should be treated as indicative because the experience of aging does not depend only on a person's age. It varies depending on the social and economic contexts of our lives. It is also influenced by historical conditions (e.g., large-scale events, such as wars, as well as dominant social institutions and policies). Reaching seventy for an African American woman born in 1930 represented a very different life journey than reaching seventy will involve for an African American woman born fifty years after the first. As noted by psychologist Frances Trotman, "African American women who lived during the first half of the twentieth century" experienced "both de facto and de jure racism and discrimination," from lynching to segregation. Many African Americans of this generation grew up with relatives and friends who had been slaves.

Furthermore, the experience of aging is affected by our individual characteristics (e.g., our sexual orientation) and the meanings and consequences of these characteristics in the communities in which we live. Consider the meaning and implications of aging as a lesbian in an urban area with a large lesbian community as compared to aging as a lesbian in relative isolation, in a rural, conservative area. Social support for being "out" would be very different in these two situations.

Historically, human development was conceptualized as a process involving universal stages and orderly psychological processes, which were assumed to always unfold in the same manner independent of context. For example, Erik Erikson, in his 1963 "eight ages of man" theory, postulated that the tasks of adolescence and adulthood involve first achieving a firm sense of identity, and then seeking "heterosexual mutuality," that is, an intimate heterosexual relationship. With regard to older adulthood, Erikson proposed a single stage and one developmental task—integrity versus despair. As the name of Erikson's theory implies, these eight ages applied to men only; in fact, they were based on a very specific male experience, that of heterosexual, middle- to upper-class, European American men of his generation. Consider, for example, the identity and intimacy stages. Erikson argued that in women, the sequence of these two stages ought to be reversed. According to him, women should wait to develop an identity until they are involved with the man by whose name and status they will be known and defined, and whose children they will bear: "a woman's identity formation . . . [is predicated on] the fact that her somatic design harbors an 'inner space' destined to bear the offspring of chosen men," he wrote in 1964. Very few people are aware of these biases in Erikson's theory because, in current renditions, the biases are hidden under inclusive language.

According to a study by psychologist Mary Gergen, in the United States, women have been assumed to be "finished at forty."

Stage theories like Erikson's are appealing and still very popular because they are all encompassing and simple. Current scholarship in life span developmental psychology, however, has moved away from grand theories like Erikson's. Basically, their very generality and simplicity makes them unfit to account for the complexity, subtlety, and diversity of human experience. Stage theories are particularly problematic when applied to older adulthood, given the even wider variability one finds in the experience of aging as compared with that of childhood. As a result, there has been movement away from grand theories of aging, with a preference for mini theories dealing with specific issues and domains, such as stereotyping or personal relationships.

My discussion here relies primarily on studies conducted in English and in industrialized countries, such as the United States. Because aging is influenced by social and cultural factors, it is important to not assume that the issues and conclusions brought up here apply to women around the world. There is also variability in women's experience of aging within countries. For example, even in the United States, older women's health and life expectancy vary greatly depending on ethnicity and income. Unfortunately, researchers have tended to focus on a narrow sample of older women (i.e., heterosexual, middle-class, educated, urban women of European American descent), so it is not always possible to articulate the diversity of women's aging experiences. Also, researchers' topics of study narrowed my view: There is, for example, more research on marriage than on friendship, so as a consequence there exists more extensive information on marital relationships than on friendships. This does not mean that marriages are more important to older women than friendships, it simply reflects a bias in the published research.

VIEWS OF OLDER WOMEN

The world of late adulthood is a world of women. And the proportion of women gets greater the older the population. In the United States, there are three women age sixty and older for every two men in that age bracket. Among those eighty-five and older, women outnumber men five to two.

Stereotypes of older women are more limiting, if not always more negative than those of older men. For example, older women are often viewed as nicer, more nurturing, and more sensitive than older men. On the other hand, older men are consistently considered more competent, intelligent, wise, and independent than older women. In addition, older men are perceived as reaching old age later than women. They also tend to be evaluated more positively than older women in terms of physical attractiveness. The stereotype that older women are nicer than older men probably enhances older women's likability. At the same time, it may put pressure on women to be forever accommodating and may interfere with women's investment in self-care.

STEREOTYPES OF
OLDER WOMEN VERSUS
STEREOTYPES OF
OLDER MEN

Older Women:

nicer, more nurturing,

more sensitive

Older Men:

competent, intelligent, wise,

independent,

more physically attractive

WORK AND RETIREMENT

A dominant topic in U.S. gerontology research is retirement. Studies of retirement have tended to focus on the experience of men from European American, middle-class backgrounds. As a result, issues and questions about retirement are still framed in terms of middle-class male experiences. For example, retirement is often defined as separation from paid employment and is assumed to bring about major changes in social status, power, income, activities, interpersonal interactions, and family roles.

What does retirement mean, and what does it involve for women? Do women retire? The answers to these questions are complex. Until relatively recently, few women were employed in the kinds of industries that offered retirement benefits. Of those women who were, few had accumulated the years of continuous employment to qualify for such benefits. Also, retirement for women is less likely to lead to major losses in status and power because women's typical jobs (i.e., sales, teaching, nursing, service, and clerical positions) or their status within those jobs already involve subordinate roles. Most crucially, women, especially working-class women, rarely experience the clear end-of-labor activities that are basic to the traditional concept of retirement.

Throughout older adulthood, women continue to do a great deal of unpaid work. Like younger women, they perform the vast majority of household work and caregiving for family and friends. A minority of older adult women is in the paid labor force.

Divorced or single women are more likely to be employed after age sixty-five than married women. These women typically work part-time and in low-paying occupations. Consider the work history of Miss Mildred, a black woman in her eighties from the rural South whose life is narrated by social scientist Annette Dula. "She has picked cotton and tobacco; she has nursed white children; she has worked as a domestic worker for several white families; she has washed and ironed white folks' laundry in her own home." As an older woman with an eighth-grade education, Miss Mildred still works for the white folks who have employed her for the past four decades: Now she only cooks and "does a bit of light cleaning." Has Miss Mildred considered retiring? We are told she thought about retirement but dismissed it as unfeasible: "Us poor colored women can't retire; that's what white folks do. We just keep on working and getting sicker and sicker. And then we die."

What do we know about the experience of retirement of women who formally retire from a paid job? The assumption has been that retirement would be less difficult for women than for men because employment is considered less salient to women's identities. In fact, women, like men, experience retirement as bringing some advantages and some disadvantages. If anything, women, more than men, report that retirement is challenging. One reason may be that women tend to retire earlier and to have lower incomes at retirement than men. Another reason is that women's retirement is more likely than men's to be precipitated by family-related events (such as a spouse's retirement or a family illness) than by work-related events, such as seniority.

What about women whose productive activity involved raising children? Do these women go through a retirement phase when their work is "done"? When their children permanently leave home, women whose primary activity involved being a parent may indeed experience some of the dynamics traditionally associated with retirement. Studies, however, suggest that the "emptying of the nest" may be stressful only for women whose self-definition and self-worth depended exclusively on being a parent. Typically, the emptying of the nest is associated with increased well-being in women.

FINANCIAL RESOURCES

Poverty is a problem for older women worldwide. According to data from the International Council on Social Welfare, older women in developing countries are often unable to fulfill minimal needs for nutrition and shelter. Women's poverty globally is the result of many factors, including barriers to education and employment, discrimination in credit, land ownership, and inheritance, as well underrepresentation in political decision making.

Is poverty an issue for older women in the United States? It is. In the United States, about two-thirds of poor older adults are women.

Consider the case of Helen. She worked part-time in low-paying jobs while raising her children but enjoyed a middle-class lifestyle until her engineer husband developed Alzheimer's disease. She ended up spending the family retirement savings to pay first for his at-home care, and then for a comfortable nursing home. By the time she was a widow, seven years later, she had to sell their house to pay for a medical emergency. She ended up in a run-down apartment in an unsafe neighborhood, isolated from friends and family, and still unable to access basic medical care.

"Sounds extreme?" ask Laura Carstensen and Monisha Pasupathi, the authors of the case study. It is not, they note. Helen was actually privileged in many ways. She was white and middle-class. She and her husband had savings. She became poor for the first time in her later years. Other women, especially ethnic minority women, struggle financially all of their lives only to become poorer in their older years.

As illustrated in the story of Helen, poverty in late adulthood reflects the accumulation of a lifetime of disadvantages for women. These disadvantages often include less education, low pay while employed, barriers to jobs with opportunities for retirement and health care benefits, family responsibilities that interfere with continuous employment, and nonpayment for household and family caregiving work. Helen's story also shows how family illnesses can place strain on older women's financial resources. Like Helen, many older women take care of their sick older husbands, a task that can keep women from working as many hours, depleting income and the family savings.

> Women, especially working-class women, rarely experience the clear end-of-labor activities that are basic to the traditional concept of retirement.

When their husbands die, women's pensions often do not include survivor's benefits. The Social Security widows receive based on their own employment is often much less than the one the couple received when their husbands were alive. Other strains on women's financial resources are women's own health problems. Because women live longer and are less likely to have health insurance, they are more likely to exhaust their resources on health-related expenses.

FAMILY AND FRIENDS

As women age, they experience many changes in personal relationships. New relationships develop as new persons enter their lives (e.g., grandchildren). Other relationships may be renegotiated (e.g., women may become caregivers for their parents). Yet other relationships end due to disagreement, distance, or death (e.g., via divorce or widowhood). Given all of this relationship variability, it is interesting that research on older women and relationships has focused primarily on widowhood.

It is true that, historically, becoming a widow was a common experience for women. In countries where divorce is less common, widowhood still is. At the same time, the intense research focus on widowhood is likely the result of a long tradition of assuming it is the greatest challenge for older women. "Widowhood is to women what retirement is to men, the conclusion of the central task of adult life," argue Elaine Cumming and William Henry in their influential 1961 book on aging.

What questions have researchers asked about women and widowhood? A major focus has been on adjustment. What has been found is that the immediate effect of widowhood for women (like for men) is negative. However, in the long run, widows do better than widowers, at least psychologically and physically. For example, widows are less likely to suffer from cardiovascular morbidity and mortality than widowers. Widows also have low rates of depression, alcohol abuse, and suicide. One reason older women adjust better to widowhood than older men may be that widowhood is more normative and occurs at a younger age for women than for men. And because women expect to outlive their husbands and spend part of the lives as widows, they have more time to adjust to the idea of widowhood and to develop other relationships.

Another reason that women adjust more easily to widowhood may be that marriage is not as important for women's well-being as it is for men's. For example, women report less satisfaction with marriage than men. They also tend to be closer than men to their children, grandchildren, and friends. And widows may be better prepared than widowers to live as single persons because of their practice in running a household. Finally, for widows, to assume responsibilities for tasks previously performed by their husbands (e.g., managing financial assets) may be psychologically rewarding because those tasks are socially valued.

While widows do better emotionally and socially than widowers, they do significantly worse financially. Widows have the lowest income of all demographic groups. The economic disadvantages of widowhood are likely the result of inequities intrinsic to marriage rather than the result of being single. Older women who never marry are better off financially than previously married older women (i.e., widows, separated, or divorced women). Always-single persons are also more likely than previously married persons to share a home

> Is poverty an issue for older women in the United States? It is. In the United States, about two-thirds of poor older adults are women.

with at least one other person, a pattern that reduces costs as well as the need for residential care. Furthermore, when compared with the formerly married, ever-single older women report the best health and the fewest disabilities.

As a consequence of widowhood as well as divorce, many older women live alone. In many cases, living alone becomes a choice. Many single (i.e., widowed or divorced) older women opt not to remarry. Only about a quarter of women age seventy-five and older are married, as compared with 70 percent of men. Older single-again women report enjoying the freedom brought by living alone. In an interview with researchers Ann Varley and Maribel Blasco, a Mexican urban woman said the following about her wish to live alone: "On my own, solita, . . . you really get some peace and quiet."

Living alone for women does not usually mean being isolated. Older women keep in touch with relatives more than older men. A particularly close relationship is the one between sisters. Sisters interact more often than any other sibling combination. For women across marital/relationship status, friendships are also significant relationships. In fact, because of other relationship losses (e.g., marriage), the value of friendships may actually increase with age: "Well, a lot of times, I'll just call her. . . . She'll be on my heart," said a widow about a friend, in an article about friendships during older adulthood by gerontologist Rosemary Blieszner. Older women have a greater number of friends and feel closer to their friends than older men. Women are more likely than men to have same-sex confidants and to have more than one confidant. Close friends are particularly important for older lesbians.

> In the long run, widows do better than widowers, at least psychologically and physically.

Yet, having a multiplicity of close ties is not always an asset for women. Relationships for women also bring care responsibilities, not just opportunities for support. Women and men depend on women for their needs. An Italian older woman interviewed by researcher Isabella Paoletti expressed concern about who will care for her since she did not have daughters: "Now when I am old what shall I do that I have two males?" she wondered.

Living alone brings advantages and disadvantages. Older women living alone spend high proportions of their incomes on housing, which leaves little money for other budgetary categories. Older women living alone are overrepresented in housing with the most structural deficiencies and the poorest maintenance. Living alone also increases the risk for institutionalization, especially after an illness or disability creates a need for assistance in daily activities. As their disabilities increase, older women living alone often change their living arrangements. Some move in with children, relatives, or friends; yet others go to extended care facilities. Women represent the majority of permanent residents of extended care facilities. Three out of four nursing home residents are women. For sexual orientation minorities, moving to a nursing home may raise grave concerns about becoming isolated. As noted by a British lesbian interviewed by social worker Jackie Langley: "If you do have to go into residential care you are going to be put into a totally heterosexual environment . . . you would not have the comfort of people who share the same understanding as you."

HEALTH

Older women have higher rates of physical illnesses and disabilities and suffer more total years of disability than older men. Women are particularly vulnerable to chronic conditions that make it difficult to get around (e.g., rheumatoid arthritis). Twice as many women as men are housebound. The gender gap in health increases at advanced stages of adulthood.

Women who survive beyond the age of eighty-five suffer from more diseases and disabilities than men the same age.

Ethnic minority women generally report worse health than European American women. For example, African American women have poorer self-rated health and higher specific mortality rates than European American women. Women of Hispanic heritage report poorer self-rated health and higher disability rates, but have similar mortality rates as European American women.

The effect of sexual orientation on health is unclear. Studies indicate that lesbians experience stigma, discrimination, and victimization at higher rates than heterosexual women. Studies also suggest that these experiences have a negative impact on health, either directly or indirectly. In either case, the consequences can be serious. Consider the situation of a lesbian who is excluded from medical discussions about her hospitalized partner because she is not legal kin. As noted by psychologist Beverly Greene, the physician is likely to miss important health information about the sick woman; and the sick woman's partner is likely to provide less effective after-care because of inadequate information about the medical plan.

> In general, older women are less likely to receive care from their spouses than older men.

Women's limited socioeconomic resources are likely to be a factor in their poor health. Individuals from lower socioeconomic classes have more health problems than individuals from higher socioeconomic strata. This is because having less income and less education often means a poor diet, insufficient exercise, unhealthy work environments, and inadequate preventive and medical care.

Women make more medical visits than older men, but the medical care they receive is often of worse quality than that of men. For example, women receive fewer therapies of demonstrated efficacy. Compared to men, women are underserved for procedures such as cardiac catheterization, bypass surgery, and renal dialysis. This is especially true for ethnic minority women. At the same time, women are more likely than men to have their physical symptoms misattributed to psychological causes and to be prescribed tranquilizers and hypnotic drugs.

Older women have lower rates of hospitalization than older men. However, they remain longer in acute-care beds and are more likely to be transferred to long-term care facilities for their recovery. The latter phenomenon is likely due to women's limited access to informal care (friends and family) compared to men, since women are usually the ones giving, not receiving, care. In general, older women are less likely to receive care from their spouses than older men. Also, having a spouse results in reduced nursing home stay for men but not for women. Finally, when women are terminally ill and dying, they are more likely than men to rely on paid assistance rather than on care from family.

DEATH AND DYING

In the United States, older women and men die of the same diseases. The leading causes of death for women and men in the United States and in other industrialized countries are heart disease, cancer, and stroke. Women, however, live for a shorter time with life-threatening conditions, such as heart disease and cancer.

There are important differences in the leading causes of mortality in women from different ethnic groups. For example, diabetes is the fourth leading cause of death among

African American, Native American, and Hispanic-descent women, but only the seventh leading cause among European American women. Suicide is among the ten leading causes of death for Native American or Alaskan Native and Asian or Pacific Islander women, but not for European American women, African American women, or women of Hispanic descent.

Around the world, with a few exceptions (e.g., Nepal), women live longer than men. One may be tempted to conclude that women's longevity is simply a function of constitutional factors. However, gender-linked behavioral factors are also influential. For example, women have lower rates of death by accident, suicide, and homicide. They also have lower rates of tobacco and alcohol use, and consequently lower rates of death due to lung cancer and chronic liver diseases.

In industrialized countries, the gender gap in longevity has increased over the past century. In 1900, women could expect to live only two to three years longer than men in most of North America and Western Europe. Currently, the age at which women die and the gender gap in longevity vary greatly depending on nationality (e.g., women live as much as twelve years longer than men in Russia) and, within countries, according to ethnicity and social class. For example, an African American woman can expect to live seventy-four years, as compared to eighty years for a European American woman and sixty-five years for an African American man. Also, the higher the socioeconomic status, the lower the risk of mortality for both women and men.

In the United States, the experience of dying has changed in the past century. Death in hospitals has replaced death at home. Also, medical interventions can often control or delay many causes of death. Dilemmas about medical care at the end of life have thus become common for dying persons and their caregivers. Very little is known on how decisions about end-of-life medical care are made. Even less is known on how being an older woman affects these decisions. One thing is for sure: The ill person is not usually the primary arbiter of these decisions. One reason is that very sick individuals are often too tired, stressed, or confused to deliberate about medical alternatives. Thus, end-of-life medical decisions are usually made by physicians, with some consultation with family members. Unfortunately, professional and family caregivers are not good at predicting the individual's medical preferences. Another complicating factor is that money plays a role in care decisions at the end of life. For example, persons with high income tend to have a private attending physician, a factor related to maintaining (rather than terminating) life-sustaining care.

What do we know about older persons' preferences for medical care, particularly about women's preferences? Research suggests that individuals are more likely to refuse life-saving treatments if they are concerned about cost. One public opinion poll found that the most frequently expressed fear about dying was the fear of being a burden to one's family. Given these findings, it is perhaps not surprising that women are less likely than men to express a preference for life-sustaining treatments under a variety of medical conditions. What may explain women's preferences for reduced care? First, women have fewer economic and family assets than men. They are more likely to rely on a publicly funded health insurance. They are also more likely to live alone or in an institution. Second, women have a lower sense of entitlement than men. Finally, women are exposed to ideologies that glorify female self-effacement. For all these reasons, women may be especially concerned about being a burden when sick and may be more likely to seek to literally remove themselves in time of need.

A finding that supports this hypothesis is that in the United States, women represent one-half to two-thirds of recorded cases of assisted suicide or euthanasia. This is despite the fact that suicide is extremely uncommon among older women, as well as the fact that when responding to polls, women (like poor, less-educated, and ethnic minority individuals) oppose assisted suicide and euthanasia. It has been suggested that killing oneself with the help of a physician may be more acceptable to women because it is death that is medicalized and packaged as gentle, graceful deliverance.

In addition, women have been found to place a higher value on having a dignified death than men. It has also been suggested that sick women may be particularly prone to seeing themselves and/or to be seen by others as good candidates for assisted suicide and euthanasia because of a societal bias against investing resources in women. Hastened-death advocates insist that assisted suicide and euthanasia are a form of personal empowerment: In hastened death, the individual determines the time and manner of her or his death, they argue. Opponents question the idea that hastened death is empowering since persons who "choose" it may not have the resources or the sense of entitlement to stay alive (as may be the case for sick older women).

Incidentally, ethnic minorities are a rarity in hastened-death cases. One reason may be that ethnic minorities have developed a healthy distrust of the medical system. As Miss Mildred put it: "Look like every time I turn on the TV, somebody's talking about euthanasia, and doctors helping kill off old and sick folks. . . . Ain't nobody going to hurry me along. You got to be careful what you tell these doctors. Even the good ones."

SOME FINAL THOUGHTS

There are many unanswered questions about older women. For example, very little is known about aging in women whose lives are less structured than those of married women, as is the case for sexual minority or ever-single women. It would be very useful to learn what aging is like for those who have had less visibility and fewer social supports and legal protections and who, at the same time, have also avoided heterosexual expectations, conventions, and institutions. Much insight could also be obtained from studying older women whose lives are more scripted than those of secular or moderately religious heterosexual married women, as is the case for married and unmarried women in fundamentalist religious communities.

It will also be interesting to see what aging will mean and what it will bring to cohorts of older women who grew up under current gender customs and values. Women who will be older adults in the third millennium were not spared gender discrimination. Yet they did experience some improvement in gender opportunities. For example, future groups of older adult women will include the largest number ever of well-educated women. They will comprise the largest-ever group of women with a stable history of employment and access to retirement pensions and benefits. They will encompass the first sizable generation of women with access to physical education and regular practice of physical exercise. One would expect their experience of aging to be different from, and hopefully more economically stable, physically healthier, and perhaps personally more fulfilling, than that of their mothers and grandmothers.

—*Silvia Sara Canetto, Ph.D.*

A Guide to Grief and Bereavement

Grief is a deeply held, even corporal, emotion. Physical symptoms such as chest pain, frequent sighing, and digestive changes are common. The recently bereaved often find their own behavior unfamiliar and their range, intensity, and variability of feeling changed. C. S. Lewis, writing in *A Grief Observed* of his own wrenching grief after the death of his wife, says, "No one ever told me that grief felt so like fear. I am not afraid, but the sensation is like being afraid. The same fluttering in the stomach, the same restlessness, the yawning. I keep on swallowing. There is an invisible blanket between the world and me. I find it hard to take in what anyone says. . . . The act of living is different all through. Her absence is like the sky, spreading over everything." Grief is also highly specific: the loss of a spouse, an elderly parent, a close friend, or a child, although carrying a common thread, can have widely different impacts.

But grief still tends to follow a course. Knowing something about the features and direction of this course may ease the pain of loss. Such knowledge can also help the grieving person decide whether, and what type of, help and support is needed.

NORMAL BEREAVEMENT

Death is one cause for grieving, but many other forms of loss may initiate grief. Loss of valued relationships or meaningful objects, loss of function through disability, or change of job may all cause grief. Change, even if anticipated with pleasure or as the result of success, may also entail losses.

When grieving, we mourn for the person we have lost and the future for which we have planned. The unfulfilled expectations, the unfinished projects, and the anticipation of shared experiences from grandchildren to retirement are all mourned. Mark Doty, recounting his partner Wally's death from AIDS in the memoir *Heaven's Coast*, writes, "Now I could cry for myself—for the pain of it, for losing what I thought the rest of my life would be like."

Normal bereavement can be loosely divided into four periods: *immediate reactions, acute responses, working through,* and *reorganization*. It is important to remember, however, that several factors shape the progress and duration of the phases of grief:

1. The age and life stage of the person who died; for example, the death of a child will have a different significance than the death of someone older who has had a full life.
2. Miscarriage or the death of a newborn may not be recognized as a major loss by friends and family but can precipitate prolonged grieving.

3. Socially disapproved deaths (suicide, secret or unaccepted relationships) may result in more social isolation and complicated grieving.

We'll take a closer look at the four periods of grief, using Doty's and Lewis's eloquence in the face of their own loss to help us through this difficult terrain.

Immediate Reactions Our initial reactions to death are influenced by our culture — by its attitudes toward the expression of grief, by its relationship to sickness and death. But some characteristics of reactions are found across cultures, including mixtures of protest, numbness, and somatic symptoms. Feelings of blunted disconnection are also common. Immediately following a death, expected or not, the bereaved usually experience shock and disbelief. They attend to funeral arrangements, greet relatives and friends, and take care of finances without feeling fully present. Intense sadness and yearning alternate with numbness and feelings of unreality. Emptiness, disorganization, and anxiety about the future are common. Grieving people may even think that the deceased is present, a belief that may be fueled by visual or auditory hallucinations. Coming on top of intense grief, this belief can cause the bereaved to worry that they're "going crazy."

> "My head feels like a vacancy; I'm a great broken space which fills alternately with weeping and with nothing."

Acute Responses As the reality of loss begins to sink in, sadness and despair become more prominent. Lack of appetite, sleeplessness, fruitless activity, exhaustion, and a variety of other physical complaints continue. Someone struck with grief may replay and remember the relationship with the deceased over and over again, particularly the events of the final illness and death. They may also ruminate over regrets and missed opportunities.

Acute grief affects every aspect of life. It impacts relationships, work, and even feelings and expectations about oneself. Mark Doty describes the fragility of everyday functioning: "I am holding myself together precariously, learning to move through the simple routines I've established for myself.... Trying to learn how to stumble through the days without falling, without falling any more than I have to. My head feels like a vacancy; I'm a great broken space which fills alternately with weeping and with nothing."

Yearning for the deceased and worries about the integrity of memory are common in this phase. C. S. Lewis, describing his frustration at his inability to see his dead wife clearly in his imagination, states, "We have seen the faces of those we know best so variously, from

---

☞ *Grief:* The feelings and behaviors that result from loss, including both physical and emotional suffering.

☞ *Bereavement:* The reaction of a person who has experienced the loss of a close relationship.

☞ *Mourning:* Social expressions, including ritual and behavior specific to religions and cultures, in response to loss. It may also refer to the psychological process through which the bereaved person tries to say good-bye to the deceased.

The progress and duration of the phases of grief is shaped by many factors:

1. The age and life stage of the person who died; for example, the death of a child will have a different significance than the death of someone older who has had a full life.

2. Miscarriage or the death of a newborn may not be recognized as a major loss by friends and family but can precipitate prolonged grieving.

3. Socially disapproved deaths (suicide, secret or unaccepted relationships) may result in more social isolation and complicated grieving.

so many angles, in so many lights, with so many expressions ... that all the impressions crowd into our memory together and cancel out into a mere blur." Feelings of guilt, irritability, hostility, and a disconcerting loss of connection with others are also part of normal grieving. The bereaved may be angry at the professionals and friends who provided care, at the deceased for leaving, or at God. Spiritual alienation or loss of faith can be for many people agonizing and isolating. As Lewis puts it, "Meanwhile, where is God?... When you are happy, so happy that you have no sense of needing Him, so happy that you are tempted to feel His claims upon you as an interruption, if you remember yourself and turn to Him with gratitude and praise, you will be—or so it feels—welcomed with open arms. But go to Him when your need is desperate, when all other help is vain, and what do you find? A door slammed in your face and a sound of bolting and double bolting on the inside. After that, silence."

And then there is the discomfort of being alone, and the equal difficulty of being with others. "Yet I want the others to be about me," Lewis says; "I dread the moments when the house is empty. If only they would talk to one another and not to me."

We should expect the reappearance of earlier feelings (numbness, intense yearning, regret, irritability), physical symptoms (exhaustion, digestive complaints, chest pain, sighing), and behaviors throughout the early and "working through" phases of grief. Grief may come in waves of sudden and overwhelming sadness that may be either spontaneous or precipitated by reminders of the deceased. Feelings of enjoyment and pleasure or planning for the future can seem to betray a loved one who can no longer share them. But by one year after the loss, these physical and emotional symptoms are much less frequent.

Working Through The length and intensity of bereavement varies. Even after acute bereavement is over, the grieving will still feel a sense of loss, although with lessening anguish and fewer waves of sadness and longing, as they confront the meanings of their loss and begin to adjust to the absence of the loved person. At this time, the grieving may feel afraid of losing touch with the deceased as grief begins to lessen. "This is one of the things I'm afraid of. The agonies, the mad midnight moments, must in the course of nature, die away," Lewis writes.

Often those who are coping relatively well six months or so after a death may experience a sudden resurgence of fresh grief. This common phenomenon can be frightening if it is un-

> ✦
> "This is one of the things I'm afraid of.
> The agonies, the mad midnight moments,
> must, in the course of nature, die away."

expected or understood as the loss of a fragile new quiet after the intensity of early grief. The events of everyday life can lead to surprising and painful confrontations with the loss. Lewis astutely observes that after a death, the many habitual thoughts, feelings, and actions one has about the deceased are frustrated, their target gone. And if the "firsts" of the first year—the first holidays alone, the first anniversaries and birthdays—are predictably difficult times, many unpredictable surges of grief occur as well. As Doty puts it, "Mostly I've been moving cautiously, numbly, steeled because I know, at any moment, I may be ambushed by overwhelming grief. You never know when it's coming, the word or gesture or bit of memory that dissolves you entirely, makes it impossible, for a while, to go on."

Reorganization Eventually the bereaved confront the task of going on. They adjust to changes in living situation and to new routines, they return to jobs, and they resume relationships. But even years later more acute sadness and longing can return.

THEORIES OF BEREAVEMENT

Several psychologists and psychiatrists articulated theories of bereavement in the twentieth century. Here we will touch on the theories most often used when speaking with people about what to expect as they grieve. Elisabeth Kubler-Ross described grief in the dying patient and lists five stages: denial, anger, bargaining, depression, and acceptance. In the 1940s Eric Lindemann observed mourning in survivors of disaster. John Bowlby documented the disruptions of attachment. Each of these authors conceptualizes and organizes the bereavement process into phases, and each names phases of grief descriptively, recognizing that different phases of the process recur and overlap.

> "I know, at any moment, I may be ambushed by overwhelming grief. You never know when it's coming, the word or gesture or bit of memory that dissolves you entirely, makes it impossible, for a while, to go on."

Sigmund Freud, in "Mourning and Melancholia," developed an influential model of bereavement. He focuses on the intrapsychic process of grief and describes the gradual withdrawal of emotional interest from the lost person. This withdrawal is emotionally painful, triggering an initial *denial* of the loss because of its overwhelming emotional implications. Denial may be followed by a time of *preoccupation* with thoughts of the dead person. Repeated *recollection* and *review* of memories allows the gradual withdrawal of ties to the deceased and, in normal grief, the eventual freeing-up of emotional energy for new relationships. Freud believed that if an individual was unable to complete grief, a pathological attachment to the lost person would drain interest away from continuing life and would result in the complication of melancholia (Major Depression).

John Bowlby viewed the need for attachment as a basic human instinct and observed children's grief when separated from their parents. His four stages include an initial *protest,* followed by *searching* behaviors in an attempt to regain the lost parent. Next, the child expresses despair and *disorganization,* and finally *reorganization* and resolution by forming new relationships.

Even this brief overview makes clear that each model uses a slightly different language or point of view to label the sequence of feelings experienced during grief. Ned Cassem, a

Table 1 THEORIES OF BEREAVEMENT

Kubler-Ross	Freud	Bowlby	Lindemann
Denial and isolation	Denial	Protest	Somatic distress
Anger	Gradual withdrawal of libido from lost object	Searching	Preoccupation with loved one
Bargaining		Despair and withdrawal	Sense of unreality
Depression	Preoccupation with thoughts of the deceased	Reorganization and resolution	Guilt and irritability
Acceptance			Disruption of normal patterns of behavior
	Libido available for new relationships		Reorganization

psychiatrist and priest who has worked for many years with dying people, summarizes these theories into three basic tasks that every mourner faces: to experience and reflect on feelings about the person during life and on the feelings evoked by death; to review the history of the relationship; and to examine the wounds inflicted by loss, attend to their healing, and confront the task of continuing without the loved person.

ANTICIPATORY GRIEF

When an individual is aware that her own death or the death or a loved one is impending, she may grieve in anticipation, experiencing sadness or anxiety, making efforts at reconciliation or completing unfinished business. Mark Doty's reflections are again useful, as he knew his lover's illness would end in death:

The grief which sweeps over me is the grief of anticipation. It is a grief in expectation of grief, and it carries with it a certain degree of guilt, since one feels that what one really should be doing is enjoying the moment, being together now while it is possible to do so, rather than giving in to some gloomy sense of incipient loss.... The future's an absence, a dark space up ahead like the socket of a pulled tooth. I can't quite stay away from it, hard as I may try.

Anticipation and the opportunity to prepare psychologically for death may speed adaptation after death, though it doesn't always feel that way at the time. But anticipatory grief can be shared by the dying person and her family. Doty notes that both he and Wally were dealing very directly with the anticipation of Wally's death a year and a half before it occurred. When death is anticipated, there is time to review memories of a life together, make new memories, say good-bye, make amends, and share some of the confusion, anger, and sadness. Anticipatory grief has a clear end in death, but any hope that the person may not leave also ends then.

Anger toward the dying person is common with prolonged illness and dying. It tends to be felt as much more dangerous and disturbing during the time preceding death than it is after death occurs.

COMPLICATED BEREAVEMENT

In general, people underestimate the time it takes to grieve. Some aspects of grief take three or more years of adjustment, depending on who has died and how. However, most of

Table 2 PATHOLOGICAL GRIEF REACTION—LINDEMANN	
1. Overactivity without a sense of loss	5. Total absence of emotional expressiveness
2. Acquisition of symptoms belonging to the last illness of the deceased	6. Lasting loss of patterns of social interactions with absence of decisiveness and initiative
3. Progressive social isolation	7. Economically and socially destructive behavior
4. Furious hostility against specific persons	8. Agitated depression

the intense symptoms of acute grief will subside in six to twelve months, although the loss stays with one always.

In what is called complicated or traumatic bereavement, the grieving person does not return to the social/vocational or emotional state that existed prior to the loss. This bereavement occurs when grief is unresolved—when the bereaved attempts to avoid or deny the loss.

Susan Block summarizes a number of risk factors for the development of complicated bereavement:

1. Lack of social supports
2. Past history of psychiatric problems
3. Past history of depression
4. High initial distress—beyond cultural/religious norms
5. Unanticipated death
6. Other major stresses and losses at the same time
7. Very dependent or ambivalent relationship with the deceased
8. Death of a child
9. Death by suicide

Common psychological patterns that indicate complicated bereavement are an absence of grief, prolongation of the symptoms of grief, and distortion of normal grieving.

When the feelings and process of grief and mourning are *absent*, the bereaved behaves as if the loss never occurred.

After a prolonged illness, Ron's wife Jean died, leaving him with their five-year-old daughter. Ron took no time off of work and immediately emptied the house of all of Jean's clothes and possessions. He then sold all the furniture and redecorated the house. When friends gingerly asked about his feelings of sadness, Ron changed the subject to his home projects.

The problem here resides in Ron's absence of normal reactions and his translation of sadness, anger, and longing into frenetic activity.

In inhibited grief, emotional suffering may be transformed into physical complaints or a mourning of only certain aspects of the relationship and denial of loss in other areas.

Rebecca was referred to a therapist by her internist, who was concerned she might be depressed. She denied sadness, lack of interest, or absence of pleasure in life. Almost as an aside, Rebecca said that her husband committed suicide one year earlier. She took care of the estate and funeral with no change in her routines. She said she did not feel particularly distressed and spent little time concerned about her husband's motivations. Within one month of her husband's suicide, she developed the stomach and bowel symptoms that have preoccupied her ever since.

Delayed grieving may occur when emotional issues or pressing obligations interfere with the initiation or progress of grief. An unexpectedly severe grief may then occur with a subsequent loss. For example, the death of a pet may initiate grief for a dead parent that has been denied or delayed. *Distorted grief* involves either the prolongation of normal acute grief reactions or a predominance of a single emotional response. It might include difficulty accepting that the death has occurred, continued searching of or preoccupation with thoughts of the deceased, auditory or visual hallucinations of the person, or extreme rage and anger directed at the deceased or at care providers. Table 2 lists some signs of pathological grief as described by Eric Lindemann.

Although prolonged symptoms can indicate complicated bereavement, some people simply need more time to adjust to major losses. In situations where it is unclear whether the bereaved is struggling with a complicated grief reaction or simply taking a bit longer to grieve, a visit to a therapist may clarify the issues.

Many people who have complicated bereavement also meet criteria for Major Depression, which is sometimes accompanied by a generalized anxiety disorder. Studies show that, in spite of this, only 17 percent of those with grief-related depressions receive antidepressant medication. This lack of treatment may reflect a mistaken belief that depression is a normal and expected part of bereavement, rather than a psychiatric disorder that should be treated.

Major Depression is one of the most common complications of grief. In the first year after the loss of a spouse, Major Depression occurs four to nine times more frequently than in the general population.

During early grief, many of the symptoms of Major Depression—crying, feelings of overwhelming sadness, occasional thoughts of one's own death, decreased appetite, and disrupted sleep—are common and normal. But in ordinary mourning, feelings of sadness are focused on the particular loss, while in depression these feelings are generalized into all or most aspects of life. During a period of mourning, although they are sad, people still experience pleasure. In contrast, Major Depression empties the world of pleasure. Grief

Table 3   GRIEF AND DEPRESSION—BLOCK, 2000

Grief	*Depression*
Focused on particular loss	Generalized to all experiences
Bereaved person continues to experience pleasure	Nothing is pleasurable
Comes in waves and then recedes	Unremitting and constant
Sense of an acceptable future	Future seen as unendurable
Sleep and appetite disturbance; decreased concentration, social withdrawal, somatic symptoms	Hopelessness, helplessness, worthlessness, as well as sleep and appetite disturbance, somatic symptoms

comes in waves. Major Depression brings with it an unremitting and constant misery with no sense of a positive future. Finally, in grieving, people often have passive wishes for death, while in Major Depression they may have active, persistent suicidal ideation (Table 3). Major Depression requires immediate treatment, which often includes medication and therapy.

HEALTH RISK AND GRIEF

Bereavement is associated with higher rates of mortality, especially among older men. Grieving people often mention decreased immune function, but its medical significance is unclear. In general, poorer health outcomes are due primarily to neglect of preexisting medical conditions and/or increased use of substances that carry health risks, such as alcohol and tobacco.

INTERVENTIONS FOR ADULT BEREAVEMENT

Most bereaved people recover from grief without need for professional help. Most often, family, friends, and spiritual or religious sources provide sufficient support. When more is required, mutual support organizations as well as psychotherapeutic and psychopharmacological providers are available.

Psychotherapy Consider individual psychotherapy when symptoms of complicated bereavement are present. Family therapy may also aid in the process of bereavement. In addition, if symptoms of anxiety or depression persist, an evaluation with a psychiatrist may be advised to clarify diagnosis and consider medication. Suicidal ideation, self-harm, or clear suicide plans should be treated as an emergency that calls for immediate evaluation.

Psychopharmacology Even in bereavement uncomplicated by Major Depression, medication with or without psychotherapy may be indicated for a limited time. During the early weeks of acute grief, antianxiety medications (Table 4) can be used for insomnia at night and tension reduction during the day. These medications can be habit-forming and are cross-addictive with alcohol. However, cautious use to reduce intolerable anxiety and ensure rest makes it easier for those grieving to deal with acute loss. Bereavement complicated

Table 4 COMMONLY USED ANXIOLYTIC (ANTIANXIETY MEDICATIONS)	
Trade Name	*Generic Name*
Ativan	Lorazepam
Valium	Diazepam
Klonopin	Clonazepam
Serax	Oxazepam
Ambien	Zolpidem
Sonata	Zaleplon

Table 5 SOME COMMON ANTIDEPRESSANTS	
Trade Name	*Generic Name*
Zoloft	Sertraline
Prozac	Fluoxetine
Paxil	Paroxitine
Celexa	Citalopram
Effexor	Venlafaxine
Pamelor	Nortripylline
Wellbutrin (Zyban)	Bupropion

by Major Depression requires treatment with antidepressant medications (Table 5). These drugs treat low mood, despair, and suicidal ideation as well as insomnia and anxiety. Antidepressants are most effective in combination with psychotherapy.

Additional Support Options Many people find it helpful to share their experiences of loss with other bereaved people. Programs may take the form of one-to-one meetings, such as the Widow-to-Widow program, or bereavement groups like those offered by hospice or community agencies. Programs are available through religious and medical organizations as well. You can also locate resources on the Internet. Some of these are listed in the Suggested Reading section at the end of this book.

—Laurie Rosenblatt, M.D.

RELATED ENTRIES

Antidepressants

Depressive Disorders

Post-Traumatic Stress Disorder

How Do We Define Sexual Health for Women?

Think about the last time you had a conversation with a friend, a partner, or a doctor about your sexuality. What did you talk about?

Too often, what we talk about is reproductive health and whether our bodies are functioning "normally." Are our periods regular or is menopause going smoothly? Are our vaginas lubricating sufficiently? Do we have "enough" sexual desire—usually meaning enough to satisfy our partner's "needs"?

What we often don't talk about is sexuality as an energizing aspect of our health. We talk about PMS, cramps, the discomforts of pregnancy, how to deal with those extra twenty pounds, overcoming the pain of childbirth, hot flashes, and different ways of communicating what we do not want sexually. We talk about negative features of reproductive health and perhaps subtle allusions to dips in our sexual desire. We rarely acknowledge or recognize that our sexuality is an essential part of who we are, a key aspect of our mental health, and fundamental to our overall health and sense of well-being. We live as if we can live without it.

Our society is obsessed with sex but gives little credence to women's sexual health. While Viagra commercials and cover stories constantly remind us that sexual potency is vitally important for men, women receive mixed messages about what their sexuality should be like. We are supposed to be sexy—that is, appealing to men; that message is clear. But the monolithic image of a sexy woman—slim, young, white, monied—toeing the invisible and elusive line that separates flirtation from sexual aggression rarely reflects what real women look, feel, or act like. More than thirty years after the sexual revolution and the women's movement, one of the greatest barriers still facing women is silence about the realities of our sexuality: silence about how we experience sexuality, silence about what women's sexual health can and should be, and silence about what being sexually healthy women means to us and for society.

In 2001, the surgeon general of the United States issued a report on sexual health that included reproductive functioning and the absence of disease and dysfunction. This report goes further than other such authoritative statements about sexuality have before by contending that sexual health is not just the absence of sexual problems or disease but should instead be understood in the broader context of "the ability of individuals to integrate their sexuality into their lives, derive pleasure from it, and to reproduce, if they so choose." Sexual health means having access to information and care that recognizes these *multiple facets* of sexuality. It also means recognizing that the barriers to sexual health are different for women and men, in large part because of society's ongoing denial and denigration of women's sexuality. Sexual health, then, is not only about having bodies that work properly. It is also about believing we have a right to our own feelings of sexual desire, whatever form they take; expecting and experiencing pleasure on our own terms and for ourselves, not simply to meet our partners' needs; and being free from violence, domination, and abuse, not only in our relationships but in society. And it is about understanding, acknowledging, and addressing how challenges to sexual health may be different depending on a woman's race, ethnicity, class, sexual orientation, age, and ableness, as well as other social circumstances in which her life is embedded.

IT'S NOT JUST "THE WAY THINGS ARE"

Psychologist Leonore Tiefer argues that "sex is not a natural act." By this she means that sex and sexuality are not merely biological functions that our bodies are programmed to perform. Rather, what we think of as normal and appro-

> ✦
>
> The monolithic image of a sexy woman—slim, young, white, monied—toeing the invisible and elusive line that separates flirtation from sexual aggression rarely reflects what real women look, feel, or act like.

priate sexuality—from feelings and relationships to behaviors and problems—reflects society's implicit agreement about what sex is and whom it is for. It's something learned, an understanding we pick up through millions of social cues. But this social contract and learning process are for the most part invisible, and so we come to believe that sex—virtually always referring to vaginal-penile sexual intercourse—*is* a natural act.

The problem with this "story" about (normal, moral, proper) sexuality is that it is based on a male perspective on sexuality: it says that male sexuality *is* human sexuality. It also implies that heterosexuality and marriage are the only appropriate contexts for sexual behavior. Think about how these assumptions make some women's sexuality either inherently problematic or deviant—lesbians and adolescent girls, for instance.

In fact, even much of the research on women's sexuality has a male perspective: it emphasizes the mechanics of performance and the physiological aspects of sexual response. When women's sexuality cannot be measured in these terms, women are more often than not thought to have a disease or dysfunction in need of a remedy. Yet, little is actually known about what a "normal" female sexual response is—or even whether there is a single model that fits most women. For instance, many women feel that having an orgasm is neither the most important, pivotal, or even most pleasurable aspect of sexual experience, nor always the purpose or goal of sexual interaction. However, the production of orgasms—reflecting the male perspective that sex ends with ejaculation—is usually how we measure sexual functioning.

> ✦
>
> What we think of as normal and appropriate sexuality reflects society's implicit agreement about what sex is and whom it is for.

Another example is the current race to find a "female Viagra," which has produced an explosion of research on women's sexual responses. The unstated assumption underlying this race is that the solution to men's primary sexual complaints, predominantly erectile problems and premature ejaculation, must also be applicable to women: increasing blood flow to women's genitals will generate lubrication, propel orgasms, and eradicate complaints. But it's likely that the contexts in which women experience sexual arousal—in a loving relationship, for instance, or on a hot date,

WOMEN'S SEXUAL PROBLEMS: A NEW CLASSIFICATION

by the Working Group on a New View of Women's Sexual Problems

Sexual problems, which the Working Group on a New View of Women's Sexual Problems defines as discontent or dissatisfaction with any emotional, physical, or relational aspect of sexual experience, may arise in one or more of the following four interrelated aspects of women's sexual lives.

I. Sexual Problems Due to Sociocultural, Political, or Economic Factors

A. Ignorance or anxiety due to inadequate sex education, lack of access to health services, or other social constraints:

1. Lack of vocabulary to describe physical or subjective experience.

2. Lack of information about sexual biology and life-stage changes.

3. Lack of information about how gender roles influence men's and women's sexual expectations, beliefs, and behaviors.

4. Inadequate access to information and services that could provide contraception and abortion, sexually transmitted disease (STD) prevention and treatment, sexual trauma and domestic violence.

B. Sexual avoidance or distress due to perceived inability to meet cultural norms regarding correct or ideal sexuality, including:

1. Anxiety or shame about one's body, sexual attractiveness, or sexual responses.

2. Confusion or shame about one's sexual orientation or identity, or about sexual fantasies and desires.

C. Inhibitions due to conflict between the sexual norms of one's subculture or culture of origin and those of the dominant culture.

D. Lack of interest, fatigue, or lack of time due to family and work obligations.

II. Sexual Problems Relating to Partner and Relationship

A. Inhibition, avoidance, or distress arising from betrayal, dislike, or fear of partner, partner's abuse or couple's unequal power, or arising from partner's negative patterns of communication.

B. Discrepancies in desire for sexual activity or in preferences for various sexual activities.

C. Ignorance or inhibition about communicating preferences or initiating, pacing, or shaping sexual activities.

D. Loss of sexual interest and reciprocity as a result of conflicts over commonplace issues such as money, schedules, or

---

or fearing violence or exploitation—are critical factors in our sexual responses. Thus, the common research practice of taking physiological measurements to evaluate women's levels of arousal in an artificial laboratory environment, paralleling the research on men, may overlook critical information. If one considers the profoundly important impact of the social contexts of women's sexuality, the "magic bullet" approach that has been seen as the answer for male sexuality fails to address many of the issues that women may face.

THE IMPORTANCE OF SOCIAL CONTEXTS FOR WOMEN'S SEXUALITY

Because society remains troubled by female sexuality, it may be easier to think about female sexual health in terms of our reproductive health or mechanical difficulties that need to be tinkered with. For instance, women are frequentlydiagnosed as dysfunctional if a couple is having difficulty with sexual intercourse because the woman is not sufficiently lubricated to make it pleasurable for either partner or because she fails to reach orgasm consistently or at all. Because the focus of the diagnosis is on the physiology of sexual intercourse rather than on what may be happening in other parts of a couple's life—economic troubles, child-

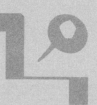

relatives, or resulting from traumatic experiences, such as infertility or the death of a child.

E. Inhibitions in arousal or spontaneity due to partner's health status or sexual problems.

III. Sexual Problems Due to Psychological Factors

A. Sexual aversion, mistrust, or inhibition of sexual pleasure due to:

1. Past experiences of physical, sexual, or emotional abuse.

2. General personality problems with attachment, rejection, cooperation, or entitlement.

3. Depression or anxiety.

B. Sexual inhibition due to fear of sexual acts or of their possible consequences, such as pain during intercourse, pregnancy, sexually transmitted disease, loss of partner, loss of reputation

IV. Sexual Problems Due to Medical Factors

A. Pain or lack of physical response during sexual activity despite a supportive and safe interpersonal situation, adequate sexual knowledge, and positive sexual attitudes. Such problems can arise from:

1. Numerous local or systemic medical conditions affecting neurological, neurovascular, circulatory, endocrine, or other systems of the body.

2. Pregnancy, sexually transmitted diseases, or other sex-related conditions.

3. Side effects of many drugs, medications, or medical treatments.

4. Inadvertently introduced by a medical treatment or diagnostic procedure, such as a hysterectomy or other necessary procedure.

rearing problems, stress at work, or simply one partner being angry at the other—the woman herself is often branded as the source of the problem. Approaches that fragment or compartmentalize women's sexuality fail to acknowledge the critical role of the social contexts of women's lives in our sexual health—that is, our ability to live fully and freely, with choice and with pleasure, in our bodies.

A group of therapists, theorists, and sex researchers collectively called The Working Group (www.ejhs.org/volume3/newview.htm) has recently argued for what they are calling a "new view of women's sexual problems." This group emphasizes the range of forces at work in determining our ability to be sexually healthy and identifies the sociocultural, political, psychological, social, and relational bases of women's sexual problems.

This multidimensional approach to women's sexual health makes it harder to treat. There are no easy solutions for having been sexually abused as a child, or for being an immigrant woman whose culture emphasizes women's sexual purity or asceticism or deems it acceptable for men to have sex with women outside of a committed relationship, or for being an African American woman whose sexuality has historically been discounted or distorted, or for being a poor woman who has no access to contraception, condoms, or HIV testing. This new view shows us how a woman's sexuality is often hobbled by her personal history with relationships and love; by powerful differences in her heterosexual relationships; by stigmatization of certain forms or expressions of sexuality; by poverty or violence; or by stereotypes about the sexuality of women of color or white women. And all of these issues are inextricably intertwined with social contexts in which we live.

HOW GOOD GIRLS CAN WANT IT BAD

Women's sexual trajectories start early and are exceedingly complex. Girls learn through sources, including friends, family, TV, books, magazines, and school, what constitute appropriate sexual behaviors and attitudes. These cultural scripts are so pervasive that it's almost impossible to escape their influence. While these scripts vary across our society—some girls get a heavy-handed version, some a version that allows for a certain amount of female sexual agency—no one escapes it entirely.

> ✦
>
> Much of the research on women's sexuality has a male perspective: it emphasizes the mechanics of performance and the physiological aspects of sexual response.

Thus, girls realize early that they are expected to react to sexual advances, not make them. Men, they come to understand, have powerful (even insatiable) sexual appetites, but girls are expected to be reluctant and resistant. They must respond to men's sexual interest with reserve and trepidation and later, in the context of a socially condoned relationship, are supposed to acquiesce willingly to their sexual requests. Alternately, they may learn to enjoy themselves within a socially condoned relationship but never quite feel that they own their sexuality.

Sexual health should promote girls', boys', women's, and men's awareness that girls and women having sexual feelings is not only normal, but something we should expect and embrace. Sexual feelings provide information about ourselves that can enhance the meanings we make about our emotions and our relationships. But the pressure to deny sexual feelings is still a key feature of the socialization of girls and women. Lacking the words to describe our sexual desires and arousal, our feelings of desire, of wanting to connect physically and sexually, these feelings are often "translated" into the more acceptable feelings of being wanted, words of romance, love, intimacy, and even enticement.

> ✦
>
> Sexual feelings provide information about ourselves that can enhance the meanings we make about our emotions and our relationships.

There is no sanctioned route for a good woman to be the seducer, for deliberating, having forethought, having her own needs and motives. Many women are thus rendered mute and powerless. They are bombarded by media images that promote sexual availability but also clear social condemnation of girls and women who express sexual agency—who act on their own feelings and think of themselves as well as their partner in sexual situations. This script is so strongly sanctioned in our society that it produces tension between being sexy but not being sexual. And so it's understandable that girls enter adulthood feeling confused and not knowing how to be sexual in a positive way. Our social scripts actually preempt basic recognition of our sexual needs or rights.

The pressure to conform to the feminine ideals held up by our culture, which can include the sexual ascetic, may lead to tremendous conflict regarding our experiences of sexual desire and interest—and their lack. Being unable or actively discouraged from acknowledging or attending to our sexual needs and interests can make us feel incapable of directing our own sexual outcomes: how can we get or know what we want sexually when actively going after it is somehow not feminine? Women feel this way because we are unlikely to be taught that we really are capable and entitled to be subjects of our own sexuality rather than simply objects of someone else's sexual desires.

But girls, as they grow up, experiment with ever-increasing levels of sexual intimacy even when faced with strong cultural prohibitions against such activity and socialized to deny their sexual arousal, desire, and needs for physical intimacy. The pressure to become sexually active and to acquire sexual experience, especially in the context of romantic relationships, is equally if not more significant in our society as those social currents championing the repression of female adolescent sexuality. Thus, many girls are at risk of being caught acting "inappropriately." And many will experiment sexually without the knowledge or skills to ensure healthy sexual outcomes. What girls have learned is how to say "no"—never how or when to say "yes."

The ramifications of defying traditional scripts are clearly communicated: Girls and women who are not monogamous, who are sexually assertive, or who have sexual encounters outside of a relational, romantic heterosexual context are all too often labeled "sluts" or "whores." Openly communicating sexual interest, arousal, a desire for sexual variety or simply denying a male partner sexual access can also bring on severe repercussions like violence (or the threat of violence) and the loss of critical material resources. Women are expected to be sexual gatekeepers and are held responsible for keeping men's sexual desire in check.

One clear illustration of this arrangement is women's long history of fighting to place culpability on male perpetrators in cases of rape and sexual assault against women and girls. Despite years of work by feminist groups, there is still no clear social mandate for male accountability and responsibility, and so women too often continue to be blamed on the basis of their sexuality for sexual and physical victimization and exploitation. We need to understand how these dynamics affect how women develop and experience their sexuality in the different contexts of their lives.

Some women, most frequently poor women and women of color, have historically been characterized as overly sexualized and have been targeted as vectors of disease, a form of severe social condemnation. Public concern about their sexuality is amplified to a near-hysterical pitch at the point when these women reach childbearing age: The media reports highlight "sky-rocketing" teen pregnancy rates and negligent welfare mothers. Well-funded local, state, and federal interventions and educational campaigns are launched regularly to control the sexual behavior of these girls, and their usual goal is to reduce childbearing and disease. Yet, almost nothing is known about the normal development of their sexual, romantic, and

> How can we get or know what we want sexually when actively going after it is somehow not feminine?

> Girls, as they grow up, experiment with ever-increasing levels of sexual intimacy even when faced with strong cultural prohibitions against such activity.

intimate thoughts, behaviors, preferences, or beliefs—a logical starting place for health intervention efforts. The focus continues to be on the negative outcomes of their sexual experiences rather than the broader context and complexities of their sexual lives.

The sexuality of white, middle-class girls and women is frequently denied altogether. They are saddled with images of a purity that must be protected at all costs against contamination by any hint of overt sexuality. An example of these efforts includes the intensive abstinence-only sex education programs in suburban public schools—frequently the only sources of sexual information available to our nation's youth. These campaigns very often spring from conservative religious groups and are clearly targeted at white, middle-class girls and young women. They often require pledges of sexual abstinence until entering a "biblical marriage relationship" and are riddled with judgmental words like *purity, innocence,* and *sin*. The clear implication, for the girls that they target, is that a woman should be asexual in thought and deed, spurning temptations to express herself sexually.

Fundamental to these programs is the promotion of the belief that there are no reliable forms of protection against pregnancy and disease other than abstinence. Unsurprisingly, when these youth become sexually active, they tend not to protect themselves. And because they have been given little or no information on how to be sexual in alternative, safe, and informed ways, they think that mature sexuality is comprised solely of sexual intercourse.

These campaigns fly in the face of a wealth of scientific evidence demonstrating that providing comprehensive sex information in schools promotes positive sexual health: Youth become equipped to make healthy decisions about their goals in life and where sexual interests fit into these trajectories, and how to meet their health needs. The United States has the highest teen pregnancy statistics among Western societies and a raging sexually transmitted disease epidemic, highlighting like nothing else how our support of ignorance among our youth constitutes an active campaign to deny their rights to sexual healthy lives.

> ✦
>
> A wealth of scientific evidence demonstrates that providing comprehensive sex information in schools promotes positive sexual health.

⌐ What are the messages that you've received about your sexuality?

    … about being female?

    … about your race or ethnicity?

    … about to whom you are attracted?

    … about your social circumstances?

⌐ What gets in the way for you in being aware of or of acting in line with your own sexual feelings or desire?

⌐ What would you do if you felt no inhibitions at all?

⌐ Who can you talk to about your right to healthy sexuality?

CLAIMING OUR SEXUALITY ON OUR OWN TERMS

RELATED ENTRIES

The Biology of Female Sexuality

Women and Trauma

When women claim our sexuality on our own terms, social change happens and injustice becomes evident. Recall how Betty Friedan's naming of the "problem that couldn't be named" led to frank discussion of sexuality and revelations that what was being said about women's sexuality and women's lives did not match their actual experiences. The recognition that marital rape could and did happen, the development of battered women's shelters, the widening availability of effective forms of contraception—all these things came about because women talked among themselves and then worked together to create change. Resistance is an important challenge to a system that undermines women's and girls' sexual health. And there is obviously a lot more resisting that we all need to do. Fears of strong social condemnation, loss of resources, and physical harm can be lessened if we work collectively toward changes in what we understand women's healthy sexuality—and the social conditions necessary for its sustenance—to be.

Key to such a movement is a positive model of sexual health that is inextricably linked to what kind of social change needs to happen for women to actually be healthy. Our efforts need to be channeled toward championing girls' and women's sexual agency and the acquisition of knowledge and skills that undermine our efforts toward healthy sexual decision making. Women and girls, boys and men need information about women's sexuality and the ways in which social contexts and social forces shape the assumptions we make about it. They also need to know about men's sexuality, itself a crucial social context for women's experiences. Society constrains women's sexuality in harmful and unhealthy ways, as we have outlined here, but men, too, face constraints and expectations, perhaps with fewer or, more likely, with different negative outcomes.

Here are some questions to think about, to talk about with other women and girls and with health practitioners to help figure out barriers to your own sexual health:

- What are the messages that you've received about your sexuality?
  … about being female?
  … about your race or ethnicity?
  … about to whom you are attracted?
  … about your social circumstances?
- What gets in the way for you in being aware of or of acting in line with your own sexual feelings or desire?
- What would you do if you felt no inhibitions at all?
- Who can you talk to about your right to healthy sexuality?

—*Deborah L. Tolman, Ed.D., Meg I. Striepe, Ph.D., and Lucia F. O'Sullivan, Ph.D.*

Female Sexuality

On her deathbed, my grandmother mentioned proudly, in the midst of a list of her other major accomplishments, that she'd never had an orgasm in her life.

On the other hand, her daughter—my aunt—had her first orgasm at the age of fourteen while sitting on the living room couch with the man she would one day marry. Although the location and company wasn't strange, what was unusual was the TV was on, her father was in the room, and she and her boyfriend were doing nothing more than furtively clasping hands. No touching anywhere else. No wiggling, no clothes off, just the simple pressure of entwined palms and the absolute power of young love.

Boom, orgasm.

This isn't as unusual as you might think. Dr. Beverly Whipple of Rutgers University has recorded cases of women who can climax by themselves, without another person or sexual device, without even touching their own body. They just sit back, close their eyes, and *think*. One pain specialist, Dr. Stuart Meloy, in an attempt to help people with chronic pain, stumbled by accident on the area in the brain that these women are stimulating. Meloy surgically inserted a neural implant in a pain center in the brain and found when he pressed the button, instead of giving pain relief, he gave instant orgasms.

Throughout her life, my aunt has been able to press that button by herself, without a doctor or electrodes. She has a six-lane highway to climax, a direct telephone line, the kind that's painted red and sits in presidents' offices.

My grandmother didn't even have smoke signals.

The range of what women experience as normal female sexuality is wide and deep. It varies not only from woman to woman, but also from one era of a woman's life to the next.

However, neither the extremes nor the norms of women's sexuality have been studied by modern science half as much as men's sexuality has. To give one example of this, the location of male genital nerves were discovered thirty years ago. Today, when operating near these nerves, doctors will even pull out magnifying glasses to make sure no damage is done to the patient's sexual function. The same is not true for women.

The location of a woman's genital nerves is not exactly known—even to the doctors who slice down through that flesh as they perform a hysterectomy (the second most common operation performed on women in the United States, to the tune of 600,000 a year). This lack of basic anatomy knowledge can lead to a postoperative patient finding her clitoris now has all the sensation of a pencil eraser.

Another example of the medical profession's disproportionate respect for male libido is that almost every medicine for faltering sexuality was originally designed for men. Viagra, testosterone, Vasomax. Women have had only one device actually intended for them from the start, the EROS-CTD, which is a handheld "clitoral therapy device" that is marketed as increasing the blood flow to the clitoris and genitalia. Any other treatment prescribed for a woman would be a (retrofitted) version of what has worked for men, with the blind hope that the same basic principles might apply.

The famous Berman sisters (Laura, sex therapist, and Jennifer, urologist, founders of two female sexuality clinics) say medical knowledge of female sexuality is thirty years behind male sexuality.

Whereas it is obvious to society, and thus to the medical profession, that a man's libido is a critical component of his quality of life no matter what his age or health status, the same is not as true yet for women.

SEXUAL DEVELOPMENT FROM CONCEPTION TO AGE THREE

All fetuses, male or female, start off with an identical primordial genital ridge. In the ninth week of gestation, unless a sufficient amount of testosterone is secreted, the ridge will fold into a vagina and uterus. If enough is secreted, it will push out into a penis and testes. Thus, the assumption is always female unless testosterone interferes.

There's a popular biological theory (called "ontogeny recapitulates phylogeny") that maintains the development of all fetuses repeats each of the major stages of human evolution. At one point the fetus has gills like the fish we all used to be, at another point a tail like a monkey. Because of this argument, and because the fetus is female unless notified otherwise, one suggested theory is that the distant precursors of humans reproduced asexually and that females came first; males are an evolutionary second thought.

Forget all that stuff about Adam's rib. He's stealing Eve's résumé.

From birth until three years old, a structure in the hypothalamus, the gonadotropin-releasing pulse generator, secretes reproductive hormones every ninety minutes or so. The ovaries respond by secreting small amounts of ovarian hormones, not enough to grow breasts, but enough to get the mind thinking. You can see it in any child old enough to explore her world. A toddler is interested in her body and the bodies of those around her. She's sexually curious, sticking her fingers into every orifice she can find. Around three years old, these hormones stop and the child becomes less curious.

AGE TEN THROUGH ADOLESCENCE

The adrenal glands, on top of the kidneys, start to secrete small doses of sex hormones at around the age of ten. Most girls begin to get crushes (whether on other girls or boys),[1] although any sexual fantasies they have tend to still be hazily romantic.

1. Homosexuality and heterosexuality have been found to be much more of a gradient than was previously thought. Between 4 and 10 percent of women define themselves as lesbians, women who are primarily emotionally and sexually attracted to women. A small percentage consider themselves bisexual. The rest are primarily attracted to men.

In this chapter, when forced by the needs of the text to name the partner's gender or sexual organ, I say "men" and "penises" because that's what the majority of women are working with. However, whatever gender or anatomy you're interested in, please insert those words instead.

At around twelve years, the hypothalamus starts to regularly spit out its hormones again. It is not really known what sets this off. Puberty and menstruation these days generally begin two to four years earlier than they did in the early 1900s. One cause for this is thought to be all the hormones the meat and dairy industries use, which end up in the consumers of the meat and dairy products. Also, body fat ratio triggers the start of menses, and children these days are fatter than children were a century ago. A pregnancy takes about 80,000 calories to carry to term. Most girls start puberty when they have about 87,000 calories of fat. Thus, puberty seems to start when a child could physically handle a pregnancy.

> ✦
>
> Puberty and menstruation these days generally begin two to four years earlier than they did in the early 1900s.

The starting up of the hypothalamus's hormones stimulate the ovaries to secrete estrogen. Estrogen makes the body put down more fat deposits, makes pubic and armpit hair grow and causes the pelvis to widen, the breasts to enlarge, and menstruation to begin.

From here on until menopause, women have three to ten times more estrogen in the bloodstream than men. Estrogen isn't manufactured only by the ovaries; it also comes from a woman's fat and muscles and liver. And estrogen isn't used by only the reproductive organs and breasts. It's needed everywhere in the body, by the bones and blood vessels and brain, by the liver and skin and bladder. Basically, it's hard to find an organ in the body that isn't deeply involved with estrogen in some way. It keeps the bad types of cholesterol away, keeps the heart strong, and sharpens the eyesight. Our bodies are female from our muscles down to the very walls of our veins.

Women also manufacture testosterone. Yes, that male hormone. Testosterone comes from the ovaries, adrenal glands, and possibly the brain and uterus. The hormone is at one-tenth the level of a male's, but it is there, perceptible, working. So far, it appears to help with libido, bone density, skin softness, and keeping a high energy level.

Many researchers have tried to prove either estrogen or testosterone as the main hormone of desire in women, studying which hormone is at its peak in the menstrual cycle when women are most likely to want sex. The results have been a bit mixed. Some studies say women's desire increases just before ovulation, while others find it is just before and after menstruation. These three points in the cycle include when estrogen is at its high and also the time when testosterone peaks.

> ✦
>
> Estrogen isn't used by only the reproductive organs and breasts. It's needed everywhere in the body.

Whatever the chemical(s) of desire turn(s) out to be, humans are not a thin veneer of civilization over the push-button power of hormones. The one fact on which all the studies agree is that the most common time for a woman to have sex is on the weekend when she has time.

ADULTHOOD

Whereas men experience their sexual peak at eighteen years old, before some of them even have gone on a good date, women's sexuality keeps climbing and climbing. We women get more than twenty years of active experimentation before our peak to learn all we can of our sexuality, to each figure out how our particular body works. Think of how widely people vary in terms of what they like to eat. If you don't sample a wide range of foods cooked in a variety of ways, you'll never discover your ultimate meal and how to prepare it.

And once you know what you want, you have to learn how to communicate that to your partner. Frequently, this takes equal parts maturity, bravery, and desperation.

Thus, it's lucky women's sexual peak hits during our thirties and forties, giving us time to find a worthwhile partner and get all we can from it.

PREGNANCY

Big changes. The blood volume in the body doubles. Every mucous membrane, from the nose to the vagina, starts working overtime. The breasts, swelling from the influence of the hormones progesterone and prolactin, generally increase two bra sizes. Estrogen levels in the blood increase six to seven times over prepregnancy levels. And in the most dramatic change to any healthy organ in the body during adulthood, the uterus goes from two ounces to two pounds (not counting the baby or placenta). Six weeks after birth, it's back to its normal prepregnancy size.

> Sex and exercise both improve the blood supply to the genitals, helping significantly with lubrication and sensation.

Many women report a lessening in desire during the first and third trimesters. The first trimester's retreat of libido might not be directly because of the tsunami of confusing hormones, but more because of the accompanying nausea and tiredness. Later, many women might simply be disheartened at the breathtaking effort necessary to heft the third-trimester body into any sort of sexual position.

Other women, because of the increased blood supply to the reproductive organs, the constant engorgement of the labia and the swelling breasts, feel unusually sexual throughout pregnancy.

MENOPAUSE AND AFTERWARD

On average, thirty-eight-odd years after adolescence, the ovaries stop producing estradiol, one of the three types of estrogen. Estrogen levels in the body decrease by 50 percent. This tends to create some weakening of the vaginal walls and a decreased ability to lubricate. These two symptoms can make sex a bit painful. Also, some women feel fewer, and occasionally painful, uterine contractions when they orgasm. Drugstore lubricants can help with the ability to lubricate. Estrogen and testosterone, applied locally, also help with lubrication, sensation, and thinning vaginal walls.

The good news is that one part of the nether regions doesn't care about estrogen—the clitoris doesn't atrophy at all after menopause.

Sex and exercise both improve the blood supply to the genitals, helping significantly with lubrication and sensation. Although this society has promulgated the idea that older women are undesirable and therefore undesiring, many women enjoy active and pleasurable sex throughout their lives. The 1993 Janus report on sexual behavior found 74 percent of women over sixty-five had sex at least once a week.

ANATOMY

Clitoris Dr. Helen O'Connell was the first to find that the clitoris didn't dead-end just under the skin. She discovered it was actually attached to a pyramid-shaped mass of erectile tissue that extended into the pelvis making the clitoris twice as big as previously thought. Believe it or not, this was discovered only in 1998. Medical researchers out there, take note. This is a field with a lot left to discover.

The clitoris has three sections: base, shaft, and crown. These sections are largely buried in the pelvis. At adulthood, the visible part, in its unaroused state, from the shaft to the top of the glans (the little button you probably thought was the whole of the clitoris), measures about the diameter of a dime.

Scientists (one of the most famous being Stephen Jay Gould) have asked again and again why women have clitorises. They often suggest that the clitoris is a vestigial penis left over from the reshuffling of the genital ridge during gestation. They've theorized alternately that the clitoris used to be useful in some way (they can't imagine how), but now, evolutionarily speaking, is on its way out, that this retreat from human anatomy is why it's currently so small.

Jealousy, I say, rank jealousy.

The clitoris is a fully functioning and healthy organ. Unlike the penis, it has no other purpose than pleasure. Forget those throbbing six inches that so much has been made of; the amount of sensation that can be transmitted through the organ is the point, the amount of pleasure it can produce. Although smaller than the penis, the clitoris has more than twice as many nerve fibers. These 8,000 nerves number more than in any other part of the body, including the lips and fingertips. The clitoris is so sensitive it has to be cushioned behind soft labial lips, only to be revealed in case of use. It can be almost painful to touch directly, which is why a circular or tapping motion is generally better than direct pressure. That way the nerves don't get overloaded.

> Although smaller than the penis, the clitoris has more than twice as many nerve fibers.

Scientists have also asked why women have orgasms. They point out, whereas a male climax transmits the sperm toward the egg, the female orgasm accomplishes nothing of evolutionary importance.

What the scientists are ignoring seems blatantly obvious to me, the owner of a clitoris: orgasms make a woman more likely to return for more. Humans are not a species that comes into heat and gets the fertilizing done in one fell swoop. We are inefficient at procreation. Even a young heterosexual couple—at the peak of their fertility—has less than a 20 percent chance of conception during a whole month of regular sex. This means we women must come back for more and come back often. And thus, we must *come.*

Every species of female primate studied so far also orgasms, so this enjoyment is obviously considered a useful adaptation by Mother Nature.

Perhaps the evolutionary importance of the female pleasure principle is why it has the potential to be so strong. The most number of orgasms ever recorded by one man in an hour in a research setting? 17. By a woman? 134. Like I said, jealousy.

> The most number of orgasms ever recorded by one man in an hour in a research setting? 17. By a woman? 134. Like I said, jealousy.

So, yes, the clitoris takes longer to get to the party than the penis, but once a woman arrives at the door, she can take off her coat and stay awhile. This longer startup time but greater endurance has led some to speculate that women were designed for serial sexual encounters with a number of partners (of both genders) instead of just one short encounter with an overeager man. The matriarchal bonobos, our closest primate relative, are like that, having sex many times throughout the day, using sex as a more intimate handshake to ease any social tensions.

An alternate theory can be suggested from the fact that when masturbating, it takes men and women on average the same amount of time (three minutes) to climax. Perhaps, during heterosexual sex, we are doing something wrong. Sexual intercourse is currently defined as when the penis is in the vagina. Everything else is waved away as unimportant "foreplay"—nice to do if you have the time. It's possible if sex were redefined as the testes rubbing against the clitoris, it would be men who take a lot longer to respond.

The clitoris is how most women orgasm. As many as 75 percent of women never have an orgasm by penile thrust alone. But, as I stated in the beginning, a climax can be reached in other ways. In a study of 300 Sudanese women who had been clitorectomized, most reported strong sex drives and orgasms.

> As many as 75 percent of women never have an orgasm by penile thrust alone.

Cervix The cervix, located at the far end of the vagina, resembles a small glazed donut. It protects the uterus against invading bacteria. It has so few nerves, surgery can be performed on it without anesthesia. Still, it has been found, with some women, rhythmic pressure on the cervix for at least twenty minutes can result in the most satisfying kind of orgasm for them, a vaginal as opposed to clitoral orgasm. This is an orgasm in which the pelvic floor and uterine contractions are very strong and there is a deep "bearing-down" sensation. Younger women who aren't as familiar with their bodies as older women are less likely to be able to orgasm this way. It's most likely to be elicited from a rear-entry or sideways position, or in the missionary position with the butt propped up.

G Spot Although many people say there's no such thing as the G spot, 66 percent of women have an area in their vagina that feels pleasurable when touched if they are already aroused. One hypothesis is that the G spot is nothing more than the foot of the clitoris, peeking up from its pelvic depths. To find it, squat or sit down and reach just a little inside the vagina, toward the front just above the urethra, and feel around. You should find a bean-sized area that's smoother than the rest of the rippled texture of the vagina. When you press firmly and rhythmically you might feel the need to urinate. When you're aroused it should increase to the size of a marshmallow and feel spongy. Pressing the G spot rhythmically brings some women to the intense vaginal orgasm.

THE ACT

Desire This is the feeling of sexual energy that makes a woman want to start sex or respond to sexual advances. In the brain, desire is located in the sites of emotion: the limbic system, the hypothalamus, and amygdala.

One fact about female sexuality of which the evolutionary scientists seem convinced is that women have a lower sex drive than men. When considering this possibility, it's good to remember that science, a mere century ago, believed the developing uterus demanded so much blood that educating a woman's brain would leach away precious nutrients and result in infertility. This theory was promulgated so much that many women considering college felt they had to choose between education and future children.

Women's desire is strong enough that almost every society in the world has spent an awful lot of time and energy trying to control it. Every mechanism has been tried from mandatory clitorectomies before adolescence to stoning a woman to death for extramarital sex. Still, no matter in what country, women get and enjoy nookie, inside the bonds of matrimony or not.

Even in the fairly liberal United States, women's desire for sex is strong enough to make them risk pregnancy, venereal diseases, sexual violence, and social disapproval. Men only have to deal with a few of these risks and none to the same level as women.

Arousal A recent survey found most couples during sex go from hugging to kissing to caressing to intercourse. Vaginal intercourse is the most common sexual activity, with oral sex the second most popular.

As a woman becomes aroused, the tissues of the inner vagina and vulva get moist from fluids secreted by the genital walls. The clitoris swells to twice its size and hardens. The vagina gets longer and expands. The uterus rises. The nipples can get erect and the breasts swell by up to 25 percent. Blood pressure and heart rate double. The pain threshold increases by 60 percent. The labia absorb blood, swell, and pull back to make access easier.

Orgasm This is the peak. The blood pressure and pulse spike. The muscles of the vagina, uterus, and sometimes rectum contract rhythmically, creating a strongly pleasurable feeling. The limbic system sends out satiation messages all over the body. The feeling varies in intensity and duration from orgasm to orgasm and from woman to woman. It can actually be powerful enough to make some lose consciousness for a moment.

On the other hand, 10 percent of women report they've never had an orgasm. One study by sex therapist Marilyn Fifthian monitored twenty of these women with machines while they masturbated. Fifthian discovered fifteen of the twenty did climax. The women just didn't think—after all the massive hype about the earth moving and so forth—that that little old thing could be it.

> Women's desire is strong enough that almost every society in the world has spent an awful lot of time and energy trying to control it.

A whole sexual experience, though, can be ruined by being too focused on attaining an orgasm. If you fixate too much on the end result, it's impossible to even enjoy what's going on. Drs. Laura and Jennifer Berman suggest that simply exploring the body of your partner in a sensual and slow way is the best way to have sex. Without all the tension and rush, you're more likely to reach orgasm, and if no orgasm happens the sex still wasn't bad or meaningless.

The average orgasm lasts about twenty seconds, much longer than the twelve seconds most women guessed it was. The subjective intensity had nothing to do with how long it lasted or the amount of blood flowing to the region.

Resolution This is the point when the vagina, clitoris, and uterus return to their unaroused states. It usually happens within seconds.

DO YOU HAVE A PROBLEM?

If you're worried about your sexual function, you should first pause and consider my grandmother and aunt again. There's a wide range of sexual normality, just as there is with height, breast size, and nose shape. We don't, under any circumstances, all have to be the same. That my grandmother and aunt were galaxies away from each other in their sexuality didn't bother either of them. They each felt their own body to be functioning just the way it should.

However, perhaps something you've read or something your best friend told you or your partner wished for makes you defensively feel your sexuality isn't all that it should be. Forget it. Sex therapists say only you can decide. Do *you* think there's something wrong? Does it cause *you* emotional distress?

There are long natural periods in a woman's life when sex just might not come first: deadlines at work, difficulties in a relationship, depression, and so forth. The majority of women go through an extended period of less sex or difficulties with sex at some point during their lives. What with pregnancy, menopause, and those sleep-deprived child-rearing years, women naturally tend to experience this more than men.

> The majority of women go through an extended period of less sex or difficulties with sex at some point during their lives.

Still, there's a lot of hype out there about female sexual dysfunction. In 1999, the *Journal of the American Medical Association* (JAMA) found 43 percent of American women had some type of sexual dysfunction as compared to 31 percent of men. Although this is a shocking statistic, JAMA defined this dysfunction by symptoms *it* considered abnormal, not by the women saying something was wrong.

However, the JAMA study was picked up by the media and publicized everywhere. Even the author of the study said he'd only intended to explore the everyday social stresses on women, not to medicalize the results.

Women already go into the doctor twice as often as men, spending three-fourths of all the health care money. Once the doctor has you on the table, she or he is more likely to recommend medical treatments than not. And women are more likely to respond to that pressure than men. Don't start this process unless you're genuinely convinced something's wrong.

Before you head to a doctor, you might want to try out some of the less medically intrusive methods. Exercise has been found to increase a woman's overall health and make her more in the mood for sex. It also increases the blood supply to the genitals, which increases lubrication, sensation, and intensity of orgasm. Dr. Cindy Meston of the University of British Columbia found that when women watched an erotic video after exercise, their genital engorgement was 168 percent greater than without the exercise.

Another method is to spend time exploring your own body and what feels good. Buy a vibrator—they're fun and they can potentially reassure you that everything's still in working order. After that, you can work with your partner to duplicate the vibrator's results.[2]

If you do decide something's wrong and a doctor or sex therapist is the best route, the tools they have are these:

• Estrogen cream, tablets, and rings can be applied directly to the genital area to increase lubrication and decrease thinning of the vaginal wall. Locally applied estrogen doesn't cause as many side effects throughout the rest of the body as estrogen taken orally.

---

2. A side note on the vibrator: During the Victorian era, women who were nervous or irritable were routinely advised to go to their doctor's office to get what was called a "hysterical paroxysm." This meant the doctor masturbated the woman to climax, which was supposed to relieve her symptoms for a while. The vibrator, invented by a British doctor in the 1880s, was a way of making this task a little less time-consuming.

And vibrators are less time-consuming. They, unlike the human hand, are designed specifically for what the neuronal impulses of your clitoris demand.

- Testosterone delivered either through oral pills or a topical cream can increase libido and the number of orgasms per sexual encounter. It can also have positive effects on skin, bone density, muscles, and energy. Too much testosterone, however, can cause oily skin, acne, facial hair growth, a possible increased risk of heart disease, lower voice, liver damage, an enlarged clitoris, and irritability.
- EROS-CTD—this device works on simple observation that the more blood there is in the genitals, the more sensation there is and the more lubrication. It gently stimulates blood flow into the area.
- Talk therapy can be for just you, or for you and your partner. A sex therapist can not only help you discuss past painful or confusing sexual experiences but can also give you "homework" assignments to try with your partner or alone. For instance, a homework assignment might be for you and your partner to explore each other's bodies without having actual sexual intercourse. Then, the next time you see the therapist, you discuss the results.

AND WHAT ABOUT LOVE?

Koko is a famous gorilla who has been taught American Sign Language. When it came time for her to breed, her researchers paraded before her a variety of possible mates. Unfortunately, like so many deeply educated females with superior communication skills, she found the dating world filled with gorillas. She rejected suitor after suitor. As it was quite expensive to truck in different primates, the researchers had zoos across the country send in videos of their prime males for Koko's perusal.

As she viewed them, Koko would lean close to the TV and study each contender—a gorilla's version of Lunch Dates. When the tape was finished, she rewound to one male and watched his segment again.

"Him," she signed, "I want him."

One of the researchers asked why. Here was a rare glimpse into what the most educated nonhuman primate had to say about the laws of attraction:

"His hair," Koko signed, "I like his hair."

For all of us, this is part of what it comes down to. One study revealed that women having sex with attractive partners tend to have more orgasms. Sure, the person could be a rotten lover, but check out that profile against your pillow.

However, having perfectly aligned facial features isn't everything. According to Dr. Martha McClintock, director of the Institute for Mind and Biology, an attractive smell trumps that of a beautiful face every time. And what's attractive nasally to one woman isn't necessarily attractive to another.

Immune molecules are released in sweat. Perhaps the importance of our mate's smell is part of the search for handing down a stronger immune system to the next generation. Each of us women is sniffing out, in our mate, immunities that won't conflict with our own.

> According to Dr. Martha McClintock, director of the Institute for Mind and Biology, an attractive smell trumps that of a beautiful face every time.

If one spouse doesn't like the smell of the other, McClintock maintains, there's little chance the marriage will last. When we press our noses deep into our lover's neck or chest, and breathe so deeply, so contentedly, we might each be reconfirming our children's chance for a healthy life.

Hormonally, love might be created with oxytocin and vasopressin. Given a shot of oxytocin, rats, voles, and rhesus monkeys will sidle over to the nearest creature—adult or baby—and start the motions of attachment as lover or mother.

Whatever happens within humans as part of the rites of falling in love, humans do it hard. In general, it's true that the longer-lived the animal, the stronger the possible attachment it can form. Humans are one of the longest-lived animals. Falling in love can make us disregard food and sleep and anything but the loved one. It can make us physically sick. *Love is one of the strongest forces in humans.*

And each of us does fall in love, and strangely enough not all with the same person. Not the best-looking person, not the best smelling. Love is individual and terrifically idiosyncratic. No matter what we look or smell like, almost every one of us loves and is loved in return. The choice of whom to love is decided upon not entirely by the eye or nose or hormones. The decision of who is the best possible mate is made, with all the other decisions, in each of our minds. This makes sense because the mind is where the sex drive is primarily located also.

As researcher after researcher has pointed out, and my aunt has proven—more than the clitoris, vagina, or breasts—the brain is the ultimate sex organ. How we perceive the sexual act is more important than the actual actions of the sex. Some people can only orgasm with a dirty basketball sneaker, some people find pot-bellied Jack Nicholson attractive. This isn't a right-or-wrong test. There is no grading. There's only the right result: love, good sex, and, if possible, happiness.

—*Audrey Schulman*

RELATED ENTRIES

How Do We Define Sexual Health for Women?

Intimate Relationships

Growth in Connection

A Relational-Cultural Model of Growth

Increasingly, we are learning that relationships are not only good for all people but are necessary for growth and well-being. For adolescents, one good connection with an adult can provide protection from the high risks of substance abuse, violence, and suicide. Scientists have long known that people with social supports are healthier and survive longer.

In most cultures women have been seen as the keepers of relationships. However, despite new evidence of the importance of connection to human life, psychology has been slow to revise its paradigm, which centers on the separate self.

WOMEN'S DEVELOPMENT

Most psychological models of human development are based on research and observation of men. These Eurocentric, male-based theories suggest that all human development ideally leads to separation. Within these models, independence and autonomy are hallmarks of mature development. Independent and autonomous functioning is particularly encouraged in the groups who are vested with the most power and privilege in the culture (the dominant groups). He who is seen as most separate, "standing on his own two feet," is also superior to others who are more dependent and vulnerable. Within these models, logical, abstract thought is lauded and seen as a sign of psychological health. By these standards, many people, especially women and other minority groups who do not typically hold the power to define worth, are seen as deficient.

New work on the psychology of women by Carol Gilligan, Patricia Hill Collins, Janie Ward, Jean Baker Miller and her colleagues Irene Stiver, Judith Jordan, Janet Surrey, and Maureen Walker at the Stone Center for Developmental Services and Studies at Wellesley College, among others, suggests that by listening to the diverse voices of women themselves, rather than generalizing about them from these models based on men, we begin to hear a different story of development. Girls and women tend to grow through and toward relationships with others. In fact, the desire to connect and participate in building mutual relationships may be a primary organizing force in women's lives. That is, they do not enter relationships simply to get something (material supplies, love, support) so they can be stronger, separate people. They participate in relationships in order to contribute to the growth of others, to the growth of relationship, as well as to further their own growth. There is interest in mutual benefit and growth.

The capacity for empathy is central to growth based on relationships. In empathy one feels *with* the other person at the same time that one better understands the other person. Furthermore, there is an acknowledgment that in any relationship, if one person is growing, both people must be growing. In a healthy relationship there is a flow of mutual empathy between people. Mutual empathy is about openness to being affected, moved, and impacted, and it involves both people contributing to the well-being of the other and to the relationship. In such relationships one literally comes alive! One feels zest, a sense of worth, clarity, and understanding, the capacity to be creative and courageous, and the desire for more connection. This new model of human development is not about the growth of the "self" but rather the growth of a sustaining relational network. At its heart it is about the growth of community.

The models of development that focus on autonomous behavior tend to glorify individual achievement and individual courage. This sadly distorts the reality of most people's lives. Furthermore, it puts forth unachievable standards of psychological growth for both boys and girls, men and women, including the false notion that we can and should stand alone in order to demonstrate our maturity and strength. Sam is a good example of this.

Until the birth of her first child, Sam was a very successful real estate agent. However, when she and her husband decided to start a family, it made sense for her to stay at home for a few years. Her husband's work schedule was not flexible, so they made a plan for Sam to stay home with their baby for a couple of years and then restart her real estate career. The plan seemed perfect—except Sam did not realize how hard it would be for her stay at home and take care of a child. She missed her colleagues, missed her clients, and missed the daily validation as a contributing member of working society. She felt increasingly isolated. When she tried to talk about this with her husband Jim, he seemed irritated and would comment that she did not understand how lucky she was to be able to stay at home, to get out of the rat race he was in. They both came from working and family environments that supported the idea that hard work would create individual advancement in the workplace. By feeling so overwhelmed, Sam felt she was letting her family down. She stopped complaining, and she and Jim drifted apart. Sam felt ashamed she could not handle the situation better; Jim felt guilty that he was so critical of his wife whom he once admired.

> Girls and women tend to grow through and toward relationships with others. In fact, the desire to connect and participate in building mutual relationships may be a primary organizing force in women's lives.

The problem with the relationship lies with neither Jim nor Sam, but rather in the belief system they both hold that functioning in isolation and not complaining are to be held in the highest regard. When Sam realized she needed support, she joined a parenting group and used her people skills to form a network of individuals who supported one another through the long days of motherhood. With this support, she felt better about herself and could again see the wisdom of the plan she and Jim had formulated.

While Wellesley College's Stone Center for Developmental Services and Studies work arose in the late seventies as an effort to better and more accurately understand the psychology of women—with specific awareness of the misunderstandings that occurred when psychological theory written from a male point of view was presented as "human psychology"—the early relational model did not adequately represent the range and diversity of women's experiences. The kind of blind spots that occur when one occupies a position of dominance or privilege were unfortunately present in these authors' own efforts to rectify inaccuracies and injustices that we experienced in the face of the dominant white male model of human development. The relational model initially also had a white, middle-class, well-educated, heterosexual bias. We now appreciate that there are many voices with which women speak; there are many experiences of advantage and disadvantage determined by race, class, sexual orientation, and other patterns of uneven distribution of power and privilege.

THE RELATIONAL-CULTURAL MODEL

Gender is socially constructed, largely determined by power and role attribution. The dominant group in any society names the values by which all are judged; there is an assumed position of center and truth. Stratification characterizes difference. Unearned privilege and advantage are made invisible as the group with power attempts to justify its right to power and material, political, and social rewards. Increasingly, the relational-cultural model appreciates the power of social stratification and controlling images to create major disconnections and disempowerment for groups of people as well as for individuals. Originally constructed to shift the paradigm of developmental and clinical psychology vis-à-vis its portrayal of women, this work increasingly seeks to shift the valuing of separation and rugged hyperindividualism that mark American culture.

What has come to be known as the Stone Center relational-cultural model suggests that isolation is the source of much suffering for people: In isolation, we often feel scared, weak, immobilized, and ashamed. Isolation comes from experiences of chronic disconnection. Disconnections occur regularly in all relationships; they involve failures of empathy, hurts, and misunderstandings. When we can represent our experience and feelings following a disconnection, when we are listened to and responded to in an empathic way by the person who hurt us, we, in fact, build stronger connection. If, in a relationship with a more powerful person, we are not able to represent ourselves (i.e., we are not listened to and/or not responded to), we learn to keep these aspects of ourselves out of relationship. We enter into less complete and more inauthentic relationships. Take the following example.

Cynthia, age ten, was being picked on by some children who lived in a different part of town. On this particular day, they had mercilessly harassed her about her "weird" skirt. She came home from school in tears and tried to tell her mother about what had upset her. Her mother was in the middle of preparing dinner and gave Cynthia a short and dismissive answer: "Don't listen to them; have you done your homework?" Hurt again, Cynthia attempted to protest, telling her mother, "You're in a crummy mood." At this point, her mother stood menacingly over her and yelled for her to go to her room "or else." This scene, repeated many times about different issues, leaves Cynthia feeling: "My hurt feelings don't matter and my anger will not be heard." She learns not to show these parts of herself to her mother and to many other people. She learns to dry her tears and hide her anger. She also begins to feel disconnected from herself and others when these feelings arise.

While the content of what caused Cynthia's feelings may not seem "big," the lack of responsiveness to her feelings has a chilling impact on her sense of herself and on her expectations of others' responses to her. She does not feel she can be effective in relationships. Had Cynthia's mother been open to her pain, asked questions, expressed concern that she had been hurt, helped her articulate what she was experiencing, and even perhaps helped her understand where these other kids were coming from and how she might protect herself in the future, she would have felt heard, strengthened in connection, and clearer about the relational forces at play. Had her mother been able to listen nondefensively to her disappointment and anger at her, she would have been giving her daughter the gift of supporting her right to protest injustice; this would have strengthened their connection to one another. Her mother would have demonstrated that she was capable of moving beyond narrow self-protection and authoritarian parenting toward a meeting that respected her daughter's feelings and needs.

Clearly, this acute disconnection can move in the direction of chronic disconnection as a result of her nonresponsiveness. While it does not have the same disempowering and violating impact as physical abuse or sexual violation of a child by a powerful (dominant) parent, it similarly pushes the child into isolation and disconnection.

Power dynamics are very important to scenarios of connection and disconnection. It is when a more powerful person does not respond to us (to our pain especially) that we learn we cannot safely share the full range of our experience; this can be a parent, teacher, boss, more financially successful partner, and so forth. A person who by virtue of an accident of birth (unearned privilege or advantage) is given more power can exercise that power in a way that leads to subordination of the less powerful person. Power differentials always hold the possibility of forcing the less powerful person into a place of inauthenticity, subjugating her or his needs to the needs of the more powerful person. The person who experiences more "need" in the relationship often feels more vulnerable to the other person and often actually is more vulnerable and dependent on the more powerful person (for material well-being).

In the case of Cynthia, she could not "make" her mother pay attention to and honor her feelings; she was forced by virtue of her mother's position of power and authority and her own need of her support to "go along" with her definition of her situation and the relationship. Cynthia's dependence on her mother and her mother's choice to exercise power in a way that denied Cynthia's emotional needs in this case clearly placed the mother in a position of dominance and Cynthia in a position of subordination.

This model not only looks at relationships between two people (parent/child, teacher/student, friend/friend) but also looks at the way power dynamics impact groups and communities. Marginalized or subordinated groups are often put in a position by the more dominant groups of having to attend to the dominant groups' needs and having to exist in a position of enforced vulnerability. Jean Baker Miller notes that it is the "job" of subordinate groups to attend to the needs of the dominant group. Dominant groups often explicitly forbid or discourage protest, authentic expression of difference, or conflict from the subordinate group. These "power over" dynamics naturally interfere with the development of mutuality and limit the growth that can happen in connection. Real growth in connection inevitably involves conflict. Protest and anger are healthy signs of authenticity and safety in a relationship. Anger is not about "venting" or acting aggressively against another; it is about representing hurt and asking directly and strongly for a respectful response, for change.

FEELINGS THAT ARISE IN CONNECTION AND IN ISOLATION

Courage We all grow in connection. We are resilient to the extent that we can turn to others in times of vulnerability and need. We find courage in the presence of others; we are encouraged to become more who we are, to grow, to move in new directions. Courage is not an internal "trait"; we bring forth courage in one another.

I remember once in a meeting being very upset about the way several hospital administrators were discussing a group of patients as troublemakers, whiners, and so forth. I struggled with my desire to speak up in the patients' defense, and I watched my sense of failing courage as I assumed I, too, would be labeled a complainer. But I caught the eye of a colleague sitting near me and I saw her anger and her struggle. In that moment of silent but clear connection and validation, I was encouraged to summon my own voice to protest the way in which these administrators were vilifying these patients. Courage grows in connection; it is not an internal trait played out by lone heroes. Growth-fostering relationships are encouraging relationships; they help us build and sustain the courage to come out of shame, into healthy authenticity and sometimes conflict.

> Courage is not an internal "trait"; we bring forth courage in one another.

Not all relationships are growth fostering. In some relationships we are neglected, injured, inadequately respected, misunderstood. Some relationships are clearly not based on mutual empathy and mutual empowerment. And people must learn to discern what mutual, growth-fostering relationships are; what nonmutual but not necessarily hurtful interactions are; and what frankly hurtful relationships are. The myths of individual achievement, "going it alone," must be questioned. The costs of hyperindividualistic models are enormous for boys and girls, men and women. The myth of meritocracy and the failure to examine unearned advantage also create hurt for many individuals. Disconnections occur at both personal levels and through societal stratification.

Shame Shame is also a significant source of isolation for people. In experiences of shame, we feel unworthy of empathic response or love from others. We feel that our very being is unworthy. In guilt we may feel we have acted in some offensive or hurtful way but we feel we can make reparations. In shame we often feel that there is something intrinsically wrong with us. Shame is a major source of isolation for individuals. The natural reaction to reach out, to heal, to repair is often shut down in shame. Shame is an interpersonal feeling; it is about our worthiness to be in relationship.

Diane was an intelligent, accomplished lawyer. She had, with the help of AA, maintained sobriety for five years, and she was developing a community of friends for the first time in her life. But she struggled with a persisting sense of isolation and shame, which largely focused on her involvement several years earlier with a partner who beat her. She had been unable to tell anyone about this abuse, fearful that respect for her would vanish. She herself felt it was a sign of some intrinsic defect that she had stayed in relationship with this partner for two years. It was not until she was able to talk about this in therapy and saw, with some surprise, that her therapist did not feel scorn for her but was empathic and even appreciative of some of the ways in which she kept herself alive during this traumatic period that she began to believe again in her own worthiness. Diane had been convinced that everyone would be disappointed and disparaging of her "weakness."

While shame arises naturally when we feel we have let people (or ourselves) down, shame is also done to us by others. It can be a very potent sociopolitical force to disempower people by isolating and silencing them. In other words, if a dominant group or individual (that is, someone with power, status, and social recognition) shames a nondominant group or individual (one without power or advantage) by suggesting that that group or person's reality is inferior or unworthy, it often will drive the nondominant group or individual into silence and isolation. As the feminist Karen Lang notes, "Isolation is the glue that holds oppression in place." All nondominant groups in any culture know the powerful and distressing impact of shaming. In shame we feel very vulnerable. Humiliation, related to shame, may be thought of as an experience of enforced and demeaned vulnerability.

> As the feminist Karen Lang notes, "Isolation is the glue that holds oppression in place."

Vulnerability and Friendship The experience of vulnerability is relevant to a discussion of power and gender. Many theories suggest that individuals gain a sense of security and safety by becoming more powerful than other people; this could be called a "power over" model. The relational-cultural model suggests that people grow and gain a sense of safety and well-being by establishing good connections with others and staying connected with their own "feeling-thoughts"(a term Jean Baker Miller uses to describe the complex reality of our feelings and our thoughts). Where competition is celebrated as the means to better functioning and higher productivity (and where productivity is king), vulnerability is not a valued or sought after condition. Where manhood is defined by the ability to resist influence from others and fear of being too open to others, vulnerability will be denied and attributed to the nondominant groups (e.g., women or people of color). Vulnerability, then, is often denied and denigrated and its expression by the "powerful" "in charge" individuals is discouraged.

Counteracting the impact of shame and disrespected vulnerability is the offer of mutual empathy and mutual empowerment, listening a shamed individual back into voice, back into hope. We all need to be encouraged, to move into connection, to feel our own strength and authenticity. The myth of heroic, disconnected individuals taking risks, acting alone in defiance of fear does not provide us with a model of strength or courage that most women can embrace. And yet a model of courage based on connection and turning to others to feel strong is often belittled by a culture that so values individual mastery.

Responding strategically to the shaming that gets done to us is a major part of the story of healing and movement back into a sense of vitality and courage. Often this involves being able to name the dominant values, see them as merely one version of reality. So often dominant groups present their values as The Values and their version of truth as The Truth. Contextual awareness and questioning the dominant myths are essential to resisting and countering what sociologist Patrician Hill Collins refers to as "controlling images." Psychologist Beverly Greene has noted that African American children learn this double consciousness, seeing the racism in the dominant groups and learning to survive in the dominant white, middle-class world without

> People must learn to discern what mutual, growth-fostering relationships are; what nonmutual but not necessarily hurtful interactions are; and what frankly hurtful relationships are.

completely losing touch with their own internal experience and the experience of their loved ones and families.

Girls and boys in general must learn this same thing in regard to gender stereotypes. Gender stereotyping injures both boys and girls, limiting their authenticity and vitality. Bill Pollack, a psychologist who explores gender roles for boys, has called the gender rules for boys "traumatizing." Gender socialization for boys and men is heavily shame laden: You're a sissy, You're a mama's boy. Boys are shamed for exhibiting any characteristics that are seen as "feminine"; girls are shamed for being too strong, too forceful, too angry (too much like boys). We are kept in line with shame.

> Research has suggested that the politicization of personal experience has been a key factor in women's resilience practices throughout the world.

Under conditions of social and economic degradation, friendship can become a strategy for counteracting the forces that victimize, divide, and condemn. Research has suggested that the politicization of personal experience has been a key factor in women's resilience practices throughout the world. The friendship between Mary and Mattie illustrates this point.

On a hot August afternoon, seventy-eight-year-old Mary was seen trudging up to her eighty-three-year-old friend Mattie's house with a lawn mower. Having completed the clearing of her own garden she decided to "help out Mattie," who lived alone in a neighborhood scarred by occasional violence and sustained governmental neglect. Mary and Mattie supported each other in their vulnerability through acts of caring and community. For example, when Mary would return from out-of-town trips visiting distant family, she knew that Mattie would keep a light on in her window waiting for her safe return. Whenever she was safely inside, Mary counted on a brief telephone exchange to learn about anything that had happened in the neighborhood during her absence and to thank Mattie for the dinner the older woman would have prepared and left on her stove. Because neither woman could drive or afford cab fare, they conducted most of their business affairs by traversing the city on public buses to distant neighborhoods where the shops, banks, and offices were located. For many years, whoever needed to "go into town" for business would take care of any business matters she could for the other. If, for example, a friend of Mattie's called to take her grocery shopping, Mattie would immediately call Mary to share the ride. Food became a part of the language of friendship; whenever one woman had some delicious treat—be it fried fish or caramel cake—she would call the other to share in the delight. In fact, it was not uncommon for one of them to spontaneously "gift" the other with some dish that she knew to be her friend's favorite. Interestingly, there was no strict accounting for their caring; neither woman felt a need to establish tit-for-tat reciprocity as the justification for their acts of kindness. Theirs was a model of friendship defined not by the standards of material valuation, but by a commitment to generosity and shared abundance.

> To live with a sense of shared abundance is to enact faith in connection.

To live with a sense of shared abundance is to enact faith in connection. In other words, Mary and Mattie's ability to live beyond the meagerness of their individual lives represented more than the sum total of their combined resources. In some sense, this model of friendship reflects both political resistance and spiritual practice.

The educator William O'Hanlon suggests that people access and nurture their spirituality through connection and contribution. Interestingly, the practice of contribution suggests a model of friendship that is larger than privatized relationship. Although each woman gained companionship and pleasure in being together, their relationship was based on more than personal satisfaction. Their relationship enabled them to partially circumvent the systems that would have physically and emotionally depleted them separately. However, the friendship was more than a matter of personal convenience or resignation to sharing a social burden. As Mary and Mattie practiced their friendship, each woman contributed to the other's well-being and, in doing so, enhanced her own sense of aliveness and purpose.

These acts of everyday resistance are nothing less than revolutionary in a culture that would regard them both as "surplus" people: elderly, black, and poor. Through their relationship, Mattie and Mary are able to express and experience compassion. In giving and receiving, each was validated of her dignity, her meaning, and her fitness for connection.

A psychology of separation, of determined, and lauded self-interest is beginning to face challenges and questions. The challenges to these prevailing models are largely coming from those at "the margin," as bell hooks, author and social activist, refers to those who are not vested in the center of power, those whose reality is underrepresented. Moving from an understanding of human beings as greedy, self-serving individuals to a new understanding that people have a desire to contribute to the growth and well-being of others, to the larger community, challenges the prevailing images of the self-sufficient, independent, lone hero. It is time to appreciate that an interest in the growth of others (so commonly associated with women) is a sign of health rather than a sign of personal inadequacy.

—*Judith V. Jordan, Ph.D., Amy Elizabeth Banks, M.D., and Maureen Walker, Ph.D.*

RELATED ENTRIES

Group Therapy for Women

Insight-Oriented Psychotherapy

Intimate Relationships

Women of Color and Relationships

Women of Color and Relationships

Relationships provide women a sense of continuity, emotional connection, and tangible support; as social beings, women seek and need relationships to sustain them. Women of color are no different. Women of color forge and manage relationships even amid a climate of hostility based on racism, sexism, heterosexism, and classism. These societal realities serve as the context in which the relationships of women of color take place and often gives them meaning and power. (For our purposes, the phrase *women of color* includes African American, Latina, Asian, Indian, Native, and other underrepresented populations of women in the United States.) Relationships are generally of great significance to women of color. Important relationships for them include family, friends, and romantic/sexual partners.

Women of color are required to constantly negotiate discrimination and marginalization on the basis of ethnicity and sex, and for lesbians of color, sexual orientation. Their lives are complicated further by their class standing and the presence or absence of any disabilities. The meaning and significance of their relationships across the relationship spectrum are shaped in the context of these variables.

For most, their culture of origin tends to use collective rather than individual ways of seeing the world and defining themselves—they define themselves in relation to others, rather than as individuals whose self is defined by its separateness from others. For example, the African proverb "I am because We are" stands in contrast to the Western Cartesian notion, "I think, therefore I am." The African proverb emphasizes a fundamental importance of one's connection to others found in tribal societies. It is as if to say that one's survival depends on the group, not the individual's personal ability alone. It also suggests that drawing support and depending on the group for help is not only supported but encouraged.

Individuals from similarly constructed cultures derive great strength and support from their connections to others. When people from these cultures live in the Western world where the ethic of the rugged individualist prevails, they may feel isolated and rootless in ways that violate the natural sense of order for them and can make them more vulnerable to mental health problems. Furthermore, individualism devalues interdependence and can make women feel that they are weak or defective if they need to depend on or look to someone for help.

Ethnicity influences the way people define family. Rules influenced by cultural values and norms dictate who is included and under what circumstances. When compared to their white American counterparts, women of color generally come from cultures in which one's family of origin is of personal as well as cultural significance. Separation or disconnection from family is a significant source of grief for women of color even when it is deemed important to avoid toxic family members. Such disconnections, therefore, are less common for women of color than for their white counterparts and are not likely to occur unless there has been a serious and extreme breach. Even when family members have behaved in a destructive fashion toward another family member, disconnection from them is still difficult.

These close family ties normal for women of color also serve to extend the boundaries of "family" well beyond the nuclear family and, for some groups, well beyond blood relationship. For many women of color, adult women friends who are emotional intimates are considered "sisters" even to other nuclear family members.

> Women of color forge and manage relationships even amid a climate of hostility based on racism, sexism, heterosexism, and classism.

Within the family context, women of color occupy critical roles shaped by the gender role dictates of their cultures and the need to adapt to a racist and sexist society. Men of color have often been denied access to the social opportunities that would allow them to assume the traditional role of the provider and head of the household. Similarly, women of color have often been required to work to help support their families in ways that the traditional gender role stereotype for American middle- and upper-class women did not include or approve, a role that is deemed defective according to the dominant cultural standard. This failure to live up to the dominant cultural stereotyped gender roles often gives rise to friction between heterosexual partners in marriage, the intensity of which depends on the degree that each has internalized these traditional standards.

Sexist constraints do not come solely from the dominant culture; they are often embedded in the gender role requirements of particular ethnic groups. Hence, for women of color, their gender and their ethnic and cultural imperatives influence the roles they play in their relationships as well as the purpose any given relationship has in their lives. African American women are often considered the "glue" that holds the family together. For the most part, it is the women of all families who maintain the ties between family members, between generations of family, and who care for family members who cannot care for themselves. Women of color are no exception. They are also more likely to be directly involved in child care. Even when they are of an age when they might be regarded as less useful, women of color play active roles in raising their grandchildren and are often relied on for essential help by their working daughters and granddaughters. We see here another example of continuity of connections in the roles older women of color play in the lives of the youngest members of families.

> The African proverb "I am because We are" stands in contrast to the Western Cartesian notion, "I think, therefore I am."

These ethnic gender role traditions reflect the tendency for women of color to be less likely to focus on self-care than to focus on the needs of family members. While it is true that women of color are depended on for many things within their families, neglecting themselves comes with a price and is usually an issue that comes up in psychotherapies with women of color.

Within the family, unmarried women are often relied on to assist with family members in need of care or tangible support. If the unmarried woman in a family is a lesbian who has chosen not to divulge her sexual orientation to family members, this complicates these relationships in ways that are not present for their heterosexual counterparts. People of color are no more accepting of lesbian relationships than the dominant culture; however, family members and connections are still very important to their lesbian members as important barriers against and safe havens from racism. When disconnections with family occur as a result of conflict over a woman's sexual orientation, it can intensify the loss for her, particularly when she desires the family to openly acknowledge her lesbian relationship; this may also lead to conflict with her relationship partner.

> Even when they are of an age when they might be regarded as less useful, women of color play active roles in raising their grandchildren and are often relied on for essential help by their working daughters and granddaughters.

Lesbians of color are challenged by the same societal pressures of heterosexism as white lesbians, gay men, and bisexuals. Add the pressures of sexism and layer on the pressures of racism, and lesbian women of color are unlikely to find support for their relationship outside of the lesbian community, and, in fact, they are more likely to find the environment directly hostile. Women of color in lesbian relationships may, ultimately, be more predisposed to a phenomenon called *merger*. Merger occurs when partners in a couple find it impossible to function autonomously from one another, which sets up an unhealthy level of dependence between them. Any romantic relationship that is required to function with little or no support, and in which partners are required to constantly defend their partner or relationship, has the potential for merger, although it would be inaccurate to say that most lesbian relationships suffer from merger or some degree of it. For women of color, for whom a high degree of connection, family, and friendship is needed fundamentally, lack of supportive networks resulting from homophobia can be additionally problematic.

It is, therefore, fair to say that women of color, because they have multiple identities, face a greater level of societal marginalization and discrimination. This can leave them at a heightened level of psychological vulnerability, making the range and quality of their relationships even more important to their survival. Our discussion here just skims the surface of this very complex issue. Consider the following.

Isolation is seen as a condition that increases vulnerability in times of stress and that can lead to depression, loneliness, and psychosomatic illness. Conversely, friendships are viewed as able to increase mental and physical well-being. This human capacity and need for connection give rise to interpersonal bonds between people that assume many different forms and that can last throughout their lifetimes, giving meaning and quality to life. Connection values cooperation, empathy, and mutual support.

> Connections between oneself and others—family or friends—have been seen as crucial to recovery from the traumas of loss, extreme abuse, protracted hardship, and other physical and mental assaults.

Connections between oneself and others—family or friends—have been seen as crucial to the recovery of individuals from the traumas of loss, extreme abuse, protracted hardship, and other physical and mental assaults. The feeling that one is not alone, that others understand and may even have experienced your dilemma is a powerful force in the process of healing and recovery. This force of connection and belonging can be seen as something that helps one person to draw strength and understanding from another and, in doing so, transforms pain and suffering.

Indeed, one underpinning of psychotherapy is connection—the relationship between the therapist and client. The feeling that you have a connection to someone who listens and who shares your joy and pain is the force behind all good and enduring friendships, and it gives all interpersonal relationships power and makes them effective.

—*Beverly Greene, Ph.D., ABPP*

RELATED ENTRIES

Intimate Relationships

Racism and Mental Health

Women and Spirituality

Intimate Relationships

The phrase *intimate relationship* means different things to different people. Social psychologist and author Sharon Brehm has labeled our interactions with friends, lovers, dates, and spouses as intimate relationships, which are characterized by interdependence, meaningfulness, caring, personal knowledge, trust, commitment, influence in many life areas, and continuity. Other theorists have noted the importance of mutuality, closeness, intimacy, warmth, openness, vulnerability, and affection in intimate relationships. Another model for intimate love relationships popularized by psychologist Robert Sternberg is that these relationships comprise varying proportions of passion, intimacy, and commitment.

But even the word *intimate* has different connotations. For many women, the word *intimate* conveys emotional expressiveness, and for many men it suggests sexual involvement. Despite different emphases in defining intimate relationships, most theorists agree that these relationships represent a basic human need to belong and a drive to connect to others.

As social attitudes have become more permissive and as women have become less economically dependent on men, women have seen a greater diversity of fulfilling intimate relationships in a variety of contexts—at work, at home, with partners, children, friends, and family members. While some women seek intimate relationships that will lead to marriage, major changes in intimate relationships can be seen in the high rates of cohabitation with same or opposite sex partners, single-hood, divorce, and marriages at a later age.

THE GENDERED NATURE OF INTIMATE RELATIONSHIPS

Feminist Naomi Weisstein has observed that it is in the dynamics of intimate relationships that stereotypes about women are most pervasive. Gender forms our earliest relationships within our families, our basic identities, and it establishes a template for our future friendships and intimate relationships. Women are expected to show love by conforming to what poet Adrienne Rich calls "compulsory heterosexuality"—that is, having children and loving and marrying men. In the United States, relationships are also expected to adhere to European American heterosexual models.

Popular wisdom seems to decree that women are uniquely wired for relationships although debate continues over whether women's interest, aptitude, and skill in relationships are more due to social development or innate tendencies. A study released in July 2002 by psychologist Turhan Canli and associates involved a very small sample size but purported to show that women's brains are in fact designed to feel and recall emotions more intensely than men, although the role of experience in this process remains unclear.

Research by Laura Cousin Klein and Shelley Taylor has shown that female friendships with other women actually trigger the release of oxytocin, the hormone that buffers the stress response. This "tend-and-befriend" response does not operate for men, but in women it decreases blood pressure, heart rate, and cholesterol—potential physical impairments associated with aging that may help explain why women outlive men.

Although biology determines that women conceive, give birth, and breast-feed, it is socially constructed gender roles that dictate that women should shoulder major responsibilities for caring for others in our society. Many women report feeling burdened by the fact that they are the emotional experts in their intimate relationships.

Women are socialized to develop the skills to enact the expected role of mother, which includes relational sensitivity, empathy, expressiveness, and caring. This mothering role can make women feel empowered because of their strong relational skills.

> Debate continues over whether women's interest, aptitude, and skill in relationships are more due to social development or innate tendencies.

But this role can also create pressure because the associated innate relational skills seem to be antithetical to the traits of independence and assertion that are highly valued and rewarded in work arenas and society in general.

The female style of sharing feelings, intimacy, expressions of affection, and self-disclosure has become the model for intimate relationships. Males are not socialized or expected to demonstrate the same qualities of intimacy as females are in their roles of friend, partner, or father. Instead, males are trained to be aggressive, achievement-oriented, and autonomous in order to prepare for the role of breadwinner. Our society, however, places greater value on the more instrumental skills of men and accords lesser status to the very necessary relational skills of women. For males, the expectations are also complex because while many women want men to be emotionally open and available, they also want men to be strong and impervious to weakness. These conflicting gender expectations can pose significant barriers for men and women in developing their close relationships.

FRIENDSHIP

Professor of psychology Susan Basow has defined *friendship* as an intimate, personal, and caring relationship involving reciprocity, mutuality, trust, loyalty, and openness. Other definitions note that friendships are voluntary as opposed to obligatory, as in kinship, and can entail varying depths of companionship, affection, and intimacy. Some individuals value friendship for the opportunity to give and receive practical and concrete support, whereas other individuals prioritize emotional support and presence as more important in friendships. These definitions are similar to our understanding of more romantic intimate relationships as well. Although many individuals believe that sexual involvement differentiates more romantic relationships from friendships, we examine the overlap and similarity that these two types of relationships can share.

Developmental Issues Two major themes are seen in women's friendships across the life span: First, friendships are important and visible from preschool years through old age and, second, the quality of these friendships is different from that of men's friendships. Women use talking to one another as a tool to develop intimacy, support, affirmation, positive self-esteem, and life satisfaction. Despite frequent assertions that women are too "catty" to have deep and abiding relationships with other women, research by many authors suggests that friendships with other women are among the most rewarding intimate relationships women have across the life span.

Early and Middle Childhood   Friendships have rules that we learn as we interact with others. As we mature, the rules of friendship shift in accord with our cognitive development. We know that from infancy, children respond positively to human faces. By the age of two, children are capable of parallel play in which they play alongside others without directly interacting. At this stage, both girls and boys prefer same-sex playmates.

Playing with others becomes important in the three- to five-year-old range, as young girls use language to play with peers and to learn about others. Girls prefer pairs, whereas boys prefer groups. In middle childhood, friendships become more complex. Loyalty, support, and status hierarchies develop. Children's friendships are marked by similarity in race and gender with girls preferring one or two close friendships of equal status that focus on cooperation and avoidance of conflict, while boys have larger friendship networks that are more status-oriented. Friends at this stage are expected to be able to help one another, share secrets, and begin to handle conflict and disagreement.

One interesting phenomenon for many female friendships is that it is often difficult for them to articulate anger or hurt when a third person enters a friendship. Susan Basow hypothesizes that unexpressed and unresolved feelings of anger about broken friendships leads some girls to be mistrustful of other females. This taboo against displays of anger can also involve negative emotions engendered by competition for male attention. It is also common for older females to limit their friendships with other females if they have the option of a "higher-status" date with a male or if they get busy with other activities.

The tendency to subvert female friends for the attention of males is most salient during the teens and twenties. Placing an emphasis on male attention over female friendships makes men appear more important than women, feeding into homophobia and serving to lessen the intensity of female friendships.

Explanations for the sex segregation of friendship are often related to differences in preferred activities. Boys tend to engage in fighting, chasing, rough-and-tumble activities, and other events that involve gross motor skills. Even when girls participate in athletic and high-energy activities, they prefer to do it with other girls, even when the girls are "tomboys."

Psychologist Eleanor Maccoby notes that prior to adolescence boys tend to play outside and in larger groups than do females, while females prefer smaller groups and fewer but more intimate relationships. Maccoby also found differences in the interaction of boys and girls that may mediate gender separations.

Girls rely more on politeness and persuasion, while boys use direct demands and dominance. It is interesting that many community and school-wide organizations reinforce the separation of genders prior to adolescence by putting girls and boys on separate teams or work groups. Theorists generally concur with the view espoused by Sigmund Freud that this preadolescent separation of the genders teaches how to form relationships without the complexity of cross-gender sexual attraction and may provide practice for romantic relationships in the future.

Adolescence   During the teen years, peers replace family as a central focus for relationships. Increasingly, friends meet intimacy needs and more time is given to these relationships. Cliques characterize adolescent girls' friendships and provide practice in handling issues of support, conflict, and peer pressure. As girls develop a greater cognitive ability to see different perspectives, they are more able to demonstrate empathy toward others and give help and advice.

Young women seek a small and intimate network of friends with whom they share the most confidential aspects of their lives and receive support. The focus of conversations involves developing a stronger sense of identity, coping with physical changes and sexual awakening, and beginning to think about career and schooling options. Peer pressures are strong and can affect decisions about sex, substance use, academic performance, clothing, and other interests and values. This pressure reaches its peak by age fifteen and then typically subsides.

Researchers Elizabeth Douvan and Joseph Adelson have pointed out that adolescent friendships demonstrate a mirroring of experiences and emotions among a small and intimate circle. These relationships are often pursued at schools and in extracurricular events. Evenings may be monopolized by frequent and lengthy telephone conversations with an adolescent's "best friend." Even boys at this stage are found to prefer to share feelings with girls rather than male peers, and both boys and girls report that spending time with girls decreases loneliness.

Males appear to learn early to fear participation in behaviors that are perceived to be "feminine" and to inhibit emotional closeness and intimacy in male relationships to avoid being labeled as homosexual. Similar constraints do not operate as strongly for women. Women can demonstrate emotional closeness and even overt displays of affection among themselves without the automatic censure associated with appearing to be homosexual.

During the college years, male and female friendships show the most similarity. Males and females report similarities in their number of friends, in the amount of time spent with them, and in their evaluations of the intimacy level. In accord with earlier trends, females still tend to spend time with other females "just talking," whereas males spent time with each other in an activity.

Researchers Margery Fox, Margaret Gibbs, and Doris Auerbach studied women's friendships in college and found that these relationships were more emotionally engaging and less hostile than were men's relationships at this age. Contrary to earlier patterns, at this stage, women were not conflict aversive. They preferred honesty in relationships even if it risked the continuity of the friendship.

Adulthood In adulthood, females continue to value the intimacy of their network of friends, while males decline in securing new friends, in wanting close friendships, and in maintaining intimacy in their friendships. The pressures of work, family, and romantic relationships seem to lead to different directions for males and females in their adult friendships. Both males and females who are married appear to devote less time to friendships than their counterparts who are unmarried and without children. During adulthood, women also seem more concerned about maintaining positive relationships with friends and seek to avoid and reduce conflict.

In marriages or committed relationships, women are typically responsible for coordi-

> Young women seek a small and intimate network of friends with whom they share the most confidential aspects of their lives and receive support.

nating friendships with other couples and families. Men receive their primary social support from their wives or partners but may engage in male-only friendships that focus on activities such as sports, card games, or repair work.

Just as serious relationships, marriage, and children may interfere with the amount of time women accord to their friendships, women use their friendships in many cases to receive support, advice, and coping strategies that strengthen their ability to parent and or to work out difficult relationship issues. Although this use of friends serves a therapeutic function, some theorists believe that the support women give to their friends in troubled relationships serves to maintain an unhealthy silence around the inequities of many relationships and may be enabling a woman to remain in a relationship that she should leave.

> Women are described as operating "face to face" by focusing on emotional intimacy, and men demonstrate "side-by-side" styles by spending time in common activities.

Frequently, separation and divorce lead to a decrease in friendships for women since women usually have decreased amounts of free time and additional financial and personal pressures. As women get past the immediate effects of a divorce, women's networks of friends increase.

Gender Differences Research consistently shows some differences in comparing male and female friendship styles: Women are described as operating "face to face" by focusing on emotional intimacy, and men demonstrate "side-by-side" styles by spending time in common activities. Both men and women seem to value self-disclosure, emotional expression, support, physical contact, and trust. However, in same-sex friendships, it appears that women prioritize self-disclosure more than men and men value shared activities in same-sex friendships and sexual contact in cross-sex relationships more than women. Theorists disagree, however, on the significance of these differences with some theorists stressing differences and others emphasizing similarities.

It appears that what may explain the disconnect in male and female friendship styles is that men are capable of the same type of intimate friendships that females demonstrate but they are less willing to engage in these type of relationships. Homophobia and cultural pressures that dictate that men should be stoic and emotionally constrained may support men's decisions to refrain from more open and intimate friendships.

Diversity Issues in Friendship We also know that culture, socioeconomic status, age, race, ethnicity, ability status, and sexual orientation influence friendship styles. During early childhood and through adolescence, interracial friendships are still rare, with most individuals choosing same-race friendships. Research indicates that ethnic minority members are more likely to have cross-race friendships than are majority members.

Ability Status Individuals with disabilities and illnesses face significant barriers with developing friendships. From childhood onward throughout adolescence, individuals with disabilities are marginalized, scorned, teased, and ignored. Individuals who are not disabled seem to be uncomfortable in the presence of people who are disabled, unsure of how they should respond and behave, and therefore have briefer interactions.

Ethnicity and Race Research has also shown that there are greater gender differences in friendships in European Americans than for African Americans. This may be related to the fact that many African American females use close family ties for friendship to a greater degree than white females and because African American men show higher levels of intimacy in their friendships than do white men.

Many African American females consider their close female friends to be part of their extended family, and these women are invited to their homes and to important celebrations and events. This network of friends often provides crucial emotional and material support. This can be particularly significant in work environments in which black women must compete and prove themselves in a predominately European American male culture. Because black women historically are not mentored as much by other males and females, they often bond in friendship to provide support and advice to survive and succeed.

Class There are also social class differences in female friendship patterns. Working-class and poor women are more likely to choose relatives as close friends, as they tend to live physically closer to one another and tend to provide concrete and practical assistance more so than middle-income women. It also appears that middle-class and more affluent women have the luxury of entertaining friends in their larger and more comfortable homes and have more leisure time and finances to participate in a variety of activities.

Age and Family Issues Researchers in the area of friendship have also observed that cross-age friendships have historically been rare, although they may be beginning to increase. Often, women choose friendships based on similarity of age, stage of life, and the fact that they are facing similar issues and challenges. Author Letty Cottin Pogrebin believes, however, that with more blending of families due to divorce; the ties of computer, television, and a common culture; and the higher educational attainment of more citizens, women are being exposed to potential friends across generations, and new friendships have developed.

Women acting as the coordinators of relationships are also apparent in family relationships, especially once children become adults. Mothers play a crucial role in efforts to maintain contact between adult children and nuclear family members. Depending on the success of these efforts, adult children and parents may develop close, emotional, and supportive relationships that are similar to other friendships. Typically, mother–daughter dyads are closer than other relationships. We are also witnessing a significant number of grandmothers who are raising their grandchildren. Despite media depictions that suggest this responsibility occurs mainly in low-income and minority families, grandmothers raising children has increased most dramatically in white households. Divorce, substance abuse, AIDS, economic stress, and other types of mental or physical illness have led to the increase of grandmothers raising grandchildren.

In elderly friendships, there is a need for practical and hands-on help and support as death separates intimate partners, spouses, and friends. Many women are forced to confront tasks that are new to them such as financial issues and the physical upkeep of property.

Financial pressures are often significant for older women, who may lose significant revenue with the death of their husbands or partners. Loneliness is also a significant problem for many older women as two-thirds of women over seventy-five in the United States are widowed and only about a third of these individuals marry again. Ethnic minority women are at even greater risk for earlier widowhood with fewer options for remarriage. Generally, for both sexes, elderly friendships involve more women because men die at earlier ages than do women and most women marry men who are older than they are. When partners are separated by death, men show a more adverse impact, as women are more able to give and receive support.

In some cases, adult children come to the aid of their parents. But aid from family members can be difficult for both the giver and receiver of assistance. Psychologists Nancy Russo and Beverly Greene have noted that the time, energy, and other financial and emotional costs of caring for parents or other family members can cause or worsen the mental and physical health problems of caregivers. Many women experience the stress of being in the "sandwich generation," in which they must confront the pressures of caring for elderly relatives while also nurturing their children and partners.

> In adolescence, many girls look for potential dates that will win their parents' approval, dates who are kind, confident, dependable, and who abstain from alcohol. Females acknowledge that they still feel pressure to not initiate dates or appear too intelligent or assertive.

There is often a great deal of pressure placed on women of color whose cultural norms oppose placing family members in nursing homes. This stress is exacerbated by the fact that daughters and daughters-in-law provide more aid to elderly parents than do sons as well as the fact that work leave, custody decisions, and calling a parent about a sick child is still more associated with mothers than with fathers. In addition, having to turn to relatives for extensive support can undermine the self-esteem of the elderly.

Women's Friendships with Men Discussions of cross-gender friendships have only emerged recently, as men and women have begun to interact more closely in the work arena and women are not exclusively relegated to the affairs of the home. One type of friendship with men that some women engage in involves either participating in or viewing a sports event or participating in some type of recreational activity like card playing together. This type of friendship is more characteristic of males and does not involve significant emotional intimacy.

Suzanna Rose, psychologist and director of the Women's Studies Center at Florida International University, in her research on cross-sex friendship has found that sexual attraction is not a factor for females in friendship with males, but it is the number one factor for men interested in friendships with a woman. This fact helps to explain the long-standing debate on whether heterosexual men and women can be "just friends."

Many researchers believe that men and women project their preferred styles of relating on each other. Females want male friends to act like their female friends and to focus on emotional intimacy and self-disclosure. Researchers believe that men, who are socialized to view females through a sexualized lens, may mistake a female's gesture for friendship as a sexual overture.

Researcher Susan Basow has asserted that the strong gender socialization males and females receive in the United States makes it difficult for both sexes to relate as friends. Basow reports that women find friendships with men to be less rewarding, less intimate, and less supportive than their friendships with women because men focus on their strengths while women self-disclose about their weaknesses.

Researcher Linda Brannon has noted that societal pressure for men and women to adopt different roles and styles of relating has stunted the relationship development of both genders. Women are placed in the roles of experts and coordinators of relationships that focus on emotional intimacy, while men are socialized to have less intense and more activity-oriented friendships. According to researcher Letitia Anne Peplau, the exaggerated gender stereotypes and traditions of society maintain power imbalances in male–female relationships that favor men.

WOMEN AND ROMANTIC RELATIONSHIPS

Until the twentieth century, financial concerns rather than passionate love were viewed as the basis for a solid marriage, and there was a long-standing tradition of arranged marriages. With the change from an agricultural economy at the onset of the Industrial Revolution, work and family duties were separated. For white females, the expectation developed that men would be in charge of the world of work as breadwinners while women would be in charge of the home and family as wives and mothers. These changes were not significant for many women of color, who have historically worked both outside of the home and in the home.

When white women started working outside of the home in the 1920s, they became less dependent on securing men's financial support, and a new model for marriage developed based on companionship. Because this model called for partners to love and choose one another rather than to have family make arrangements, dating became a major tool for partner selection.

Dating Dating has evolved from being a tool for formal courtship to being a means for achieving status, fun, socialization and relationship skills, sex, companionship, and self-knowledge and identity. In adolescence, many girls look for potential dates that will win their parents' approval, dates who are kind, confident, dependable, and who abstain from alcohol. Females acknowledge that they still feel pressure to not initiate dates or appear too intelligent or assertive. This perception is accurate because males see women who initiate dates as "pushy." Boys seek dates based on physical appearance and whether the partner is sexually active. There appears to also be a predominant social script that males and females follow on dates, in which males are expected to initiate and females to react.

Hook-Ups Some theorists believe that due to high involvement with video games, movies, and the computer, a new generation of young people has emerged with limited social skills to prepare them for dating relationships. As a result, many young people participate in group dates rather than in one-on-one interactions. Researchers Elizabeth Paul, Brian McManus, and Allison Hayes have noted that the trend for "hook-ups" has developed perhaps because this new generation possesses limited social skills and an unwillingness to slowly develop dating relationships over time. Hook-ups are sexual encounters that may or may not advance to intercourse that occur on only one occasion between people who are strangers or briefly acquainted. These spontaneous encounters often fall in the category of high-risk sexual behavior.

Gender Roles and Stereotypes Again, popular stereotypes suggest how quickly women fall "head over heels" in love with their partners. The reality is that men fall in love more easily, report greater love, and hold more romantic beliefs about the ability to love at first sight, for love to last forever, and for love to overcome all odds. Women tend to be much more practical and objective about their emotions since they look for mates who will earn a good income.

The literature on intimate romantic relationships well supports Susan Basow's view that gender role mediates such relationships between men and women. Support for this view also comes from the fact that lesbian relationships are generally less gender role stereotypic than are heterosexual relationships. Letia Anne Peplau has noted that although both men and women want intimacy and support from their intimate relationships, society dictates different dating, partnering, and marital relationships for men and women, placing women at a role of lesser power in their relationships.

In 1984, researchers Kay Deaux and Randel Hanna analyzed personal ads for lesbian, gay, and heterosexual partners. They found that heterosexual women were more interested in the financial security, occupational status, and the psychological qualities of a potential partner, while men were more concerned with physical attractiveness and objective characteristics. Lesbian women were most interested in offering information on their own sincerity and interests. Other researchers have consistently found that heterosexual women in general use the gender role stereotype of occupational success and that heterosexual men focus on physical attraction.

These differences between men and women in dating preferences have been linked to evolutionary and social role explanations. In the evolutionary theory, men seek attractive and healthy-looking mates, using these characteristics as indicators of fertility. This will ostensibly lead to greater success in reproduction. There is no evidence, however, linking attractiveness to fertility. From a parental investment model, women are more invested in protecting their children than men are because they have more limited opportunities to reproduce. Because of some of the weaknesses in this evolutionary model, other theorists support an explanation involving social roles for male and female preferences. In the social roles model, women seek partners high in income and education in cultures in which they are disadvantaged in their social roles and opportunities.

Research by Howard, Blumstein, and Schwartz shows that across sexual orientation, people desired partners who were caring, kind, and physically attractive, while individuals across gender in same-sex relationships expressed an interest in individuals who were athletic and emotionally expressive. Despite the gender differences that can be seen across individuals, research has shown that both men and women seek affection, warmth, pleasant personalities, and being liked in return in their intimate relationships. Popular stereotypes that "nice guys finish last" are not true.

Also, contrary to popular stereotypes, people gravitate more to people who are similar to them rather than following the adage that opposites attract. Most individuals look for commonalities in potential partners in the areas of religion, race and ethnicity, socioeconomic status, and adherence to traditional gender roles. Individuals tend to "match" each other in level of attractiveness, personality, interests, and tastes. Even in the area of interracial dating and relationships, beyond the racial differences, these individuals are similar with respect to age, educational status, and attractiveness.

Within different racial ethnic groups, gender differences and sexual orientation mediate interracial relationships. Interracial relationships are more common in lesbians due to difficulty in meeting and connecting with extended networks of other lesbian women.

There are higher rates of interracial dating and committed relationships for African American males than for African American females, although interracial relationships for these women are increasing. More Latina and Asian American women are involved in interracial relationships than are their male counterparts.

Research shows that interracial relationships may be at a higher risk for dissolution. It appears that this may be due to the fact that all couples with areas of dissimilarity (including gays and lesbians) have to work harder in relationships, and couples who are interracial usually do not enjoy the same societal and personal support as do heterosexual same-race couples.

Gender role stereotypes pressure men to be successful breadwinners and women to achieve high standards of physical attractiveness, which many women, especially women with disabilities, can never meet. The male stereotype disadvantages men who face impediments in being successful breadwinners, such as race, ethnicity, culture, education level, or ability. Men are discouraged from showing gentleness, being nurturing, and practicing self-disclosure because these behaviors are considered feminine; they are reinforced for being sexually aggressive and for treating women as sex objects. Meanwhile, females are reinforced for being attractive, submissive, and not too intelligent so as not to threaten the success or self-esteem of men.

> Contrary to popular stereotypes, people gravitate more to people who are similar to them rather than following the adage that opposites attract.

Although these gender stereotypes are based on middle-class white culture, racial and ethnic minorities typically feel pressure to adhere to both societal gender standards as well as to stay within bounds of cultural gender norms. These sometimes-conflicting standards cause significant stress for many individuals and couples.

The different role pressures and strains that society places on men and women have led author Lillian Rubin to describe men and women in intimate relationships as "intimate strangers." Women focus on self-disclosure in intimate relationships, while men focus more on physical proximity and sex.

COMMITTED RELATIONSHIPS AND MARRIAGE

Relationship Types and Power Dynamics Committed relationships include marriage as well as cohabitation among gay, lesbian, and heterosexual partners. Happy and stable relationships fulfill the emotional needs and enrich the lives of both partners. Characteristics of these relationships include high levels of trust, communication, positive feedback, support, flexibility, equity in tasks and decision making, and effective problem-solving skills.

In the case of marriage, research reports newlyweds having high levels of satisfaction. After several years, however, satisfaction decreases, a trend that is usually associated with women resenting the heavier responsibilities for the home and children placed on them. It is often not until children leave home and conflicts over parenting decrease and economic resources increase that an increase in marital satisfaction occurs.

Committed relationships often fall into one of three patterns: companionship, interdependence, and independence. In the companionship model, there are well-defined gender roles with women maintaining responsibility for the love relationship and men assuming a more major responsibility as the breadwinner. In the independent model, both partners endorse a more equal, more androgynous, and less gender stereotypic relationship that emphasizes individual self-development. In the interdependent model, flexible gender roles exist, but there is an overt recognition that the partners are still dependent on one another for emotional and financial support.

Letitia Ann Peplau and her colleagues have developed another model for classifying relationships. This system involves egalitarian, traditional, or modern marriages. Traditional marriages subscribe to stereotyped gender roles with the husband as the dominant partner in terms of power. In egalitarian relationships, partners share power. Egalitarian relationships can be subdivided into those that are syncratic, in which the couple shares decision making in all areas, or autonomic, in which each individual is in charge of separate domains.

> Research also shows that when women earn more money than their husbands, both partners work to portray to others that the husband is dominant and the wife is dependent on him.

In modern relationships, there is less adherence to strict gender roles, but males are still more dominant and powerful than females. In all but egalitarian relationships, the partner who makes the most money also has the most power.

In 1994, Diane Felmee found that men were twice as likely as women to be seen as the most powerful individual in the relationship. In addition, less than half of the college-aged individuals she studied believed that they were in egalitarian relationships. Men held the most power, made lesser emotional investments, and were judged to have the more ideal position in the relationship.

An interesting finding from research conducted by both Diane Felmee and Bernadette Gray-Little is that satisfaction in relationships decreases when women hold the most power. The theory is that since these relationships are more rare and do not comply with cultural norms, the lack of social approval increases relationship distress.

Research also shows that when women earn more money than their husbands, both partners work to portray to others that the husband is dominant and the wife is dependent on him. In a study completed in 2000, researchers found that even in egalitarian relationships, women who had higher incomes than their husbands reported more relationship discord, negativity, and distancing behaviors than did women in traditional relationships. It is also interesting to note that most women still adopt their husband's name after marriage as a marker of the fact that their identity is now fused with his.

In contrast, research has consistently shown the majority of lesbian relationships to be egalitarian. Linda Garnets has observed that rather than adhering to rigid masculine or feminine gender stereotypes, lesbian women tend to be more androgynous, confident, assertive, sensitive, and unconventional than heterosexual women. Perhaps this strong array of strengths undergirds lesbian women's ability to parent their children effectively despite confronting issues of discrimination and homophobia. Because many lesbians must cope with societal hostility, these women often establish strong and supportive communities to safeguard their lives, values, and rights.

Again, contrary to popular stereotypes, women are less traditional than men with respect to marriage and love and are less romantic. Although men actually have more romantic ideas about marriage than do women, they are also taught that women target or trap men for marriage.

The view that marriage is something that men should try to avoid because it is so desired by women is interesting. Jessie Bernard, in her highly publicized research, has found that marriage actually benefits both men and women. But it benefits them in different areas, and the advantages are greater for men. Married men demonstrate higher levels of mental and physical health than unmarried men while married women show lower levels of mental and physical health than unmarried women do. Married men also report greater happiness and life satisfaction than unmarried men, but this does not hold for African American men, who report less life satisfaction than unmarried men.

Although there have been long-held stereotypes presuming that African American marriages accord more power to women, research consistently shows that these relationships are generally egalitarian. African American women have frequently been characterized as less "feminine" than European American females. This negative slant may best be explained by the fact that African American women have been socialized to be less deferential and passive to men because of the challenges in their life circumstances. It is interesting that researchers have found that in African American and Hispanic cultures, both males and females embrace an ethic of collectivism, communalism, and caring that is portrayed as feminine in the European American culture.

COMMUNICATION ACROSS GENDER

While most professionals in gender relations do not believe that men and women truly act as if they are from different planets, the same differences that are evident in male and female friendships appear in communication styles. In communication, women strive for intimacy by talking and self-disclosing, while men try to connect by activities and by sexual contact. Correspondingly, women try to relate with the use of empathy and consensus, while men are more competitive and hierarchical.

Communication styles seem to also affect how men and women assess the success of their marital relationship. Men tend to rate their satisfaction with marriage at higher levels than do women. Because women have been socialized to be attentive to communication and relational issues, they are more perceptive about identifying these issues as sources of dissatisfaction. Deborah Tannen has noted men's need to be instrumental and women's need to be nurturing. As men and women reach middle age, "sex role crossover" often occurs, whereby men and women begin to incorporate more of the opposite sex's communication patterns into their own.

Males and females also differ in how they handle conflict. Most women have been socialized to use indirect ways of expressing conflict in accord with their lesser power relative to men and proscriptions against their direct expression of anger. Hence, women use compromise, deference, and accommodation, whereas men are likely to withdraw or deny the conflict or use power strategies to assert their views. Women's tendency to try to face and talk about conflict and men's preference to pull back and avoid this type of discussion have been called the "demand–withdraw pattern." It has been hypothesized that the disadvantaged status that women face in the wider society may motivate women to try to elevate their status at home with partners, while men are more invested in maintaining their higher power status. Both men and women appear to want to eradicate the conflict, although their preferred methods differ. Many women report simply wanting partners to listen and empathize, while men seem to prefer offering problem-solving advice. If both males and females offer what they want rather than what their partners want, frustration can result. Unfortunately, failure to resolve conflict in productive ways can lead to violence.

WOMEN AND WORK

Intimate relationships at work are complex. Research has shown that when some women first entered predominantly male arenas, they demonstrated the "queen bee" syndrome. These women liked being isolated from other females in their positions of power and were unwilling to reach out with friendship and mentoring toward other women. Although the queen bee syndrome is less evident today, women in executive positions often suffer from an inability to develop and sustain friendships.

For high-level executive women, there are usually few if any other women in comparable positions, which makes status and power issues salient with nonpeers. The demands of their position, in turn, leave limited time to devote to friendships outside of work. An encouraging trend has been seen as many professional women have begun to develop networks and caucuses of female friends both on the job and outside it that provide them with support and encouragement in their careers.

A problem that many women in the workforce must cope with is sexual harassment. It appears that the same issues that affect male–female intimate and friendship relationships also affect work relationships. Men at work often view women through sexual lenses and believe that their greater power in the workplace allows them to participate in both overt and more subtle types of harassment of women. Despite laws, training, and monitoring, many women suffer physical and emotional damage due to harassment and are still vulnerable to retaliation if they attempt to protect themselves or report this behavior.

> ✦
>
> Because most psychological theories advocate independence and autonomy as defining characteristics of healthy adulthood, women have been denigrated for wanting attachment and intimacy with others.

Males and females have different relationships with peers, clients, and supervisors at work, even when they have the same job titles. Women are expected to be more sensitive and concerned about the needs of people and more tolerant of inappropriate and even abusive behavior from clients. Men are often intolerant of female supervisory or peer authority. Men seem to expect to be dominant and for women to be deferential.

LOVE AND INTIMACY

Love is often considered a basic emotion involving trust, intimacy, commitment, passion, devotion, and sexuality. In the past, distinctions were often made between the passionate love associated with intense arousal and companion love involving affection and friendship. Despite societal stereotypes to the contrary, both the new-in-love and long-term lovers report high levels of both types of love throughout the different stages of their relationships.

Because most psychological theories advocate independence and autonomy as defining characteristics of healthy adulthood, women have been denigrated for wanting attachment and intimacy with others. Newer theories espoused by Carol Gilligan, Nancy Chodorow, Jean Baker Miller, and others view women's ability to connect with others as a strength in their developmental quest to be independent, empathic, caring, and responsible. These theories assert that women build on their similarities to their mothers and learn early to value connection, whereas males are often socialized to push away from their mothers to establish autonomy.

Some research shows women to be more focused on practical and friendship-based love, while men prefer more romantic and game-playing scripts. The male gender role seems to encourage more sexual and romantic exploration, while the female gender role seems to be more oriented toward stable and long-term monogamous relationships. Although men seem to endorse sexual permissiveness in love relationships more than women, differences in love styles seem to be small with both men and women valuing passionate and altruistic love.

RELATIONSHIP CONFLICTS

Despite major changes in family and work life, with the majority of women in the United States working outside of the home, few changes have occurred in who does the work in the home. Although two-thirds of families with children under eighteen include working mothers, women continue to do two to three times the amount of domestic and child care work in the home that their husbands or partners do. Only about 20 percent of men in dual-worker relationships share equally in the care of the home and family. Women still assume responsibility for gender-specific and time-specific household tasks, and men still do chores that are more flexible with respect to when they must be completed. Women's tasks tend to be more repetitive, mundane, time-intensive, and involve multitasking. In addition to doing more work, women also typically bear the psychological pressure of coordinating and managing the jobs of other family members and the social responsibilities for staying in contact with friends and extended family.

Only in relationships in which both partners hold egalitarian values is there an equitable sharing of household responsibilities. This appears to be true for gay and lesbian couples for which household responsibilities are shared more equally. The issue of shared responsibility for household tasks is a major source of conflict for many couples and is unlikely to be resolved unless individuals are able to commit to more egalitarian relationships. In couples in which household tasks are equally shared, higher relationship satisfaction is evident in higher levels of intimacy, communication, joint decision making, women's happiness, and men's greater satisfaction in fathering.

Similarly, child care still resides mainly in the domain of women. Men's limited exposure to infant care makes them more comfortable with protecting, providing for, disciplining, and playing with their children rather than the day-to-day feeding, bathing, dressing, and nurturing activities that are associated with mothers.

WHY REMAIN IN, WHY LEAVE A RELATIONSHIP?

In general, women are less satisfied in relationships than are men. This seems related to the facts that women have higher standards and that men get more of their needs met in relationships than do women.

Couples' problems most often involve arguments about money, balancing work and home life, and fidelity. Cohabiting couples are more likely to end a relationship than are married couples, and cohabiting couples have a higher rate of divorce once married than couples who have not lived together.

Individuals are willing to stay in relationships in which they feel a sense of equity—that is, when they are getting as much out of their relationship as they have invested. What is significant is an individual's perception of equity, not other more objective indicators. Once an individual believes that the relationship is inequitable, if change does not occur, a breakup can result. Unfortunately, social exchange theories state that it is the person who needs the relationship least that typically holds the most power, and for many heterosexual relationships, men have greater power. As a result, women often work in relationships to alter their needs and perceptions and to make accommodations and compromises to maintain relationship stability.

Evolutionary theorists have hypothesized that men and women handle jealousy in different ways in relationships. For men who are concerned about paternity issues, sexual infidelity of women is a major issue. For women who are dependent on the financial resources of men, emotional fidelity, concern that the male will leave, rather than sexual fidelity, is the issue.

Again, contrary to social stereotypes, women often are the initiators of breakups. Work by Vickie Helgeson indicates that even when a male partner initiates a breakup, women report more positive emotions than do men. Although both males and females report similar negative feelings of anger, anxiety, and sadness following the end of a relationship, women also report joy and relief. It appears that because women tend to be the caretakers of relationships, they are more attuned to the problems that exist. Women seem to be attentive to both the verbal and nonverbal dynamics that may suggest a potential end to the relationship. As a result, they may already have felt a sense of the inevitable demise of the relationship, whereas a man may be shocked. Both men and women may feel ambivalence, guilt, and blame at the end of a relationship. It is interesting to note that women blame men more than men blame women for failed relationships. Researchers hypothesize that this may be attributed to women feeling that they have worked harder to maintain the relationship and feeling angry at what they perceive to be lower commitment to the relationship from men.

SINGLE-HOOD VERSUS MARRIAGE

Increasing numbers of women are remaining single or marrying at later ages despite societal pressures that assert that a woman has no value unless she is attached to a man. In 1960, about 94 percent of all people married at some point, but by the end of the twentieth century, this figure dropped to 85 percent. These days, women do not marry for the first time until an average age of twenty-five; for men, it is twenty-seven. In society, there are higher ratios of women to men, which may make finding a marriage partner difficult for some women, especially African American women. Marriage rates also tend to decline in periods of economic sluggishness. One-third of all individuals delay marriage until their thirties, and 53 percent of African Americans are unmarried at the age of thirty-four.

For some women, remaining single is a conscious and positive choice. Many women have enjoyed greater educational and financial resources, making them less dependent on and interested in marriage as a source of economic or psychological support. Technological advances and support for adoption and single parenthood have further freed some women from marriage.

For other women, single-hood is based on an inability to find a suitable partner. *Single* does not mean solitary, however; single women often live with male or female partners, parents, siblings, children, or friends. One-half of the American population lives with a partner without marriage at some time in their lives. One-third of all households in 1999 consisted of cohabiting couples, and one-third of all babies born at this time were to unmarried couples. The fact that almost half of all marriages end in divorce has also increased the number of single women. As a result, many single women particularly value, depend upon, and nurture their friendships with other women.

Claire Etaugh's research indicates that societal disapproval is still associated with women remaining single. Single-hood in women contradicts such notions as women need men and that all women should be heterosexual and married to men in order for civilization to continue. As a result of social pressures for women to marry, single women are perceived to be less attractive, less skilled interpersonally, less likable, and less well adjusted than married women. Etaugh reports that single women view themselves as more assertive and autonomous than married women and enjoy higher levels of education, earnings, and career status. Some women have decided that they prefer to remain single and focus on their careers rather than marrying and focusing on a family. For some women, negative experiences in their family of origin have discouraged them from getting married.

THE CONTROVERSIES IN FEMALE INTIMATE RELATIONSHIPS

It is clear that many women establish their strongest and most meaningful intimate relationships with other women, irrespective of sexual orientation. Women have noted that they experience more trauma in the end of a close friendship with another female than they do in their romantic relationships.

The expressive and communal models of relating that women have developed that center on talking as a rich and mutual form of affirmation, communication, and exploration has become the standard for intimate relationships. This pattern has been regarded as more valuable than men's models, which are deemed less relational, more independent and focused on shared activites. But Steve Duck and other researchers assert that males also value talking, although they may do so in the context of an activity.

It is believed that women's high levels of self-disclosure foster interpersonal intimacy and distinguish deeper relationships from more casual friendships. But it is often difficult to draw the line between "friendship" and "romance." Some sexually and romantically intimate partners are each other's best friends, and some friends have sexual chemistry that may or may not be acted on.

Males generally are less likely to separate friendship from sexual involvement and are more likely to view women from a sexual versus a relational perspective. Although some women are also comfortable with combining sexual contact with male friendships, most women make clear demarcations between behaviors that signal interest in sexual involvement versus what they consider harmless flirtation.

We have already noted that for lesbians, friendship can be a precursor and a follow-up to an intimate sexual and romantic relationship. It appears that the perspectives of the participants can only accurately determine the meaning and the level of intimacy in a friendship. Unfortunately, the heterosexual focus of our society often devalues and is suspicious of platonic relationships between males and females as though the only acceptable relationship is a romantic and sexual one. Don O'Meara has noted that in the absence of rules, models, and scripts to guide female–male friendships, each gender either slips into a path of romance or tries unsuccessfully to impose the behaviors used in their same-sex friendships.

Theorists have noted that women often remain in intimate relationships and friendships with men despite their belief that they are doing most of the work and making the more

> ✦
> Many women establish their strongest and most meaningful intimate relationships with other women, irrespective of sexual orientation.

significant sacrifices. Because women are often deemed the relationship experts, they have more work to do than men and are often blamed by others, and by themselves, when relationships don't work. Again we see a power imbalance because men are allowed to not develop their relationship skills. Psychology professor Susan Hendrick has noted that the collusion of men and women to let men off the hook for relational skill is a disservice to both sexes. Again, it appears that the status, power, and financial resources of men lead women to tolerate relationship inequities.

Theorists have also noted that women have many rules and high standards with respect to what constitutes being a good friend. These rules and expectations can impose more stress on females. For example, research on African American women has shown that for some of these women, having such an extensive support system of friends and family, can actually increase rather than decrease stress.

Most of what we know about intimate relationships has been based on white and middle-class samples. It has been a relatively recent phenomenon for researchers to try to understand the experiences of diverse individuals and the barriers to friendships across diverse groups. Researchers of female friendships note that these relationships often restrict friendships across race and class and reinforce societal pressures to uphold gender stereotypes. In this way, female friendship can reinforce white and middle-class values, power, and privilege.

There have also been long-standing concerns that many women buy into cultural stereotypes that trivialize female friendships, that teach females that they should compete for male attention and should withdraw from commitments with females if they receive a more "attractive" offer from a man.

The supportive and therapeutic value of female friendship has also been criticized, as noted earlier, when it encourages the perpetuation of gendered relationship inequities. In examining this criticism, however, many theorists have come to conclude that female friendships are more enriching than divisive. Women receive validation, liberation, empowerment, and a greater sense of their own worth and ability to be self-determining in spite of societal pressures.

Letty Cottin Pogrebin has defined *feminist friendship* as a type of caring that helps women function in the world as it is while making it better. Recent research is alerting us to the fact that women are right about how vital intimate relationships are to their lives. Although controversies and barriers still exist, these intimate relationships shape, define, nurture, preserve, and protect women from stress, and add years to their lives.

People in satisfying relationships report greater happiness than individuals who are not in such relationships. Individuals with unfulfilled needs for closeness and intimacy are at higher risk for alcoholism, depression, eating disorders, and serious mental disorders. When others value their relationships with us, our self-esteem is enhanced. When we are unable over time to connect and feel a sense of belongingness in an intimate relationship, we feel undesirable, unworthy, and suffer from low self-esteem. Despite the costs and challenges of intimacy, we need intimacy. Intimate relationships for women are not luxuries. They function as vital necessities in our lives.

—*Janis V. Sanchez-Hucles, Ph.D.*

Adjusting to Divorce

As a clinical psychologist with a specialty in marital, family, and divorce therapy who therapy who has been in practice for three decades, I have seen an increasing number of couples choosing to divorce. The United States has the highest divorce rate of any country in the world. The rate leveled off in the late nineties, but the chances of a new marriage ending in divorce in the next half of the new millennium are likely to remain between 40 and 50 percent.

Many popular and scholarly books have been written about why contemporary marital relationships are more likely to end than they did fifty to a hundred years ago. Sociologists clearly document the weakening of marriage and the family as cultural institutions. Economists point to the decline in women's economic dependence on men. More women than men initiate divorce today, since they are more able and willing to leave unhappy, inequitable, or abusive marriages.

Divorce can also be seen as a form of women's resistance to the marriages of the past. Other analysts cite factors such as less punitive laws, diminished cultural and religious sanctions, and lowered expectations of childbirth and parenting as reasons for high divorce rates. Almost any cultural observer will also point to the effect of Western individualism. The belief that one should be free to pursue personal happiness above all other values has made divorce more acceptable.

In the past, marriage was undertaken largely for economic necessity and the preservation of lineage. Today's expectations for emotional fulfillment in marriage have no parallel in history. With the high incidence of divorce, more people are realizing that the psychological expectations of marriage are unrealistic. Significantly more couples all over the world are choosing continued cohabitation as an alternative to marriage, though dissolution rates for cohabitation are even higher than legal divorce. It seems to have become much harder to sustain a long-term commitment to a lifetime partner and to provide the family stability and continuity that are helpful to childrearing and child development.

One positive outcome of the high incidence of divorce is that most of us, including therapists, public policymakers, and clergy, have become more compassionate and less judgmental about divorce. We realize that even if you are not divorced, you are very likely to experience intimately the consequences of divorce as a friend, colleague, parent, grandparent, or stepparent. More people are also willing to seek counseling as a relationship dissolves, and many states require some proof of counseling before a divorce is granted. Yet, as any therapist will tell you, couples almost always come into therapy too late, making marital change more difficult and divorce perhaps more inevitable.

A marriage or long-term relationship will not get better on its own. Do not ignore problems; seek help quickly, but be a very good consumer. Not just any psychotherapist will suffice. Marital, couple, and family therapy are perhaps the hardest of all psychotherapies to do well because the therapist must become the ally of all parties. Ask many questions about the therapist's qualifications, experience, and specialized training and seek recommendations and referral to very experienced professionals.

Insurance is another matter. One would think that because marital and couple problems are so prevalent and are frequently accompanied by symptoms of depression and anxiety, that third-party payers would cover this area of mental health. Yet the tragic catch-22 is that insurance providers refuse to pay for marital therapy, terming it "not medically necessary."

Patient and therapist must give evidence of an individual psychopathological diagnosis in order to be seen and to use insurance coverage.

> If you don't complete this critical process of analysis and insight, the chances are increased that you will go on to repeat the pattern, acting out old conflicts and unresolved personal issues and familial deficits in succeeding relationships.

The acute distress, depression, and anxiety that people feel in the throes of a marital breakup are for the most part normal and not pathological. With time and healing, these feelings are replaced by hope, acceptance, and positive change. Because divorce has become a predictable part of many people's lives, I wrote a book for therapists on divorce therapy, outlining how divorce needs to be integrated into the stages of the normative individual and family life cycles. It is important to see divorce as part of a developmental process. Like all important life events and changes, it has the potential to allow for important growth and gain as well as for significant distress and loss.

CHANGE AND MAKING THE DECISION TO DIVORCE

The final decision to divorce is rarely one that is made quickly. Fantasies of leaving, expressed or not, may have been in the mind of one or the other person for months or years. Sometimes a person feels he or she had made a mistake from the day of the wedding but sticks it out, hoping for a change or a miracle, a "personality transplant" that never happens. While partners desire change in the marriage and spouse, they fear changes brought about by separation. The divorce decision also may be delayed because of important economic impediments or concerns for the children. In my own experience, people finally call it quits when they see no hope of change in the relationship, when the same conflicts occur over and over again. It feels like being on a merry-go-round; you always come back to the same place you started.

You will feel more vindicated and, in the long run, less regretful about the divorce decision if you can honestly say to yourself that both of you tried everything you could to make the relationship work, including some individual and couple therapy. Irrespective of the length of the marriage, it is very critical for you to understand why the marriage ended and the "dynamics" of the marriage; that is, what you consciously or unconsciously desired from your spouse to feel complete as a person, and how that interaction played itself out for better or worse. It is important also to understand and acknowledge your own personal hangups and problems that contributed to the marital dissolution.

If you don't complete this critical process of analysis and insight, the chances are increased that you will go on to repeat the pattern, acting out old conflicts and unresolved personal issues and familial deficits in succeeding relationships. The divorce rate for second

The information about the decision to divorce must be adjusted to the age and maturity of the children, but three bases need to be covered:

1. the strong statement that the children are not to blame,

2. stating that you love them and that both of you will continue to be their parents and involved with them for the rest of their lives, and

3. stating that, insofar as possible, their lives will not change (e.g., same house, same school, same friends).

marriages is even higher than it is for first marriages. To some extent it is possible to learn through self-reflection, reading, and talking with trusted friends, family, or your ex-spouse. Often, however, you and these people cannot be objective, and a skillful therapist can be very helpful. Together you unravel the causes of the conflict by doing a "marital autopsy" of sorts to prevent repeated dysfunctional relationships and marriages.

Bringing in lawyers too quickly can exacerbate the adversarial process of legal divorce. Many couples do not want to see themselves as enemies or to escalate the anger inherent in feelings of rejection and failure. They want to move beyond blame, anger, and hurt to a more compassionate, neutral, and rational position, one of the most important goals of divorce therapy. The alleviation of these negative feelings can also help spouses break the news of divorce to family, friends, and children. Telling children about divorce is one of the hardest things parents have to do. Rarely do parents appreciate that even very young children know that there is unspoken distance and/or conflict in the marriage. It is best when both partners together can sit down calmly with their children and relate this news as a mutual decision that does not put blame on one parent or on the child. The information about the decision to divorce must be adjusted to the age and maturity of the children, but three bases need to be covered: (1) the strong statement that the children are not to blame, (2) stating that you love them and that both of you will continue to be their parents and involved with them for the rest of their lives, and (3) stating that, insofar as possible, their lives will not change (e.g., same house, same school, same friends). They are losing the family they know as "the family." You are losing the person you knew as "the wife" or "husband," but they are *not* losing a father or a mother. It may be necessary to have repeated conversations and assurances.

The essence of what we know about divorce and children is that it is often hard on them but that the process is much easier if their parents do not put them in the middle of their divorce. This means that the ex-spouses co-parent peacefully and cooperatively and that they always put the needs of their children first. They *never* speak to their children about the ex-partner with any anger or blame, and the child is *never* used as a go-between for communication, convenience, or revenge. If these guidelines are followed and the parents themselves model successful, peaceful separation, children also are more likely to adjust and recover from a divorce in a family and to grow up happier and psychologically healthy.

THE STAGES AND DEVELOPMENTAL TASKS IN DIVORCE

Self-help books about adjusting to divorce commonly compare the process in terms of the stages that we go through when someone close to us dies; that is, an initial period of denial and confusion, then a more intense stage of anger against the deity, fate, ourselves, or the person the loss of whom we acutely feel. There may be feelings of blame or regret that we could have done this or that and certainly grief over the loss. The period of grief and mourning may be brief or lingering, depending on the circumstances of the death. Helped by the passage of time and the tides of life, hopefully, we reach the final stage of acceptance, reconciliation, and of letting the past go.

There are parallels to these psychological stages in the process of divorce adjustment. Denial, anger, grief, and acceptance, however, are far less likely to come in sequence. One can feel an intense mixture of these feelings almost from the time one begins to think about leaving an important relationship. What also makes the process so different from a death is that the person you are losing is still around to remind you of the loss. This makes wounds harder to heal, especially if you must continue to see your ex-spouse because of children or other obligations. It is also much harder to heal and to move on if you did not want the divorce or did not make the initial decision to divorce. You are likely to feel shocked and rejected, but your partner may have been distancing, grieving, and preparing for some time before announcing the decision to divorce. A spouse's healing and adjustment process is likely to seem shorter and be less traumatic than yours.

In divorce counseling, I explain to people that there are two kinds of significant losses with which they must cope, adjust to, and hopefully transcend. The first is obvious, and it is the person loss, the significant other with whom you imagined a lifetime of commitment and love. Accompanying this personal loss is what is called an "ego injury." By *ego* I mean your sense of who you are. A divorce can damage your self-esteem; your feelings of attractiveness, confidence, and self-worth; and your belief in your good judgment. This is true no matter how much you wanted out of the marriage and even if the reasons for leaving were obviously good, as in cases of physical and psychological abuse. In divorce, it's hard to escape some sense of loss, failure, rejection, and wounding that must be healed to move on effectively. Thus, the first developmental task in divorce is *ego reparation,* the process of striving to repair the wound to your ego.

The second major developmental task in divorce is *role restructuring*. This task stems from another loss you are likely to experience in divorce. You not only lose a *person,* you lose a *role.* You were part of a couple identity, a dyad, a twosome presented to the world, your family, your friends, and your co-workers. Losing or changing that role can involve many adjustments from no longer being a homeowner to being a lone parent, a single head of household, and a question mark in a network of couple friends. You are thrust into a single world again, not necessarily knowing the rules of navigating that world. You may also have to take on new roles that are undefined and vague, like ex-stepmother or ex-in-law. Role loss and role disorientation in divorce are a usual part of the stress and adjustment process. The positive opportunities, however, are also important. They involve great possibilities for change and for learning new things about yourself and the freedom to try on and even enjoy new roles and behaviors.

HEALING, ADJUSTING, AND REBUILDING AFTER DIVORCE

The initial period of adjustment to divorce can be extremely difficult psychologically, especially if the marriage was long lived or the divorce complicated and contested. You may have problems with sleep, appetite, motivation, and/or concentration. You may find it extremely difficult to make countless necessary small and large decisions. Some medication can help the extreme anxiety or depression that is natural in this period. Individual therapy can also be very useful in the process of ego repair, helping you understand that a difficult loss can be transformed into an opportunity for growth. To do this, you need to appreciate both your own and your former partner's contributions to why the relationship ended. You also need a firm understanding of how you may have to change some of your attitudes, values, and/or behaviors to ensure successful relationships. These rational understandings help us let go of the great guilt and prevalent "blame mentality" in divorce, to move from anger and personal rejection to more compassion for oneself and for one's partner. Guilt and blame must be replaced by trust and hope—trust in the belief that one will be all right and eventually in an even better place, and hope that one will make better choices in the future because one has learned and changed.

The process of transcending loss and seeing it transform into new learning, new behaviors, and a happier life is not brief nor is it easy. The key behavioral task after gaining insight into the whys and wherefores of a divorce is to be able to make some personal transformation that will enable you to reach out and to rebond. Some people become experts at developing an impenetrable suit of armor toward intimate relationships so they will never be hurt again. You may decide that you don't want or need marriage again, but almost everyone—except, perhaps, the most extreme loner—needs people and needs to love and be loved. This is the essence of what makes life meaningful.

I advise people that after a divorce it is wise to have an introspective period with no significant relationships, to learn to be alone, particularly if you are trying to become more independent. Being alone, however, does not mean lonely and/or friendless. The more you see and talk with friends, make new friends, and practice what you learned about yourself in the process of divorce, the quicker you will heal. Men, in particular, need to reach out to friends, as they often belatedly realize that the only real friend they felt they needed or had was a "wife."

> I advise people that after a divorce it is wise to have an introspective period with no significant relationships, to learn to be alone, particularly if you are trying to become more independent.

After or during separation and divorce, people may enter a "transition relationship." This is usually a fairly quick and short-lived experience with a person who helps you heal ego wounds by conveying that you are attractive personally and sexually. At least superficially, this new person may look different, even be opposite to your ex-spouse in terms of personality and style. The differences, however, are commonly surface ones. You are not likely ready yet for a lasting commitment, and eventually the relationship ends. Yet transition relationships help, sometimes a good deal, in healing and in paving the way for future healthy relationships by helping you reaffirm that you are worthy and lovable. However, if a transition relationship becomes a second hasty marriage, it may be destined to end. (Affairs are most often transitional relationships, although sometimes the other person does represent a better match and a healthier partner.) A high level of personal transformation is achieved if, in this period, you learn and truly believe that you are a good and worthwhile person irrespective of whether you are in a relationship.

The desired period of self-reflection and personal growth may not be possible in the initial period after a divorce. A myriad of practical adjustments may take precedence, like a residential move, an economic downturn, a job change, and/or children's pressing needs.

The complications of separating lives, finances, and families sap available energy for a while. Supportive friends, families, therapy, and divorce adjustment groups can also aid you in accomplishing these practical tasks. Such groups perform an immensurable service in helping you understand that your problems are not unique, that countless others have transcended this difficult passage of divorce, and that there is abundant hope for better times.

Being open to change is key. Hanging on to the past and to what was or what might have been will not help you, but will intensify your grieving and delay your adjustment. Realizing and accepting that you cannot control your ex-spouse are also necessary in order to move beyond obsessive efforts to force him or her to do what you want. A lesson of divorce is that people will make decisions you ultimately cannot control, but that intimately affect your life. You can control, however, how you react to these decisions and changes. The enemy is anger, not the ex-spouse. Anger will cloud your judgment and escalate the conflict. You are working to forgive. Forgiveness is the healing process that enables you to have compassion for your mistakes and those of your ex-spouse and to love yourself again and to wish your ex-spouse goodwill and better times. That may include a new partner, the acceptance of which is often the hardest part of letting go and truly completing the process of forgiveness. When you have found and built a healthier and happier relationship yourself, it is easier to wish that same happiness for your ex-spouse.

Successfully transcending a divorce means being able to love again and to give wholeheartedly again, to rebuild trust in others. Trust is so critical in relationships, and divorce often shatters trust. Trust is most easily regained when you don't permit yourself to wallow in pity, blame, and regret, but instead work toward feelings of compassion, understanding, and forgiveness. You don't withdraw in fear and shame; instead, you reach out for friendship and understanding. You don't resist change, but work toward accepting change and positively using the opportunities it offers. If these psychological tasks are accomplished postdivorce, many individuals report that they feel freer, more confident, and more independent than ever before in their lives. They are less fearful about taking care of themselves and more willing to try new things and take on new jobs, explore new interests, meet new people, and generally expand their vision and lives.

Men are likely to remarry sooner than women, and women with young children sooner than women without young children. Another marriage may or may not be the next life passage or mark the next significant relationship. Some people find they are happiest living alone; some may choose cohabitation without marriage. A majority still finds that marriage offers special and unique opportunities for intimacy, satisfaction, and family life. A second marriage in a blended family presents a host of special opportunities and difficulties that are a topic in and of themselves. Yet part of divorce recovery and transcendence is wisely educating yourself about how such a subsequent marriage and family will be a significantly different experience. Again, embracing change is key, for a second marriage is not a first—nor perhaps a last.

—Joy K. Rice, Ph.D.

*That Most
Unfeminine Emotion*

Anger is a complicated emotion for women. Cultural rules and norms dictate when and how both men and women can express anger and who is allowed to display their angry feelings openly and directly. Women's anger is typically seen as unnatural, dangerous, and aggressive, in part because women are socialized to be mothers and caretakers, and in part because women have less physical and social power in most cultures. Their anger can be taken as a sign of insubordination or transgression of what's considered to be normal.

Anger is different from aggression. Anger is an emotion that is accompanied by an accelerated heart rate, elevated blood pressure, and a release of adrenaline. This physiological arousal prepares a person to take action. One can choose to act aggressively in a destructive and hurtful way or constructively, fostering self-definition, increased communication, and even social change. Anger is a very common emotion, a natural response to a perceived wrong or to an assault on one's sense of self-worth or personal pride. Anger suppressed over a long period of time can lead to physical illness, depression, or self-harming behaviors, such as eating disorders or self-mutilation.

DEVELOPING ANGER

Across race and class lines, girls experience and express anger as a necessary part of relationships. The capacity for young girls to be openly angry—to be "really mad," to cry "unfair!"—reveals a simple, straightforward desire to speak and to be listened to. Young girls assert their strong feelings when something is wrong in their relational worlds. This is the hallmark of a healthy, embodied anger, an emotion distinct from the more destructive, controlling forms of aggression that, as psychiatrist Jean Baker Miller explains, "may or may not follow from anger."

As we might expect of young children, girls follow their impulse to respond to things that hurt them, and this impulse is usually tied to self-righteous demands that their hurt be taken seriously, that unfairness toward them be addressed. As a result, their anger toward others often quickly dissipates. Relationships have a free-flowing quality—girls move together and apart, between harmony and conflict, almost daily. In this way, young girls appear to have a healthy resistance to those experiences and messages that would pull them away from their lived experiences, their feelings and thoughts, and thus they have a basic protection from psychological trouble.

Psychologists Lyn Mikel Brown and Carol Gilligan observe how girls gradually learn that anger is an emotion heavily laden with judgment, especially for girls and women, and that open and assertive expressions of anger by the female sex are inappropriate and unacceptable. Over time, then, what was once a sign of girls' strength and resiliency—their capacity to feel their anger, to know its source, and to respond directly—becomes a liability, at least in those places where white, middle-class values and definitions of femininity as nice, kind, caring, loving, and smiling prevail. Along with these messages of what to say, how to speak, and what to feel and think, if they want to be the right kind of girl or young woman, if they want to be listened to, accepted, rewarded, included, girls receive voice training from those adults who, themselves, have uncritically bought into this fiction: good girls, nice girls are calm and quiet, they speak softly, they do not complain or demand to be heard, they do not shout, they do not directly express anger.

> Girls gradually learn that anger is an emotion heavily laden with judgment and that open and assertive expressions of anger by the female sex are inappropriate and unacceptable.

Although there is cultural pressure for all girls to bury, disown, or redirect their anger, girls' understandings and expressions of anger and aggression are greatly affected by class, race, and ethnicity—that is, by the definitions of appropriate femininity communicated to them through their communities, families, and friends. Such contexts define the contours of anger, the degree and form of its expression. Brown and Gilligan observe that while the expression of direct anger may be strongly discouraged in girls from white, middle-class families, for example, anger is more likely to be valued in girls from low-income, white communities, or from some communities of color in part because it prompts children to act quickly and forcefully to protect themselves. Parents in such communities may, in fact, encourage their children to express their strong feelings when they are hurt or treated badly, and they may value anger as a call to constructive action. These girls may find themselves in trouble when they bring their anger to school, however, where they are judged against white, middle-class norms of femininity. This can be a real struggle for some girls and it may feel like a loyalty test. Do they follow the ways of communicating that are encouraged in their home communities or the values and means of expression encouraged in school? Not surprisingly, the unfairness of such a choice can increase a girl's frustration and anger. Some girls in this situation choose to live a kind of double life; others experience sadness and loss from distancing themselves from their home communities, choosing to "act white" because it is the perceived avenue to school success.

THE SOCIAL CONTEXTS OF ANGER

People most often become angry in interpersonal situations. Theorist John Bowlby, who investigated attachment behaviors in humans and other animals, describes anger as a response to disconnection or obstacles in a relationship. Positive anger expression, an "anger of hope," as Bowlby calls it, requires a belief that one can communicate and be heard and that anger and conflict can have positive benefits to relationships. In contrast, an "anger of despair" often arises from a feeling of being powerless to restore a relationship, or when hostility over separation has replaced the bonds of attachment. Women's anger of despair most often finds expression through hostile aggression toward others or toward oneself.

Women describe their anger primarily in relational terms, placing their anger squarely in stories about relationships and focusing on the interpersonal effects of their anger. And women tend to react to interpersonal events with more anger than do men, perhaps because they tend to be more sensitive to the quality of their close relationships, have a greater desire to achieve intimacy in them, and derive self-esteem from them. People who feel secure in their relationships are able to use their anger to remove barriers to relationship and express their anger in ways that create positive dialogue. However, the ability to express anger positively is related to more than feeling secure. It's also related to a person's equality with respect to power and place in the social hierarchy.

Within cultures, social rules indicate who gets to be overtly angry, in what situations, and with whom. These rules allow those with more social power and dominance to express anger more directly and openly than those who are less powerful. Women's struggle with expressing anger arises, in large part, as psychiatrist Jean Baker Miller argues, because "the problem is a situation of subordination that continually produces anger, along with the culture's intolerance of women's direct expression of anger in any form." In fact, for many women, anger falls into the category of what philosopher Allison Jagger terms "outlaw emotions."

At odds with expectations of caretaking, when women express strong feelings such as anger it can feel unacceptable and often dangerous. As philosopher Elizabeth Spelman argues, while women and other members of subordinate groups "are expected to be emotional, indeed to have their emotions run their lives, their anger will not be tolerated." Such anger is likely to be called irrational, "redescribed as hysteria or rage." This is so, she argues, because the expression of anger is intimately tied to self-respect, to the capacity to fully realize and control one's life. For this reason, women's anger is often considered not only inappropriate but threatening, an act of insubordination: to express her anger means that she takes herself seriously, that she believes she has the capacity, as well as the right, to be a judge of those who treat her unfairly, who might exclude, silence, misname, stereotype, or betray her.

ANGER AND ITS RELATIONSHIP TO WOMEN'S PHYSICAL AND MENTAL HEALTH

Studies of anger in daily life find that when recognized and acknowledged by others as appropriate, anger does not present problems and more often leads to positive rather than destructive changes in relationship. On the other hand, when anger is suppressed or held back over a long period of time, it can have serious psychological and physical health effects. Anger suppression has been linked to depression, eating disorders, irritable bowel syndrome, hypertension, cardiovascular disease, and suicide. How one's expression of anger is associated with specific health outcomes for women is not clear since, as author Sandra Thomas observed, behaviors women often use to deal with anger, such as crying, physical activity, reflection, prayer, writing, or planning for a problem-solving discussion with the offender, are often overlooked by researchers. Research does suggest a relationship between racial discrimination and higher blood pressure in African American women due to arousal and subsequent suppression of anger. Racial and gender contexts affect whether or not people choose to reveal their anger, as well as the psychological and physical consequences of that choice.

The emotion of anger has been linked to women's eating disorders in a number of ways. On the most basic level, food is used to alter moods (overeating, not eating, or bingeing and purging), which may become an addictive behavior. An estimated 30 to 85 percent of women who are bulimic have been physically or sexually abused and experience problems with depression, anxiety, interpersonal relationships, and anger. Numerous studies report that overweight women use food to deal with depression, anxiousness, or anger. The bingeing and purging of bulimia often relate to crises and upsets involving anger. Suppressing anger, or self-silencing, has also been tied to eating disorders.

The relationship between women's anger and depression is complex. The popular belief is that anger turned inward can lead to depression. Yet, depressed people are often outwardly angry. In fact, increased irritability is one of the symptoms of depression. Also, depression may result from the ineffective use of anger, as when anger does not accomplish its intent of changing an ongoing situation, or fails to remove obstacles to relationship or barriers to achieving one's goals. After anger has been ineffective, it is easy to feel more hopeless about having any control over one's life.

Psychologist Dana C. Jack notes that social realities including poverty, violence against women, and women's general social inequality, as well as their inequality in intimate relationships with men, affect both women's anger expression and women's vulnerability to depression. Women's fears about the negative consequences of expressing anger, which many equate with aggression, appear to be related to the inhibited behaviors and styles of thinking that have been associated with female depression. Research suggests that when anger cannot be expressed, it often finds an outlet in depression-related actions such as negative self-talk and self-deprecation. Whether a woman's anger is related to her depression in any given instance depends on a number of factors: the social situation that caused her anger and depression, the woman's understanding of the situation, the social supports she has available, and her perception of the choices she has in response to the situation.

Dana C. Jack has found that self-silencing, or keeping anger and other vital feelings out of the relationship, appears particularly linked to depression, because anger demands positive, interpersonal expression; its function is to regulate relationships, restore connection, and have an interpersonal effect. Silencing anger doesn't change what aroused anger in the first place. And self-silencing can make a woman feel separated from others and from herself and can present a "false self" to others. Her anger over this disconnection can contribute to depression, as can hopelessness about changing the conditions that instigate anger.

On the other hand, uncontrolled, explosive anger expression does not protect women against depression. The critical issue regarding anger appears to be how a person brings it into a relationship; whether doing so facilitates dialogue and connection, and whether the situation that relates to the anger is open to change.

As well as suppressing anger, women often turn their anger against themselves. If a woman perceives some aspect of her *self* as the barrier to what she desires—positive relationships, inclusion, success—then she may direct her hostile anger against herself for not being pretty enough, smart enough, or lovable enough. Culture plays a vital role in women's tendency to self-blame and self-attack, providing images of how they "should" be and look, and holding them responsible when relationships fail. In self-attacks, social factors contributing to women's feelings of powerlessness become converted into hated personal deficits as a woman perceives herself as creating the problem. Studies show that directing angry hostility inward creates depressed feelings.

ANGER AS A POLITICAL EMOTION

Women's anger is deeply affected by a context of inequality relative both to men and to a culture that values certain groups of people over others. When heterosexual couples engage in violent, physical arguments, women tend to fear men's anger and aggression; men do not fear women's. While men are more likely to display anger and contempt in conflict situations within heterosexual relationships, women are more likely to express sadness and fear. This fear is a major gender difference, but power is often at the heart of the matter. In lesbian couples that engage in battering (which occurs at a rate similar to that of heterosexual couples), fear of the partner's anger is also associated with fear of the partner's physical attack. However, one study revealed that jealousy and power imbalances, including economic inequality, predicted abuse more than anger did.

"My response to racism is anger," poet Audre Lorde once wrote. "I have lived with that anger, ignoring it, feeding upon it, learning to use it before it laid my visions to waste, for most of my life. Once I did it in silence, afraid of the weight. My fear of anger taught me nothing. Your fear of that anger will teach you nothing, also." Anger is a vitally important emotion because it recognizes a violation and motivates a person to make personal and political change, to oppose oppressive circumstances and discrimination.

Anger, *because* it is tied to self-respect, because it signals a sense of entitlement and clear thinking about bad treatment, must be available for girls and women to use positively. The pressure for girls and women to split off their anger is enormous and the rewards are clear. Those who do so, however, risk losing the capacity to locate and clarify the source of their pain and thus to do something about it; they risk losing the capacity for a once ordinary, healthy resistance to turn political. Without anger there is no embodied impetus to act against wrong treatment or violation or injustice done to them. There becomes, as feminist scholar Naomi Scheman argues, "an inability to interpret ... [to put] feelings and behavior in the proper political perspective." If we take away girls' and women's anger, then, we take away the foundation for their political resistance.

> "My response to racism is anger," poet Audre Lorde once wrote. "I have lived with that anger, ignoring it, feeding upon it, learning to use it before it laid my visions to waste, for most of my life. Once I did it in silence, afraid of the weight. My fear of anger taught me nothing. Your fear of that anger will teach you nothing, also."

Responding to racism, sexism, classism, heterosexism, able-bodyism, ageism—any form of relational or systematic unfairness or oppression—means responding to anger. This is why philosophers refer to anger as "the essential political emotion." Anger, according to psychologist Carol Gilligan is "the bellwether of oppression, injustice, bad treatment, the clue that something is wrong in the relational surround." Indeed, "reasoned anger" (the ability to engage conflict effectively and constructively) is critical not only to the healthy psychological development of individual women, but to women's capacity to recognize injustice and organize for change.

THERAPEUTIC INTERVENTIONS FOR WOMEN'S ANGER EXPRESSION

Therapists working with women's anger use a number of approaches. Feminist therapy works toward facilitating empowerment, on both a personal and social level. Empowerment means validating women's experiences, fostering awareness of power imbalances within personal relationships that reflect imbalances in the wider society, and facilitating the woman's ability to control her own life, define her own goals, and make the changes that she desires for her own well-being and circumstances. Women who have been victims of destructive anger and aggression can fear the consequences of anger expression, making them fearful of exploring their own anger.

Women rarely name anger as the problem for which they are seeking therapy. More often, anger comes up as it relates to the issue for which a woman seeks help, such as depression, eating disorders, anxiety, or physical illness. Women have often tried anger-control strategies or have been ordered (by a court or other official body, particularly school-aged children or mothers) to attend anger-management sessions. A number of different feminist approaches to anger-related conflicts exist that can help women identify the sources of their anger and find constructive ways to respond.

Jean Baker Miller and her colleagues at the Stone Center for Developmental Services and Studies associated with Wellesley College take a relational and psychodynamic approach to women's anger. Not only does anger remind a woman of her separateness, it brings to the fore a seemingly unresolvable conflict between autonomy and intimacy, which needs to be addressed in therapy. Miller and Janet Surrey suggest helping women rethink the common assumption that anger is a destructive and negative emotion. Those in power have an investment in women's perception of their anger as something negative to be feared; such a belief can be used to maintain positions of power and subordination. Within relationships, the signal of anger serves a communicative function and is a necessary part of dynamic relationships. Therapy can be aimed at deconstructing a woman's fear that expressing her anger will cause conflict that may threaten her connections. It can also focus on helping a woman find positive, direct ways to communicate her anger.

Miller suggests reframing anger as a signal, an emotional response to having been wronged, and as a powerful motivation to bring about change. If, for example, anger is tied to trauma, such as rape or battering, the client can not only work through the trauma, but can also connect her anger with appropriate trauma-related groups working to create social change.

Cognitive behavioral approaches to anger management consider that anger is triggered by irrational thoughts in response to situations, especially thoughts related to unconscious demands and expectations. People are able to control and change their thoughts, which allows greater freedom of response to anger-provoking situations. Cognitive behavioral techniques can be used to help women with a range of difficulties, from uncontrolled, destructive anger to habitual suppression of anger. Goals are set by the client and revolve around identifying sources of anger (both external situations and irrational thoughts) and developing cognitive behavioral coping techniques to deal with anger. Com-

> "Reasoned anger" (the ability to engage conflict effectively and constructively) is critical not only to the healthy psychological development of individual women, but to women's capacity to recognize injustice and organize for change.

monly used techniques include thought stopping, self-talk to prevent the escalation or suppression of anger, time-outs or other self-calming techniques, changing negative self-talk to positive self-talk, and disputing irrational beliefs about anger expression. Since physiological arousal is part of anger (both suppressed and expressed), techniques may also include relaxation methods such as muscle tensing and relaxing, deep breathing, and self-guided imagery.

Many cognitive behavioral therapies also focus on values clarification, in which the client identifies the source of her anger and assesses what actions she can take to resolve the situation, including addressing or leaving it. Role-playing scenarios help practice assertive, constructive expressions of anger rather than aggressive or passive responses. In situations in which expressing anger will make the problem worse, such as in certain work situations, a woman can actively choose alternative outlets such as exercise or creative pursuits to dispel the energy generated by anger. Joining groups working for social change on the issue that is causing the anger is also an alternative.

Rather than "anger management," psychologists Deborah Cox, Sally Stabb, and Karin Bruckner advocate a method of therapy that involves two dimensions. First, the revelation of anger to self—the release of anger in a safe and empowering manner so that anger becomes a less threatening emotion. And second, the revelation to others—the appropriate and respectful expression, or clarification, of anger to others. These revelations of anger require safety from a risk of loss of control or shaming by others. Becoming acquainted with one's anger in these ways allows for its integration and for its creative, positive expression.

Anger awareness can be linked to body awareness, and women can learn to integrate feelings of anger with positive actions. Possible avenues include martial arts and self-defense training, as well as practices that teach one to recognize bodily sensations and physicality, such as yoga and tai chi. The body gives signals about health, safety, and emotions as well as being a source of force; many women have become so split from their bodies and emotions that they do not recognize their anger. Knowledge of one's power includes knowledge of one's potential for both creativity and destruction.

Women face many obstacles to using their anger in positive ways, yet positive anger expression is necessary to define one's self and goals and to oppose conditions that are oppressive. The changing norms of today's society regarding women's behavior allow more freedom for women to utilize this powerful emotion in positive ways for personal and societal change.

—Lyn Mikel Brown, Ed.D., and Dana Crowley Jack, Ed.D.

RELATED ENTRIES

Depressive Disorders

Eating Disorders and Disconnections

Insight-Oriented Therapy

Cognitive Behavioral Therapy

Intimate Relationships

Women and Trauma

A much-wanted pregnancy ends too early in miscarriage. The occupants of a house return home to find their sanctuary broken into and ransacked. A woman is sexually assaulted. A beloved relative is discovered to have molested children in the family. A plane smashes into an occupied building. A flood devastates a community, sweeping away homes and shops.

What do all of these disparate events have in common? Each is potentially traumatic for the person who experiences it, witnesses it, or feels emotionally connected to it in some way. Traumas are hugely variable. They run the range from public disasters of overwhelming size, like the terror attacks of September 11, 2001, to personal, private events like a miscarriage. Each of these events may, in turn, differ in how they affect people. But traumas occur in the lives of almost everyone. Their impact on us, our lives, our relationships, and our networks of support and community can be destructive or transformative.

Women's lives are diverse, complex, and varied, and generalizations about all women's experiences are to be avoided. The scientific study of trauma now acknowledges that trauma is highly subjective—that one person's traumatic event may be the next person's exciting experience, and that even in the face of shared experience mutually defined as trauma, each person will have a unique reaction.

One of the main struggles in the field of trauma studies over the past several decades has been to move beyond a common, fixed, supposedly objective definition of what constitutes a trauma to the embrace of a more diverse, subjective criterion. The specifics of women's lives—their cultural backgrounds, economic resources, physical and emotional health, spiritual practice—can create both special resilience and special vulnerabilities in the face of a traumatic event.

But there are some aspects of living in a female body with female biology, and with the responses of the people and culture around us to our inhabiting that body, that may affect what trauma means to women, and how women experience it. Women who are exposed to trauma develop problems afterward at rates higher than men. Some traumas that are specific to women's lives, such as sexual assault, have been found to have worse and longer-lasting impacts than other, gender-neutral traumas, such as physical assault by a stranger.

In fact, in some studies of the general population, more than 60 percent of women reported post-traumatic problems occurring at some point in their lives. Several aspects of the things that women share due to biology and culture help shape our responses to trauma—and some differences may arise because of our personal and cultural histories; we touch on some pathways to dealing with those unique personal reactions in this chapter.

MYTHS ABOUT TRAUMA

Many factors can either ease or complicate a woman's recovery from trauma. A complicating factor is that Western society, and particularly mainstream U.S. culture, has a number of harmful myths about trauma and the people who experience it. Many of us have internalized these myths unconsciously, then torment ourselves with them when we or someone we're close to is traumatized. Exploring the myths can explode them.

Myth 1. People will have fewer symptoms from a trauma if they just "put it out of their mind."

The first myth reflects what Judith Lewis Herman has called our culture's history of "episodic amnesia" about trauma. This myth expresses the wish that trauma will not happen by silencing those who have experienced it.

Ruth, a nurse who served in Vietnam, came home to a family and society that preached this myth. For more than a decade, she used increasing amounts of alcohol to keep the trauma out of her mind. When she got sober, her experiences in the war zone came back to her with shattering impact. Not thinking about a trauma can worsen symptoms.

Myth 2. People who seem calm and functional at the time of a trauma are "handling it" well. Strong emotions in response to a trauma are "hysterics" or "overreaction."

Our scientific data say otherwise. This second myth parallels the first, and also reflects mainstream cultural norms that reward nonemotionality. People who are traumatized often experience something called peritraumatic dissociation (PD). Persons who experience PD appear calm and functional, but are in fact numb, shutdown, and acting on automatic pilot. When people have PD at the time of a trauma, they are more likely to experience serious post-traumatic problems in the following months and years.

Trauma is terrifying. Strong emotion at the time of a trauma, and at those times when we recall it, is a reasonable response to the unreasonableness of horror, betrayal, or helplessness, not a sign of weakness or "losing it."

Anna was coming home from work when a man followed her up her apartment stairs, pushed her in the door, and raped her. Afterward, she told no one and tried to get on with her life, telling herself that she was a strong woman who could handle difficulties. She felt numb, but she functioned. Six months later she read a story about a similar rape and her terror returned in full force. She spent the next three years dealing with flashbacks, nightmares, and the overpowering sense of unsafety that she had been numb to.

Myth 3. People enjoy playing the role of victim when they are angry, scared, or unforgiving. A "good" trauma survivor is like Nelson Mandela, Elie Wiesel, or Oprah Winfrey—transcendent, articulate, and highly functional.

This myth is particularly cruel. Often, when people have experienced a trauma, it has an impact on their identity and how they understand who they are in the world. The rest of life experience may, for a time, be filtered through the mud-colored lenses that trauma has splashed over their eyes.

What is true is that sometimes trauma happens in the lives of extraordinary human beings, just as it does in the lives of ordinary people. Extraordinary humans may have extraordinary responses to trauma, too. Most people do not have transcendent experiences as their first, second, or tenth response to trauma. It is only well down the path of trauma recovery that most people can transform terror and helplessness into spiritual growth or social action.

Charlene's child died from leukemia. Six months later, she learned that her home had been built on a toxic landfill full of chemicals that were known to cause cancer. She spent the next several years in a state of grief and outrage. Finally, after she had had a chance to move through her feelings, she started what became a full-time career as an environmental policy activist "so that no more children would die like mine did."

The truth about trauma is that traumas scare and can hurt us. They are not experiences that we voluntarily seek out, even though they often happen to us in the midst of everyday life. They wrench away control over bodies, feelings, safety, and lives. Being scared, angry, unforgiving, and focused on the trauma are all normal reactions, particularly in the immediate weeks and months after the trauma occurs. When trauma survivors begin to see their responses as signs of simply being human, they are often taking an important step in recovering from the harmful effects of trauma.

WHAT IS A TRAUMA?

In the *Diagnostic and Statistical Manual of Mental Disorders,* 4th Edition (*DSM-IV*), a trauma is defined as "Experiencing or witnessing or being confronted with an event or events that involved actual or threatened death or serious injury or a threat to the physical integrity of self or others, and to which the person's response was one of intense fear, helplessness, or horror."

This definition fits with many of the large-scale traumatic events that are easy for people to recognize as traumas—earthquakes, combat, disasters. It also fits into many women's experiences of being sexually or physically assaulted.

Yet, many women who subjectively know themselves to have experienced a trauma don't fit into this definition. So let's look at some other descriptions of what constitutes a trauma, which will assist us in expanding our understanding of how certain events can lead to the emotional and physical responses that fall under the general term of *trauma response.*

✦

One person's traumatic event may be the next person's exciting experience.

The first additional concept of trauma comes from the work of a social psychologist named Ronnie Janoff-Bulman. She has studied how people think about themselves and the world after traumatic events. Her model for what makes something traumatic says that a trauma is an event or experience that *violates a person's expectations of a just or safe world.* So, for example, having a much-admired professor and mentor begin to pressure you for sex would fall within this concept of trauma. Sexual harassment at school and in the workplace, which happens to more than half of all women, usually doesn't meet the *DSM* definition of trauma. Nonetheless, many women who have been sexually harassed have symptoms very much like women who have been through a *DSM*-variety trauma.

Reproductive losses often fall into this kind of trauma, too. Losing a wanted child at any point in a pregnancy can be devastating to a woman's sense of control and her ability to predict what will happen in her life. Although for some women this kind of loss is experienced primarily as grief, for some women it leads to post-traumatic responses instead or as well.

Janoff-Bulman's concept helps to explain why these experiences and others like them are traumas for women. If you have admired and respected someone, your expectations are that they will continue to act in admirable and respectable ways. If you have trusted someone to act in your best interest, you generally will expect him or her to continue to do so. When such a person's behavior changes radically, your expectations of the world and your sense of the world's safety and predictability can be challenged and sometimes shattered. If you have believed that you were about to become a mother, and then had that taken from you by forces beyond your control, the world ceases to feel as safe as it once did.

Yet another definition of trauma comes from the work of Jennifer J. Freyd, a cognitive psychologist. She has coined the concept of *betrayal trauma*. Her model is particularly relevant to the traumas that arise in the context of betrayals of trust in relationships of extreme dependency and caretaking, such as those that occur between parents and children, therapists and their clients, or clergy and members of their congregations. Freyd has found that the traumatic component of these situations, even when no physical harm is done to the dependent person, is the betrayal itself. She discusses how it is that people who have experienced betrayal traumas, such as sexual abuse at the hands of a parent or priest, may be unable to even recall what happened to them until they are no longer dependent on the betrayer. Freyd argues that the pain of betrayal is so great that it, if acknowledged, can threaten the security of the person's attachments to others.

Another model of trauma is Maria P. P. Root's paradigm of *insidious traumatization*. Root, a clinical psychologist who has specialized in studying the life experiences of racially mixed people, has observed that for many people who live their lives in marginalized positions in a culture, trauma is not the single-blow, overtly dangerous event that is described by the *DSM-IV* definition of trauma. Instead, she suggests, many people have small, persistent, sometimes daily encounters with things that are symbolic threats to their existence. For example, many women of color encounter daily reminders of racism—and may also be subconsciously reminded of the fact that racism can sometimes turn violent or deadly. Lesbians, disabled women, and any woman who belongs to a group that is targeted for lesser or dangerous treatment in our culture may experience this insidious traumatization.

This continuous encounter with reminders of what could occur, says Root, leads to an ever present vulnerability for some people, even as they continue to go through life looking well. When this vulnerability develops, the most recent apparently small thing can lead to the development of posttrauma symptoms, even though that latest small event meets none of the *DSM* criteria. When the cumulative effect of these small things is added up, however, their potential to be traumatic to an individual becomes more apparent.

What is thematically common to all of these definitions of trauma?

1. Betrayal of trust. Whether it is our trust in the stability of the physical world (earthquakes, floods), the political world (terror attacks, war), social world (harassment, discrimination), or intimate world (sexual abuse, violence in intimate or family relationships), each definition of trauma describes the experience of no longer being safe and at home in places that formerly felt so.

WHAT IS THEMATICALLY COMMON TO ALL OF THESE DEFINITIONS OF TRAUMA?

Betrayal of trust.

Existential challenges.

Intense emotion.

Subjective experience.

2. Existential challenges. Death, danger, betrayal, all of these can call into question our beliefs about the meaning of life. Our spiritual selves, our sense of what gives order to the chaos around us, can shatter or transform when in the context of experiencing trauma.

3. Intense emotion. Trauma occurs at the high end of the emotional spectrum. The terms used by trauma researchers—*shattering, betrayal, horror*—convey the intensity of the experience.

4. Subjective experience. The traumatic part of a trauma may occur privately and internally. Many traumas leave no obvious physical mark that is visible to the outside world, although most traumas do have both acute and lasting impacts on our brains, hormonal systems, and immune systems.

THE EFFECTS OF TRAUMA

The effects of trauma are hugely variable. Each person responds to trauma in her own way. There are no right or wrong ways to react to a traumatic experience, either while it is happening or in the months and years afterward.

However, there are some common responses to trauma that, when understood as such, can help a person feel less overwhelmed or isolated after experiencing a trauma. As described earlier in the discussion of cultural myths about trauma, many women who've experienced trauma think that they are overreacting, being "weak" or "hysterical, terms that have often been used in Western cultures to describe women's entire emotional experiences. In fact, *much of the emotional response to trauma is due to physiological changes that occur involuntarily* when we are in situations of threat or betrayal.

In the *DSM-IV*, there are two specific posttrauma diagnoses: Acute Stress Disorder (ASD) and Post-Traumatic Stress Disorder (PTSD). Research on trauma recovery has also shown that several other disorders are likely to have their roots in trauma exposure. Dissociative Identity Disorder (DID), a diagnosis once known as "multiple personality disorder," most probably is caused in large part by repeated exposures to severe trauma in early childhood. Borderline Personality Disorder (BPD), a disorder that leads to difficulties in managing emotions and attachment, has been shown in much research to emerge from childhoods in which both severe repeated trauma and emotional neglect occurred. Depression in women also has trauma, particularly interpersonal trauma, as one of its possible sources. Later in this chapter, I discuss the specifics of ASD and PTSD as well as some of the more effective treatments for these disorders.

WHY SOME ARE MORE AFFECTED THAN OTHERS

Research on trauma, and on these disorders, has uncovered some of the factors that contribute to a woman developing posttrauma problems, as well as some suggestions about what factors might be protective against these difficulties.

Age The younger you are at the time of a trauma, the more likely it is to have long-term consequences for you. This is due to several factors including the following:

• Children simply are too young to have developed the cognitive and emotional coping mechanisms for dealing with extreme terror and loss. When children experience trauma, they often blame themselves, due to their normal tendency to assume that everything that happens around them is in reaction to them personally. Their neurological systems are still immature and may be flooded and overloaded with sensory information. All of this may, in turn, interfere with a child's ability to complete the jobs of childhood, such as learning to read, to relate to others, to soothe oneself. This cascade of impacts has large, lifelong consequences that are less likely to happen when a trauma occurs to an adult who has already successfully accomplished the tasks of growing up.

• For many traumatized children, primary caregivers are the sources of trauma. Parents who physically, sexually, or emotionally abuse their children are not available as sources of love or comfort when they have hurt a child. Children are more likely to be traumatized by those they know and trust than by strangers.

Source of the Trauma Traumas that are caused, or believed to be caused, by the uncaring or malevolent actions of other humans have much bigger effects in general than those that are seen as random acts of nature. It's hard for a person to say, "The earth must hate me" when an earthquake destroys her home. The quake is terrifying and disruptive, but she knows it had nothing to do with her. It was an impersonal moving of the earth's tectonic plates.

In contrast, interpersonal traumas, like rape, assault, and hate crimes, or disasters that appear to be due to human cause (such as terrorist attacks or industrial accidents caused by corporate or government negligence), are felt much more as direct attacks on our relationships with the world and our abilities to trust others. We may also be, or feel, personally sought out or preyed upon when the human perpetrator of a trauma is known to us and/or when something about who we are—our sex, culture, race, or sexual orientation—is the perpetrator's rationale for violating us. The consequences of these traumas in general are more intense and harder to deal with than the consequences of traumas not of human design.

Biological Vulnerability Not everyone is born with the same temperament. Some people are more nat-urally calm and even, others more easily agitated by daily life. It appears that temperament has some bearing on whether a person will develop post-traumatic symptoms, although the exact relationship between biology and trauma is not yet clear. What is known now is that for every hundred people exposed to a given trauma, about twenty-five will develop PTSD, the most clearly trauma-related disorder. The rest will develop some other problem or no long-lasting problems at all. Because these same vulnerabilities also function as sensitivities that we value in other contexts, they are not flaws or signs of something wrong.

Resiliency Resources For many people, trauma is an alienating, isolating experience that disconnects them from their communities and the people they love. When a trauma survivor does have such connections, their presence helps. Having family, friends, and community that will not ignore us or leave us alone after a trauma, even if we say we want to be left alone, can reduce symptoms for many people. Having a social network that does not silence us can assist in processing the trauma.

For some, but not all, women, spirituality or religion can be factors that reduce the impact of a trauma. However, not all spiritual practices are equally useful to trauma survivors.

Beliefs that blame the victim or frame the trauma as "God's will," or worse, "God's punishment" can make it harder for people to come to terms with a trauma. The best spiritual supports are those that give the trauma survivor the permission, like Job, to rage against the Divine as well as seek Divine comfort.

PERITRAUMATIC DISSOCIATION

Research on trauma has found that for some unknown percentage of people, an internal process occurs *during* the trauma, called "peritraumatic dissociation." In these instances, the person experiences an involuntary alteration in consciousness while the trauma is happening. People describe this many ways—feeling as if time has slowed down to a crawl, feeling as if they are watching themselves in a movie or from the side or above themselves, feeling as if they are dead or numb inside even though they may be walking around or smiling.

People who peritraumatically dissociate are more likely to develop PTSD within six months after the trauma. Why this happens is unknown, although some researchers who have studied this phenomenon think that Peritraumatic dissociation by numbing a person, makes it more difficult to fully integrate and process the emotions of terror and helplessness that usually accompany a trauma. What's most important to know is that this is an involuntary response—and that if a person has had it in response to a trauma, he or she is likely to need some professional help in dealing with the aftermath of the experience.

Gender Women are more likely to have mental health consequences of trauma than are men, all other things being equal. Why is this? No one knows for sure, but there are several theories that have been explored to explain it.

First, it appears that women in general may gain self-esteem from being able to connect with and be helpful to others. Trauma interferes significantly with this capacity, and thus trauma may be more threatening to women's core identities than is true for men.

Second, women are often targeted for traumatic experiences due to our sex. Rape and childhood sexual abuse are crimes primarily aimed at women. Sexual harassment, similarly, mostly occurs to women. Research indicates that rape, of all traumas, has the longest lasting negative results, and that childhood sexual abuse, of all childhood experiences of trauma, is the most disorganizing and disruptive to normal development. Because the threat of rape in women's lives never entirely disappears, women may experience the kind of insidious traumatization that increases vulnerability.

Finally, there are questions about how women's biology may contribute, in terms of both vulnerability and resilience, to our risk for developing posttrauma emotional difficulties. We know from general research on trauma that exposure to trauma affects hormonal systems that regularly interact with sex-based hormones such as estrogen and progesterone. However, direct effects on women's sex hormones have yet to be studied. So, while it is possible that women's cycling may play a part in this picture, that part is yet to be well understood.

COMMON POST-TRAUMATIC RESPONSES

As mentioned earlier, there are two diagnoses that describe common emotional responses to trauma—Acute Stress Disorder (ASD) and Post-Traumatic Stress Disorder (PTSD). There are also common responses to repeated, chronic exposure to trauma, described by Judith Lewis Herman as Complex PTSD.

Acute Stress Disorder ASD describes the feelings and behaviors that occur during and in the immediate aftermath of exposure to a trauma—feelings of disorganization, feeling outside of oneself, being disoriented, easily tearful. The symptoms may also include some of the symptoms of PTSD, including nightmares, disturbed sleep, irritability, and having intrusive thoughts about the trauma. ASD is expected to last no more than a month after a trauma and usually appears only within the immediate time period following trauma exposure.

Post-Traumatic Stress Disorder PTSD describes the complex of problems that can develop in some people in the weeks and months following a trauma. Delayed-onset PTSD can also occur, when a long-ago, forgotten trauma emerges into consciousness, and symptoms develop at that time. PTSD consists of the following:

1. An exposure to a traumatic stressor
2. Symptoms of intrusive reexperiencing of the trauma, including:
   a. Flashbacks (not simply recalling the trauma but reliving the trauma as if it were happening in present time)
   b. Intrusive thoughts (images of the trauma that show up in the mind and won't go away)
   c. Nightmares (often of things that symbolize the trauma rather than the specific detail of the trauma)
   d. Fear of being around anything that resembles the trauma
3. Symptoms of emotional numbing, including:
   a. Trying to avoid thoughts or feelings about the trauma
   b. Feeling numb inside
   c. Avoiding or being unable to participate in things that used to give pleasure
   d. Withdrawing from people
   e. Difficulties remembering all or part of the trauma
   f. Feeling bleak or hopeless about one's future
4. Symptoms of high, chronic anxiety, including:
   a. Being very jumpy and easily startled
   b. Being angry, irritable, or impatient
   c. Constantly scanning for the possibility that a trauma might recur (called "hypervigilance")
   d. Getting sweaty, shaky, or nauseous when reminded of the trauma
   e. Difficulties sleeping
5. Symptoms having a significant impact on your life, making it hard to work, love, play, and develop spiritually
6. Symptoms lasting for more than a month past the time of the trauma, although in delayed-onset PTSD, they may not begin to emerge until long after a trauma occurs

Complex PTSD Complex PTSD is not a formal diagnosis, but it is a concept that is well accepted by those in the field of trauma studies. Complex PTSD arises when a person is repeatedly subjected to traumatic experiences, usually in childhood. In addition to the symptoms of PTSD described previously, persons with Complex PTSD often experience some of the following difficulties:

- Problems with trust, being either overly trusting or unable to trust when it is appropriate
- Difficulties with managing emotions, becoming easily emotionally overwhelmed
- Difficulties in caring for oneself, including engaging in behaviors that are intentionally hurtful to oneself
- Pervasive feelings of distrust of the world and hopelessness about the future
- Feelings of alienation, disconnection, and disenfranchisement
- Experiences of identity confusion or alteration
- Experiences of dissociation (feeling "outside of yourself," feeling weird, odd, or not yourself)

WHAT TO DO IF YOU'VE EXPERIENCED A TRAUMA

In the immediate aftermath of a trauma, there are many things that a person can do that may ameliorate the impact of the trauma on their well-being. These include the following:

- Connect. Talk to the people who care about you. If you've been the victim of a catastrophe or disaster, take advantage of the free emotional support services made available by groups like the American Red Cross, which has a network of trained volunteer therapists. If you have a clergyperson, health care provider, or other trusted individual, talk to him or her.
- Focus on what's right in front of you. Trauma makes it hard to think about the future. Don't try to. Instead, pay attention to what you need to do in the moment. Over time, this will restore to you some of your sense of control, because you will have had multiple experiences of making things happen.
- Focus on self-care. Eat as well as you can. Engage in physical activity. If you have a spiritual practice, make that important. Pet your dog or cat. Some people find it helpful to be in nature, listen to music, or make contact with something that reminds them of hope, beauty, and the joy of being alive.
- Don't scare yourself about your symptoms. Most people will have some symptoms, if not a full-blown picture of ASD, in the time immediately following a trauma. This is scary for most people, but can be more tolerable if you know it's normal. Talk to yourself about how it's reasonable to be having nightmares or terrible thoughts, or feeling numb, or tearful. Normalizing things can reduce the secondary problems that arise when people see their posttrauma reactions as a sign that something is terribly wrong with them.

WHEN SYMPTOMS DON'T GET BETTER

Most people who experience a trauma begin to feel some symptom relief within a month or so. But if your symptoms persist or worsen, then it makes sense to seek professional advice. Some things to think about in looking for a therapist are these:

- The therapist's degree doesn't matter. What does matter is whether he or she knows about treating trauma. Ask potential therapists about what they know. Have they read books by people like Judith Herman? Do they belong to, or attend the meetings of, professional organizations for trauma practitioners? Therapists who don't know about trauma may not know where to focus and how to help. Treating trauma is not part of standard training in any mental health profession yet.

- Your therapist should know that trauma is a body–mind experience. She or he should know to suggest some kind of somatic assistance for you. This could include antidepressant or antianxiety medications; exercise, yoga, tai chi, or similar sort of structured movement program; or referral to an alternative health care provider if that is your preference.

Research has shown that there are some specific therapeutic approaches that are helpful for people who have experienced a trauma. One, which is especially helpful for people who have had a one-time trauma and which has been specifically studied for its helpfulness to women who have been raped, is called *Exposure Therapy* (ET). ET works through the behavioral principle that helping a person to tolerate the reexperiencing of feelings over an extended time frame will reduce the overall anxiety associated with the trauma. Most people who are knowledgeable about ET are trained in cognitive behavioral or cognitive therapy.

A second treatment that has been found helpful for trauma survivors is called *Eye Movement Desensitization Reprocessing* (EMDR). EMDR involves a process whereby bilateral stimuli, such as side-to-side eye movements or sounds alternated in each ear, are presented to a trauma survivor while she visualizes, thinks about, and feels about the trauma. EMDR practice requires specific training, which is available to therapists through workshops. If a therapist suggests EMDR, ask whether she or he has at least "level-one" training. If you are asking for help with repetitive childhood trauma, your therapist should have had "level-two" training. EMDR therapists have a wide range of theoretical orientations.

CONCLUSION

Trauma can happen in the life of any woman. If we refuse to allow the myths about trauma to control our response, and if we empower ourselves to seek support in the face of trauma, we are more likely to recover from its impact.

Recovery from trauma does not mean going back to who we were before the trauma, however. Trauma changes us. Our view of the world, ourselves, and the meanings that we give to life will always take into account the reality of trauma and this intimate knowledge of the way in which life can skew out of our control. We can regain our sense of hope and efficacy—a hope and efficacy that are grounded not in illusions of safety but in our knowledge that we can heal from traumatic experiences.

—*Laura S. Brown, Ph.D., ABPP*

RELATED ENTRIES

A Guide to Grief and Bereavement

Anger: That Most Unfeminine Emotion

Domestic Violence

Sexual Abuse and Rape

Terrorism: Another Form of Violence

Domestic Violence

Domestic violence is a term used to name abuse that occurs within an intimate relationship, whether it is emotional, physical, or sexual abuse, or any combination of these. Women of all races, socioeconomic backgrounds, and national origins are victims of domestic violence. And it happens all too often: the Bureau of Justice Statistics estimated in the mid-1990s that by the most conservative approximation, each year one million women suffer nonfatal violence by an intimate.

Alexandra was twenty-eight when she followed her sister to the United States from Mexico. Her family was not poor, so she wasn't seeking to escape poverty; she had just always dreamed of living in America. Her older sister had arrived two years earlier and had quickly found a job in a cleaning service; Alexandra joined her there. The hours were long but the pay was stable. She started taking night courses at the community college.

Alexandra's plan was to stay beyond her visiting visa. She would deal with getting a green card eventually, if everything else worked out. Initially, she stayed with her sister but then she met a nice guy. He was so attentive—he seemed interested in her day, in almost her every move. They moved in together after just a few months.

Their romance was passionate, filled with both love and anger. She began to suspect his passion was too much after one evening out. He had seemed obsessed with her, jealous of the friends she talked with at the bar—both men and women. She decided it was alcohol talking.

At times, Alexandra thought she loved him, but increasingly he made her afraid, which left her feeling sad, confused, and anxious. Within six months of their moving in together, he began to beat her—on places on her body where no one would notice. She was too ashamed to tell her friends and family. She wondered if it was her fault.

Linda grew up in the suburbs of Boston; she attended a private high school where she excelled in academics and sports. She was admired by many, but she often wondered if they would be as admiring if they knew she was gay.

After graduating from an Ivy League college and falling in love with a woman for the first time, she came out to her family. They were accepting of who she was, though they never wanted to talk about the details of her life or her relationships. She and Pam moved in together, and she secured her first job. Linda felt life should be good, but she and Pam fought often. Then the fights began to end with violence. Pam would lose it and threaten her. Recently, Pam had pulled a knife.

Linda knew about domestic violence—she had worked at a shelter during college—but it never dawned on her that she was caught in an abusive relationship with a woman. Since her family didn't want to talk about her relationship at all, certainly these details could not be shared with them.

Abuse of any kind at the hands of a loved one can be particularly traumatic and confusing. It can result in long-lasting changes in your mental health, damaging your sense of yourself physically, sexually, emotionally, socially, intellectually, and spiritually. It can make you feel as if you're crazy. To make matters worse, family members, well-meaning friends, and even institutions often blame women for the abuse they endure. Abusers use certain behaviors that it's important to be aware of.

COMMON ABUSER BEHAVIORS

Isolation An abusive partner may try to control his partner's contact with other people. He may be judgmental of friends and suspicious of her loyalty to him. As he cuts her off from outside relationships, she is left with his view of the relationship and its problems—and in his view, she is the problem. As she spends a lot of time trying to fix the relationship, she may become worn out emotionally. Of course, the relationship is not the problem. The *abuser* is the problem, and nothing she does will change that.

She needs to break her isolation any way she can. Also, if it is safe, she needs to reconnect with family and friends, educate herself about domestic violence, and contact a domestic violence hotline or support group to begin to understand the cycle of abuse, rebuild her self-esteem, and see that she is not alone. She may have to be secretive about these efforts. If it is unsafe for an abuse victim to follow through on any of these suggestions, then starting a diary (in secret) can help get the feelings out of her head and may give some emotional relief.

Control Most abusers believe they have a right to control their partners. The abuser may control with whom the partner can speak, what she can wear, the family finances. Some abusers feel entitled to their partner's full servitude and expect their partners to wait on them hand and foot. Being controlled in these ways can lead to self-doubt. Over time, self-doubt can progress to emotional and mental immobilization.

Alexandra called the domestic violence hotline one evening after a fight she and her partner had while they were at a friend's house for a birthday celebration. She had met him at his office at the end of the workday wearing a recently purchased red dress. He glared at her when she entered his office building. By the time they got to the car, he was calling her a tramp and a whore. He accused her of sleeping around on him. The argument ended with him throwing her to the ground. She was humiliated and confused; she had bought the dress to look good for him.

The person on the hotline began to talk with Alexandra about her boyfriend's long history of controlling and abusive behaviors. She suggested that when Alexandra felt safe she should do a "controlling behavior inventory" on her boyfriend.

Taking an inventory of controlling behaviors, focusing particularly on verbal and emotional abuse, is an important first step—it helps uncover the particular pattern of control an abusive partner has instituted. Understanding these controlling behaviors can help to counter self-doubt.

COMMON ABUSER BEHAVIORS

Isolation

Control

No disagreement allowed

Apologizing for abusive
    behavior

Each year one million women suffer nonfatal violence by an intimate.

No Disagreement Allowed   The mind-set of an abuser makes healthy arguing impossible. An abuser usually believes that an argument should only last as long as she says it should; that if the issue is important to her, then she should get what she wants; that she knows what is best for her partner and the relationship; that her partner is wronging her if she disagrees; and that the abuser has the right to leave or threaten to leave if she doesn't get what she wants. In the short term, an intimate relationship based on these principles—one that doesn't allow for disagreement or conflict—can feel frustrating. In the long term, it often generates feelings of helplessness.

> Most abusers believe they have a right to control their partners.

Linda could remember the fights with Pam, the feeling of frustration as Pam twisted her words and belittled her needs. Over time, Linda could read Pam's moods the minute she walked through the door. If Pam's brow was wrinkled, it would be a long night, with Pam lashing out at any little thing. Linda felt as though she were constantly walking on eggshells. Under such intense scrutiny, Linda felt trapped and irritable but unable to let anyone in to her pain. She began to have nightmares, stomach pains, and fatigue. It is important to remember that an abuser's anger or argumentative nature does not cause him or her to be abusive. Contrasting the experience of the abusive relationship with a nonabusive relationship can be helpful. Healthy relationships resolve conflicting needs and differing opinions by negotiating, compromising, and processing each other's feelings. This type of healthy exchange leads to open communication, trust, and satisfying interactions.

With the help of a trusted friend, Linda began to weave herself back together. She told herself that she had a right to express her opinions and to have them be respected. She was not the problem; Pam's abusive behavior was the problem, and Linda began to realize she could not change that. With this realization, Linda began to redirect her energy from understanding and pleasing her partner to understanding, changing, and pleasing herself. Though she did not immediately leave the relationship, being able to escape the cycle of self-loathing was an enormous relief.

APOLOGIZING

One of the most powerful forms of manipulation an abuser uses is following abusive behaviors with apologies and promises of change. An abuser may show a dramatic range of emotions after an episode of abuse. He may cry, beg for forgiveness, or berate himself for treating his partner so badly. These feelings are usually short lived and do not represent real change. Within a few days, he may be complaining that his partner is not yet "over it." For an abuser, there is only one goal—to get his way all the time. Even remorse, genuine or false, shifts the attention back onto him. These feelings of remorse may lead the abused partner to forgive the abuser or to recant threats to leave. The seemingly sincere feelings of guilt the abuser has over his actions may even lead the partner to cover up his actions, hiding them from other family members or children.

> Taking an inventory of controlling behaviors is an important first step—it helps uncover the particular pattern of control an abusive partner has instituted.

The combination of abusive behavior and remorse is extremely confusing. Hoping against hope that this time things really will change, remorse may trap a woman in an abusive relationship. Unpredictability and crisis become the center of the relationship and the abused partner comes to crave any positive treatment from the abuser. This desperation makes it even harder to leave.

Other subtle and not-so-subtle abusive behaviors include the following:

- Blaming the partner for the abuse, that she provokes it and deserves it.
- Undermining the partner's progress in life by such things as not allowing her to take classes or work outside the home in an attempt to limit her interactions with others and keep her dependent on him.
- Denying what he has done to harm his partner by making his actions seem less severe, her fault, or even not having happened at all.
- Insulting his partner, demeaning her to boost himself and to make her feel insignificant and deserving of his abuse.
- Coercing his partner into having sex with him perhaps by threatening abuse or perhaps by promising not to be abusive.

MENTAL HEALTH EFFECTS OF DOMESTIC VIOLENCE

Abusers get worse over time. The longer an abusive relationship lasts, the harder it is for the abused partner to feel she deserves better treatment. The end result may be depression, substance abuse, anxiety, or post-traumatic stress disorder.

The batterer may use these feelings to threaten or control his partner, suggesting that his partner is crazy and cannot take care of her kids. The reality is that many women who are battling with depressive symptoms continue to get up each day, see their children off to school, and work to support their families.

Constance, a forty-three-year-old Caribbean woman, worked many hours in a factory to support her family. Her substance-abusing husband physically and sexually abused her, leaving her depleted and depressed.

For a period of time, Constance's anxiety was so high when she anticipated seeing her husband that she thought she was having a heart attack. A violent assault left Constance with increasing traumatic symptoms. She was often anxious and jumpy, she lost motivation and interest in life, and withdrew from family and friends. She "numbed out" often through alcohol or sleep. She avoided any painful re-minders of the abuse. The nightmares and flash-backs of the violence intruded into her days and nights.

Sara, a thirty-four-year-old African American woman, felt afraid and denigrated in her own home. Despite being smart and competent within her profession, her husband led her to believe she couldn't succeed without him. Sara numbed herself from the pain of her partner's verbal abuse and threats by drinking alcohol when she got home from work and throughout the evening. With the support of friends, Sara was able to decrease her drinking once the batterer was out of the house.

> Healthy relationships resolve conflicting needs and differing opinions by negotiating, compromising, and processing each other's feelings.

Like Sara, many women being violated at home turn to alcohol to cope with difficult feelings. Drinking may become a habit or a dependence; in either case, it causes further problems in a woman's life. A woman who is drinking before entering into a relationship that turns abusive may drink more once the battering begins. She may lose everything she has and/or require rehabilitation.

Marie, a forty-eight-year-old Caucasian professional woman, had a history of paranoia that became worse from suffering verbal and physical abuse from her husband. She left him, but her mental state deteriorated until she was unable to hold a job and depended on Supplemental Security Income (SSI) to sustain her. Marie became homeless and had to give up custody of her beloved young son. Being worried about going home because of potential threats of violence, experiencing an increase in heart rate, or feeling shaky when you're an abusive partner begins to yell are all examples of anxiety. For some, it may be possible to shake off anxiety, but for others counseling and/or medications may be needed.

> For an abuser, there is only one goal—to get his way all the time.

The effects of domestic violence may be short lived or may stay with the abused person for a long time. Regardless of the duration of the abuse or the effects of the abuse, hope and help are always available.

RECOVERY

The Victims of Violence Program, which is directed by Mary Harvey and based on the work of Judith Herman, used information from survivors to understand how they healed. They determined that recovery proceeds in three recognizable stages.

1. Safety The first stage of recovery focuses on physical and emotional safety—developing a safe home, secure finances, safe relationships, stable physical health, and healthy strategies for dealing with stress. For a victim of domestic violence, developing a feeling of safety in all aspects of her world can build confidence. During this phase, it is essential to establish an internal sense of safety and ability in managing one's own emotional states and in comforting oneself (and one's children) in the face of pain and fear.

2. Remembrance, Integration, and Mourning With safety established in her physical and emotional life and strategies in place to deal with stressful life events, a survivor can move on to the next phase of healing. This involves exploring the impact of the traumatic events.

Some women are surprised that they do not feel better after establishing safety in their lives. An abused woman has usually been so busy trying to survive that she does not fully comprehend the impact of the abuse. Once she has some distance from the abusive relationship, the process of deeper acknowledgment may begin.

> For a victim of domestic violence, developing a feeling of safety in all aspects of her world can build confidence.

It is important to grieve the many losses involved in domestic violence. Giving up the dream of a happy marriage or acknowledging the betrayal of friends and family members can be devastating. Anger and self-blame often surface as the profound impact of the abuse sinks in. Moving through grief and anger can free up a sense of hope to move on. Reestablishing the ability to care for oneself and the presence of safe relationships can help buffer this mourning process.

3. Reconnecting with Others Stage three of recovery is marked by new understanding of the effects of abuse and personal transformations that were unimaginable at the beginning of recovery. Relationships are now built based on the expectation that the survivor deserves and is capable of nonexploitive and nurturing connections. Confidence grows. The survivor realizes that even when things aren't going well, she can cope using new strategies rather then relying on old patterns of behavior. Some women confront family members or even an abuser (if it is safe to do so), hoping to transform these relationships. Life goals may have changed dramatically from the beginning of the healing process.

For example, although she always dreamed of being a seamstress, after she moved through the healing process from abuse, Sylvia decided she would teach English as a second language for new immigrants. She realized how much she liked and wanted to help others in the ways she was helped.

Though these stages of healing are common to most survivors, recovery is highly dependent on each person's unique personal, familial, and cultural background and happens for each person at her own pace. Claire's story illustrates this complexity.

Claire is an African American woman who endured many years of domestic abuse. She felt alone with her pain and feared that talking with her family about a separation from her husband would be a betrayal of their religious values. Because of the assumptions that might be made about her culture, she felt she could not get help from the white mental health system. She wasn't sure if a therapist could understand the traumatic effects of racism as well as the effects of the abuse. Claire also had a strong personal belief that she should be able to help herself. During Claire's recovery, she has to explore all of these questions and many more.

THREE STAGES OF RECOVERY

Regain feeling of emotional and physical safety

Grieve losses

Reconnect with others

GETTING HELP

Getting help is the first step in getting free from an abusive relationship. Reaching out for help breaks the bonds of isolation, denial, and self-doubt. It is always a sign of strength and courage.

Ironically, there can be so many forms of help available, it can be confusing to know where to start. Help can come from family and friends, a spiritual community, a battered women's program, a court advocate, a community service organization, even the World Wide Web. A good place to start is with a local women's domestic violence program or a program that specializes in the treatment of abuse survivors, which you can find by looking in the Social and Human Services section of the most local phone books. Not only can these specialized programs help sort out what kind of further services are needed, they may also be better able to help with practical safety issues. Most domestic violence programs have advocates on staff that can help access other community

> Getting help is the first step in getting free from an abusive relationship. Reaching out for help breaks the bonds of isolation, denial, and self-doubt. It is always a sign of strength and courage.

resources. They often will have peer support groups, a twenty-four-hour anonymous hotline (often with teletypewriter [TTY] and multilingual access). Many have access to shelters and safe homes. Domestic violence programs are usually free and confidential.

At some point in the healing process, a woman may consider seeking professional therapeutic help. Here are a few answers to some basic questions that often come up about therapy for survivors of domestic violence.

What is therapy?

Psychotherapy for victims of domestic violence offers a safe environment to explore the impact of the abuse, to heal from its effects, and to access and build on inner strengths. Therapy is often weekly and can happen with an individual therapist who understands the impact of domestic violence or within a group context. Group therapy with other victims of domestic violence can be important in breaking the isolation that is at the core of the abuse experience. Therapy should be a supplement in your recovery process to the other community resources mentioned previously.

How does one find a therapist?

Psychotherapists are everywhere, so the first thing to consider is affordability. Some clinicians have sliding scale fees, some clinics have a free-care system, other places have grants to support free care, and most insurance plans have some mental health coverage. In some states there may be victim compensation benefits through the state attorney general's office. Once a location for services is identified, the survivor must understand how to evaluate what is the right treatment.

How does a survivor pick the right therapist?

Mental health professionals receive various types of training and not all have been trained to treat victims of domestic violence. At a minimum, anyone treating individuals involved with domestic violence shoÅuld have

- an underlying philosophy that domestic abuse in and of itself can cause severe mental distress, above and beyond other complicating factors that a survivor may have (i.e., addiction or other psychiatric illness);
- knowledge of safety issues and local domestic abuse resources;
- an understanding of the stages of recovery, the factors that influence the recovery process, and the multiple approaches needed in the healing process;
- the ability to support a survivor in developing new coping strategies and to make appropriate referrals for additional help such as group therapy or medical assistance;
- an awareness of the effects of racism, homophobia, sexism, and other forms of oppression on a woman's mental health; and
- an understanding of the importance of assisting a survivor in connecting with supportive social networks.

It can feel intimidating to interview a potential therapist, but therapists do expect to be screened by potential patients. Once the screening process is completed, it is important to reflect on the experience. Did the therapist and the environment feel warm and supportive? Was the therapist respectful? Because having the right to make choices based on experience is in direct contradiction to the abuse experience, choosing—or learning to choose—is part of the healing process.

COMMON QUESTIONS ABOUT DOMESTIC ABUSE THERAPY FOR SURVIVORS

☞ What is therapy?

☞ How does one find a therapist?

☞ How does a survivor pick the right therapist?

☞ If I go to a therapist will they hospitalize me?

☞ If I see a therapist, will they take away my kids?

☞ If I am an undocumented immigrant and see treatment, will my therapist report me to the authorities?

☞ Do therapists understand the needs of lesbians in abusive relationships?

☞ If I want to improve my relationship with my partner, wouldn't couples therapy be better than individual therapy?

☞ Are therapy records confidential?

☞ I understand about the therapy process, but then what? How long does it take to feel better?

I already feel crazy. If I go to a therapist will they hospitalize me?

The experience of abuse can leave the survivor with a distorted self-image. She may feel crazy. But therapists only recommend hospitalization as a last resort, in situations in which a client is a danger to herself or others, or if she is unable to care for herself. Abuse survivors can develop strategies to cope with overwhelming feelings that are harmful—such as an eating disorder, substance abuse, or self-mutilation. If these harmful behaviors are not controlled in outpatient therapy, a therapist may recommend hospitalization to help the victim stabilize these symptoms and learn healthy coping strategies. Some victims of abuse also already have other psychiatric conditions such as bipolar disorder or schizophrenia, which can be exacerbated by abuse. If the symptoms of these disorders become too destructive, hospitalization may be needed. If hospitalization is necessary, the therapist should work with her abused client to educate the inpatient unit about the effects the abuse has had on her mental health.

> ✦
> An abused woman has usually been so busy trying to survive that she does not fully comprehend the impact of the abuse.

If I see a therapist, will they take away my kids?

Many survivors worry about losing their children, especially since abusers often accuse them of being inadequate mothers. A good therapist will help her client work on parenting skills and as long as a therapist is convinced that the client's children are physically and emotionally safe, the kids should be able to stay with the mother. However, if a therapist has exhausted all strategies in helping to keep a child safe, she is obligated by law and by her professional code of ethics to file a report with the local child protection agency. This agency will have additional resources to assist a survivor in keeping her children physically and emotionally safe. Domestic abuse can harm a child emotionally, even if the child him- or herself has not been physically hurt. Understanding the impact domestic violence has on children and finding help for the children involved is an important part of the therapy for survivors.

If I am an undocumented immigrant and seek treatment, will my therapist report me to the authorities?

Absolutely not! Therapists have no legal obligation to report an undocumented immigrant to the authorities. A survivor is always entitled to seek help for emotional and physical problems. If the abuser threatens disclosure to the authorities or forbids his partner to seek care as part of his controlling behavior, consultation with a lawyer or an advocate can be reassuring.

Do therapists understand the needs of lesbians in abusive relationships?

This is an important question, particularly if the abuser has used sexual orientation to discredit the survivor in any way. Many clients wonder whether their therapist will understand them if they are "different." For lesbians, it is important to select a therapist who understands that popular culture and institutional laws and policies may not protect them. In some places there are programs that focus exclusively on the needs of lesbian and bisexual domestic abuse survivors and their children.

If I want to improve my relationship with my partner, wouldn't couple's therapy be better than individual therapy?

Many women hope that if they change themselves or identify the abuse as a problem in communication, then the abuse will stop. This is a myth. The abuser must acknowledge responsibility for his behaviors and he must then choose to get help to change these behaviors.

Many states have batterer intervention programs that may include some contact with the abused partner. Anger-management programs are less comprehensive and may not be as effective.

Often, domestic abuse happens in the context of drug or alcohol abuse. If this is the case, the abusive partner will need to get treatment for substance abuse as well. Substance abuse and battering may coexist, but they are two separate problems and need two different types of treatment.

If the relationship is free of coercive behaviors, then couples counseling may be considered. A survivor should discuss this decision with her advocate, therapist, or even a staff member at a certified batterers treatment program before entering into couples' therapy.

Are therapy records confidential?

By law, all mental health records are confidential. In general, a third party can have access to mental health records only with a signed release from the person being treated. However, in domestic violence situations, if a child is being treated for abuse by a parent, confidentiality can become more complicated. For legal proceedings, a judge can subpoena records. A mental health provider's records should be focused on the impact of abuse on the client's ability to function. And every client has the right to see her own records.

I understand about the therapy process, but now what?
How long will it take to feel better?

Trusting another person after being a victim of abuse is not easy. Restoring physical, emotional, mental, relational, and spiritual health takes much energy and some creativity. Keeping track of the small steps can help. A relationship with a therapist or within a group may be a good place to explore relationships that include conflict, anger, and joy without the controlling responses of the abuser. The recovery process is rarely quick or easy. Therapy should include regular evaluations of progress with the therapist.

One definition of mental health is the ability to love, work, and play. As an abused person regains her ability to love and care for herself and others, to work or participate in meaningful activity, or simply to be able to enjoy herself (and her children), her healing is a success. Some, however, are tempted to drop out of therapy after relief of some of the initial symptoms. The healing journey must be paced so that the survivor is not chronically overwhelmed. With support, survivors typically find the strength to face the pain and fear that is uncovered during the course of therapy. The abuse experience is never forgotten, but with determination and support, survivors can create a life that is directed by their own inner wisdom.

—*Carole Sousa, Lisa A. Tieszen, M.A., LICSW, and Janet Yassen, LICSW*

RELATED ENTRIES

Women and Truma

Sexual Abuse and Rape

Cognitive Behavioral Therapy

Dialectical Behavior Therapy

EMDR

Post-Traumatic Stress Disorder

Women and Addictions

Antidepressants

Antianxiety Medication

Polypharmacy

Group Psychotherapy with Women

Sexual Abuse and Rape

Thriving After Sexual Assault

When people think of what a rape survivor looks like, they may imagine a woman dressed all in black, crying hysterically, isolated and alone, depressed, unable to connect with men, and incapable of success. While rape has many negative effects on one's spirit, body, heart, mind, and relationships, it does not eliminate the possibility of healing, strength, and success. As a rape survivor myself and as a therapist, I know that life does not have to end after rape.

I find that many survivors have come across no images of rape survival that speak to their hope for transformation. Their questions often include: "Will I ever be happy again?" "Will I ever be able to be a good partner, spouse, or parent?" "Can I ever trust again?" and "What hope is there for my future?"

As a rape survivor, I found myself looking for role models of women who have not only survived but who are thriving. I discovered that there are numerous miracles among us; those who have survived and gone on to be lights of hope and inspiration. The rape of yesterday does not determine the possibility and beauty of tomorrow. Traditional therapy and nontraditional therapeutic techniques can assist women in finding greater voice and power after a sexual assault.

WHAT IS SEXUAL ASSAULT?

Definitions of sexual assault vary by nation and by state. For our purposes, *sexual assault* is any unwanted physical sexual contact, including fondling of genitals, breasts, and buttocks, as well as oral, anal, and vaginal penetration. This contact may be achieved by physical force or coercion. Sexual assault also is defined as sexual contact with a person who is unable to give consent; this inability may be a result of being intoxicated, being asleep, or being under the influence of "date rape" drugs or other drugs. In the United States, 15 percent of women report having been raped in their lifetime.

WHAT ARE THE EFFECTS OF SEXUAL ASSAULT?

From individual testimonies and from well-documented research, we know that sexual assault has devastating effects. Sexual assault affects people's emotions, thoughts, actions, and relationships. The array of possible effects can mostly be categorized around the following emotional symptoms: anxiety, fear, depression, and general mood swings. Symptoms related to one's thoughts may include dissociation or blanking out, low self-esteem, learning problems, attention problems, and Post-Traumatic Stress Disorder. Physical behaviors that may result from sexual assault include physical complaints, aggression, sexualized behavior, and self-destructive behaviors. Spiritual effects may include disruption of faith and spiritual beliefs and practices.

> ✦
> Thriving refers to using the trauma itself as a motivation for personal positive outcome and psychological growth.

THRIVING

While the term *recovery* usually refers to the resilience needed to overcome the symptoms related to sexual assault, *thriving* is a step beyond overcoming symptoms. Thriving refers to using the trauma itself as a motivation for personal positive outcome and psychological growth. The areas of growth may include the development of new skills and knowledge, the improvement of interpersonal relations, the increased use of personal and social resources, and the capability to make meaning of the past. Examples of thriving are varied and may include focusing on one's own needs for the first time, seeing possibilities for one's future, getting actively involved in a social movement, becoming critically aware of oppressive forces, and making decisions to re-create one's life. While *victim* refers to anyone who is violated and *survivor* refers to anyone who is able to gain control over the symptoms that were caused by the violation, *thriver* refers to a person who is able to experience psychological growth after an experience of trauma.

Violence, including sexual violence, is about power, force, and dominance. With this in mind, any survivor of violence must regain her personal power to thrive. The real-life experiences of women who have been assaulted and who have thrived include both growth and struggle—periods of transformation, stagnation, and setbacks. To assume that recovery means permanently eliminating trauma-related symptoms is simply not based in reality. Thriving is a process that leaves room for the true growth and despair that characterizes the short-term and long-term aftermath of sexual assault. It acknowledges the ways in which women are forever changed by sexual assault and how some of these changes, with work, can include growth and transformation.

> ✦
> When we gain wisdom or empowerment, it is not because of the assault but because of the choices we have made. A person is not strong because she was raped, but she has strength based on the work she has done after the rape.

All women have the potential to have a positive outcome and sense of empowerment after working through the issues of loss, power, and identity integral to sexual assault. Certainly, those who are violated need to gain the skills necessary to reduce post-traumatic symptoms; however, after these symptoms are under control, it is important to address the issue of growth and empowerment. While the reduction of symptoms through therapy, medication, and personal work is essential to the recovery process, survivors, and those who care about them, must also pay attention to strategies that promote growth and positive transformation. True healing or recovery for thrivers must include coming to a place of self-reliance, strength, and power over one's body and life.

If you have experienced sexual assault, think about the following:

1. In what ways did the assault affect your emotions, thoughts, behaviors, and relationships?

2. What has helped you to address some of the negative effects of the assault?

3. In what ways, if any, do you feel you have grown as a person in the aftermath of the assault?

Whether traditional or nontraditional, the paths to thriving have to address the empowerment, psychological growth, and social connection of survivors.

If you have experienced sexual assault, think about the following:

1. In what ways did the assault affect your emotions, thoughts, behaviors, and relationships?
2. What has helped you to address some of the negative effects of the assault?
3. In what ways, if any, do you feel you have grown as a person in the aftermath of the assault?

When we do gain wisdom or empowerment, it is not because of the assault but because of the choices we have made in our recovery process. In other words, a person is not strong because she was raped, but she has strength based on the work she has done after the rape.

TRADITIONAL THERAPEUTIC PATHS TO THRIVING

Individual Therapy "I'm seeing a psychiatrist. My job sent me to therapy because they could see it was affecting my work. It's made me a stronger person as far as learning not to blame myself. I had to learn where to put the blame. I've been going to different therapists for over the past five years and it's been really helpful."

Some sexual assault survivors choose individual psychotherapy. Some of the primary therapeutic needs of survivors striving to be thrivers are focused on feelings, safety, self-care, building positive relationships, problem solving, and self-reliance. Survivors require therapy that can assist them in making use of their own healing power.

A variety of therapeutic approaches may assist women in psychological growth in the aftermath of assault. These include crisis intervention therapy, supportive psychotherapy, insight-oriented therapy, cognitive behavioral therapy, dynamic therapy, and exposure therapy. Two individual therapies that have been documented as effectively transforming sense of self and sense of empowerment are crisis intervention therapy and cognitive behavioral therapy.

Crisis Intervention Therapy Crisis intervention therapy is short-term work with a counselor immediately after an assault. Receiving a supportive initial response when you tell people about the assault is important to your recovery. It is important for you to talk with someone you trust about your experience, and it is also important for the person to provide you with information on available resources and self-care strategies. You should only talk about the assault with someone with whom you feel comfortable and include only the level of detail with which you are comfortable.

True healing or recovery for thrivers must include coming to a place of self-reliance, strength, and power over one's body and life.

Cognitive Therapy Cognitive therapy is focused on transforming thought and behavioral patterns that are disserving the survivor. Cognitive therapy has not only been shown to be effective in the reduction of symptoms, but it may also assist in the psychological growth of survivors by allowing them to face the memories of their experience and thus take power over their experience as well as their thoughts. Cognitive therapy also assists survivors in processing and reframing their experience, therefore giving an opportunity to gain wisdom about themselves, the perpetrator, and the assault. For child survivors, this work is also empowering when it involves parental treatment—growth in the lives of caretakers of survivors maximizes growth and life appreciation in the survivor.

Cognitive therapy also assists in the growth process by teaching the survivor new skills and strategies that allow her to reach specific treatment goals. These new skills may be taught through psychoeducation for child, adolescent, or adult survivors. By gaining new skills and knowledge, the survivor is able to exercise power and control in her life. In assisting survivors' capacity to get in touch with their healing power, cognitive therapy helps provide knowledge and skills related to self-esteem, power, trust, safety, faulty thinking patterns, and intimacy.

Group Therapy Group therapy provides an opportunity for survivors to gain knowledge about themselves and other survivors. It lets the survivor know that she is not alone, that her responses are normal, and that learning to trust others again is a possibility. Group therapy may follow a variety of approaches, including but not limited to providing education, using ritual ceremonies, focusing on support, or addressing thoughts and feelings associated with the assault. In addition, feminist groups that focus on the use of narrative and social context can help women gain empowerment. Groups are helpful with not only controlling symptoms, but also with issues of identity, self-esteem, and relationship. Dealing successfully with these issues is key to becoming a thriver.

Things to think about:

1. If you have experienced sexual assault and you are not in therapy, what are the barriers that keep you from going to therapy? What are the possible gains you may make from trying therapy?
2. If you are in therapy, what have you found helpful about it? What has not been helpful?

ALTERNATIVE PATHS TO THRIVING

For many people, there is still a social stigma attached to traditional psychotherapy. This stigma is particularly relevant for survivors who have experienced classism, racism, homophobia, and discrimination based on religion or disability. There are alternative ways in which people have found healing and transformation; when possible, these methods should be included in traditional therapy.

Arts *"What writing does is make you think. Um, I spent some years not thinking because of the violence. You know. 'Cause if you think you may have to feel. Writing makes me feel. . . . What I write I've been exploring in my mind and thinking about and, you know, contemplating for a time."*

Use of the arts, in and out of traditional therapy, has the power to help survivors give voice to their experiences. The arts may be used to explore themes related to sexual assault and to release negative affect and beliefs precipitated by sexual assault. The arts may include visual art, drama, dancing, storytelling, music, and poetry. In working with child survivors, all of these artistic approaches may be incorporated in play therapy.

The use of the arts with adolescent survivors has been found to give them the opportu-

Things to think about:

1. If you have experienced sexual assault and you are not in therapy, what are the barriers that keep you from going to therapy? What are the possible gains you may make from trying therapy?
2. If you are in therapy, what have you found helpful about it? What has not been helpful?

nity to resist the stereotypical depictions of rape by having them create their own depictions that are more authentic and related to their own experience. The arts are also a powerful tool because instead of silencing women and girls, they provide the means for affective expression, including expression of emotions that are usually restricted such as anger and shame.

Drawing is an effective tool for sexual assault survivors that may help to break the silence and secrecy imposed by the perpetrator of the abuse. Poetry has also been discussed as a tool for the exploration and transformation of self-esteem. Dance and movement may be used to gain a sense of self, strengthening body image and developing personal strength and trust as well. Writing can be used as a way to name the horrors and pain of rape.

> The arts may be used to explore themes related to sexual assault and to release negative affect and beliefs precipitated by sexual assault.

If you have ever experienced sexual assault, try writing a poem, drawing a picture, making a collage, or dancing as a way to express your feelings.

Activism *"I get my immense feeling of importance from places like Rape Crisis and stuff like that . . . and being involved with helping other survivors. The only thing is, again, I never see really a whole lot of black women come in, that way, so, you know, I think there's a lot of fear in that. Going to places like Rape Crisis. I never thought about it. Never thought it applied. Never thought they knew what I was talking about, being a black female, you know. So I'm there now and it makes me feel good to be there helping."*

Engaging in community work to decrease the likelihood of others being violated, to gain a sense of empowerment, to counter feelings of self-doubt, and/or to make sense of the trauma by finding ways of taking the negative experience and using it for the good of others is a method of using activism as a coping strategy. Whether they educate their communities about rape, volunteer at rape crisis or battered women shelters, or lobby to improve rape laws, many women find the act of helping others an integral part of their recovery. Whether through formal or informal involvement, finding ways to have voice and power through action can be a key component to thriving for sexual assault survivors.

> Many women find the act of helping others an integral part of their recovery.

Consider volunteering at a rape crisis center, battered women's shelter, or other agency that either helps those in need or educates the community about violence against women.

Spirituality *"My mom tried to get me to go to therapy but I didn't want to go. I've been dealing with it through my spirituality, growing closer to God and talking every week with my pastor. There is still physical tissue, scar tissue down there, so there is damage, but I'm dealing with it. I talk with my pastor to search, heal the hurt, and gain peace. I know that counseling and therapy work, but God is the actual answer."*

"I would say that praying was probably the most helpful because there is someone so loving and so benevolent that's really listening to you. It helps you sort things out in your head and to understand that touching your body doesn't mean touching your soul."

Strong religious beliefs have been found to have positive effects on coping and serve as an important tool for some families in responding to crisis. For some survivors, faith and psychological well-being are quite connected. Along with individual belief systems, membership in a spiritual or religious group may serve the purpose of increasing the survivor's support networks. Some survivors of violence use spirituality as a tool of growth, meaning making, and empowerment in the aftermath of violation.

Try meditating, praying, reading a spiritual text, or talking to your spiritual leader about your recovery from sexual assault.

Social Support *"I knew my parents would take care of it. I talked with them about it and I had other siblings that we were able to talk about it and relieve some of the stress and emotion and get it out of the system. And I remember it very vividly to this day. I always had someone I could talk to and I really had a close-knit family."*

Talking with members of one's community to explore themes and issues raised by the sexual assault and/or to actively problem solve conflicts created by the sexual assault is an important use of the survivor's social support network. Building and sustaining community networks serve an integral role in women's empowerment. The existence and effectiveness of social support networks must be established in a survivor's life; when these networks are weak, women should make an attempt to build them in order to decrease isolation and increase connection and sense of strength.

> The existence and effectiveness of social support networks must be established in a survivor's life.

Think about who among your family and friends may be a safe person for you to talk with about your sexual assault.

NEEDS OF VARIOUS WOMEN

All women are unique and require individual strategies during the recovery process. Traditional therapy as well as alternative forms of healing must take into account context and must aid survivors in regaining power and control in their lives. Violence against women happens within a specific social-cultural context, and the psychological growth of survivors requires a respectful recognition of that context, including race, ethnicity, class, sexual orientation, gender, and disability. Addressing issues of power, dominance, and oppression, as well as the response of family, community, and social institutions, must be a part of the road to thriving for women of various backgrounds.

WOMEN OF MARGINALIZED RACIAL AND/OR ETHNIC BACKGROUNDS

Sex assault survivors who are members of racially and ethnically marginalized groups have to cope with multiple traumas simultaneously. Along with the issue of sexual assault, there is the trauma of racial oppression in all of its forms. The historical and contemporary oppression that racially and ethnically marginalized women experience must be a part of any empowerment activity. When stereotypes held by legal, medical, and clinical personnel lead to lack of support for Asian, Latina, African American, and Native American sexual assault survivors, the effects can be devastating.

Your practitioners should be knowledgeable about the specific symptoms of survivors of ethnically marginalized groups. Oftentimes, even when the violation has been severe, survivors of color may not exhibit extreme symptoms. Working on recovery and thriving is valuable regardless of the evidence of symptoms. It is important for marginalized survivors to be empowered with knowledge of their rights and value and to explore their cultural and individual understanding of rape and the meaning they attribute to being a rape victim or survivor. For racially and ethnically marginalized women, treatment approaches must attend to the intersection of racism, sexism, classism, and homophobia, as well as include coping strategies that have historically been effective such as humor, activism, spirituality, social support, and the arts.

> Rapists are less likely to be convicted when the survivor is a black woman.

African American female survivors often experience silencing both within and outside of their communities. Rapists are less likely to be convicted when the survivor is a black woman. Therefore African American women have to address not only the violation by the perpetrator but also the violation by a society that sees them as unworthy of protection. In addition, African American survivors often find a silencing of their experience within the African American community because of presumption that once must choose between self-preservation and community preservation. Silencing factors within and outside of the community must be acknowledged for African American women to find voice and power in the presence of institutionalized and internalized racism.

Cultural context is key to the process of moving from survivor to thriver. The healing process for Latina survivors must include attention to silence, cultural ideology, social construction of gender, experiences of racial-ethnic discrimination, and cultural values, including the value of family connection and loyalty. While social support may serve as an effective empowerment tool, the support networks of many Hispanic immigrants are small and have limited resources. Available resources must be explored in order to devise an effective intervention.

Asian American girls and women who are survivors of sexual assault must be empowered for psychological growth in areas of sociocultural ideology around a number of issues, including but not limited to collectivity, conformity, inconspicuousness, shame, sexuality, mental health systems, and self-control. In order for work with Asian American survivors to be effective, therapists must be aware that the premigration trauma experiences of different Asian ethnic groups, such as Cambodians and Vietnamese, vary greatly. Therapists should also understand the specific spiritual principles to which an Asian survivor may adhere.

> Indigenous women, such as the Inuit of Canada, have been guided toward thriving with restorative justice models.

Promotion of psychological growth for American Indian women who have been sexually assaulted should address not only issues of individual empowerment, but also the empowerment and transformation of the community. Indigenous women, such as the Inuit of Canada, have been guided toward thriving with restorative justice models that incorporate issues related to silence, education, needs of the woman or girl, power in relationships, role of elders, cultural values, and community resources.

To truly aid all survivors of racial and ethnically marginalized groups, there must be an eradication of systemic oppression based on race and gender within the education system, media, and criminal justice system. There also must be an acknowledgment of the negative and positive uses of coping strategies by members of the group for dealing with such issues from substance abuse to spirituality.

Consider how your race or ethnicity has affected how you and others think about your recovery process.

REFUGEE AND IMMIGRANT SURVIVORS

As with all survivors, empowerment and transformation of refugee and immigrant survivors must be put in the context of their individual experiences. This context includes the survivor's culture, religious beliefs, experiences as an immigrant or refugee, as well as race, class, and sexual orientation. Presentations of physical complaints for which no cause is found may be an indication of the stressful experience of migration and refugee status, as well as the stressful experience of violence, including sexual violence. An awareness of the physical and emotional connections of symptoms and experiences can help survivors themselves gain a greater sense of personal understanding and power.

How has your immigrant status or nationality affected your recovery?

> In one study of attempted and completed rapes occurring at the workplace, only 21 percent of women complained through appropriate channels and only 19 percent quit their jobs.

SOCIOECONOMIC STATUS

"And at the time, I guess thinking back now, I didn't realize that we were a poor family. And I don't know if it's a cultural thing or not, but we didn't go to therapists and things like that. We went to church and then we went and talked to each other. And if there were things like child molesting or whatever in the community, it was taken care of by the community."

While sexual assault occurs across economic lines, poverty does increase vulnerability to violence. Some survivors experience sexual assault at the workplace; financial coercion is a factor used for intimidation. In one study of attempted and completed rapes occurring at the workplace, only 21 percent of women complained through appropriate channels and only 19 percent quit their jobs. When women are dependent on their job for the basic necessities of life, they are more vulnerable to those in power at their workplace. Having compassion and sensitivity to the conditions under which women are subjected to sexual violence is important to aid in the transition from self-degradation to empowerment. This requires an honest analysis of the systems in which women work, not just the choice patterns of the individual woman. It is essential to find paths to thriving that are time- and cost-effective. One of the strengths of cognitive behavioral therapy for survivors has been its capacity to assist survivors in attaining growth in knowledge, skills, and sense of empowerment in a brief number of sessions.

How have your financial resources affected your recovery process?

LESBIAN AND BISEXUAL SURVIVORS

Sexual assault early in life disrupts the development of identity and the capacity for intimacy. Lesbians who are raped in adolescence or early adulthood by men need to relinquish self-blame, establish the capacity for intimate relationships with women, and develop a positive lesbian identity.

STRATEGIES FOR THRIVING

Important strategies to help women on the path to thriving include the following:

1. Understand that the sexual assault was not your fault. Do not minimize or dismiss your experience. Sexual assault, in any form, is a serious violation for which there is no justification or excuse.

2. Make use of your personal skills and community resources as well as effective therapeutic approaches and/or medication to address posttrauma symptoms.

3. Remember that reducing your symptoms is one step in your recovery process. The next step is building positive self-esteem, healthy connections to others, and meaning in your life.

4. Know that you have the right to have power over your body and mind.

5. Know that you are a person of worth and value.

6. Know that there will be moments when issues surface that you thought you had already addressed. This is a part of the life journey of thrivers, so try not to be discouraged. New life situations may trigger old difficulties related to the assault. There are skills and resources available to help you handle those issues when they arise.

7. Remember that thriving does not mean a life without struggle. Thriving means having access to the skills, knowledge, and self-empowerment to make it through the times of struggle.

Lesbian and bisexual youth are generally at higher mental health risks than their heterosexual peers. This discrepancy is due to a number of factors, including but not limited to family rejection, homophobia in society, internalized homophobia or self-hatred, and lack of appropriate resources that are sensitive to the issues of lesbian and bisexual youth. These issues must be explored to effectively bring about psychological growth in lesbian and bisexual rape survivors. For these reasons, lesbian and bisexual survivors must go beyond simply controlling symptoms to thrive; cognitive skills and knowledge of resources must be provided with sensitivity to issues of identity and oppression. Lesbian and bisexual survivors, whether assaulted by men or women, have to explore and address the following issues: self-blame caused by internalized self-hatred for lesbianism; lack of support from family and community resulting from prior rejection based on sexual orientation; feelings about the men in their lives, if the perpetrator was a man; sexual intimacy with their partners regardless of the gender of the perpetrator; and, often, feelings of shock and betrayal, if the perpetrator was a female. Lesbian and bisexual survivors must utilize their social support networks and must draw upon the ways they have coped with homophobia in the past to deal with those who discriminate against them as sexual assault survivors. Similarly, they must remember that one's sexual orientation does not provide justification for assault, violation, and violence.

How has your sexual orientation affected your recovery process?

> ✦
>
> Perpetrators tend to seek out girls and women in vulnerable situations, making physical and mental disability a risk factor for sexual assault and other forms of violence.

PHYSICAL AND MENTAL DISABILITY

Perpetrators tend to seek out girls and women in vulnerable situations, making physical and mental disability a risk factor for sexual assault and other forms of violence. The social and cultural context of disabled survivors must be taken into account in addressing issues of thriving after sexual assault. Disabled survivors' ability to understand and accurately describe their abuse experience is often questioned, leaving them open to discrimination. Most disabled survivors, however, are able to disclose their experience when confronted with sensitive and compassionate people. Instead of a reliance on the verbal and cognitive focus of traditional therapy, the arts can serve as an empowering tool to help learning-disabled survivors have a sense of control, power, and connection. Key issues for disabled survivors' empowerment include independence versus dependence, accepting help versus distrust, existing survival skills versus the need to acquire new skills to deal with an increased sense of vulnerability.

Have physical and mental disabilities affected your recovery?

—*Thema Bryant-Davis, Ph.D.*

RELATED ENTRIES

Child Abuse, Neglect, and Maltreatment

Domestic Violence

EMDR

Post-Traumatic Stress Disorder

Women and Trauma

Child Abuse, Neglect, and Maltreatment

Sharon is forty-seven years old, but she might as well be seven. Her life has been frozen in time for as long as she can remember. She often "zones out" for hours at a time, not eating, talking, or sleeping, just staring at the wall. She eventually snaps out of this "mood," as her mother calls it, but she is usually tired and listless and lacks the motivation to go on with her daily tasks.

Sharon's uncle sexually abused her as a child, and the effects of his abuse have been traumatic and life altering. Making it even more difficult is the fact that he died a few years ago; it is now impossible for her to confront him.

Like thousands of other women who have suffered the effects of sexual, psychological, and other types of abuse, Sharon feels she cannot move on. She is often overwhelmed by intrusive thoughts or spends large chunks of the day dissociating with real life as an escape from these intrusive thoughts, leaving her unable to keep a steady job. Intimate relationships have failed; she has been accused of being "too needy" and "constantly distrustful." Friendships have also been rare for Sharon; she has often been described as "blowing too hot or too cold," and potential friends have not been able to keep up with her constantly changing moods.

Children, the most vulnerable of human beings, come into the world helpless and dependent on the adults around them for their emotional and physical well-being. When children become subject to neglect, sexual abuse, and other forms of maltreatment, the trajectory to a well-balanced adulthood is not possible.

Abuse in childhood can leave indelible scars and have effects that reach far into adulthood, yet individuals have unique ways of reacting and coping with the trauma. Some adults experience the effects of childhood abuse only many years after the original event has occurred. They may have repressed the memory as a way of coping; but the memory may be recalled much later in life, usually triggered by some new event.

In general, adults describe six areas that are affected by childhood trauma: psychological (the way we feel); cognitive (the way we think); physical; behavioral; relational (the way we relate to others); and spiritual (the way we think about the world).

Psychologically and emotionally, survivors of childhood abuse describe a core sense of disconnection and a feeling of powerlessness. They feel a violation of trust, a reduced sense of autonomy or independence (they are usually not given a choice), lacking in initiative (violators thrive on control), and a reduced sense of competence (perpetrators usually make victims feel like they cannot get anything right). Childhood abuse damages an individual's sense of identity and intimacy. It is not unusual for victims of childhood abuse to experience a sense of isolation (feeling that they are the only ones that have experienced such a trauma) or like they are on an emotional roller coaster, feeling sad and depressed one day and angry and full of rage another.

A behavioral change that a survivor of childhood abuse may experience may be an overwhelming need to withdraw from others, a forced isolation, since the burden of the trauma is too distasteful to even talk about. They experience themselves as being tarnished and not a whole person. Some survivors may avoid being with others because of a fear of being judged or feeling guilty that they "allowed" the abuse to occur.

Impulsiveness can also be a common reaction to trauma—a feeling of not caring about the consequences of one's actions, not having anything to live for. Living life "on the edge" is not uncommon among survivors of childhood abuse, and so abuse of drugs/alcohol/medication becomes a new way of life and a negative way of coping with past abuse.

Trauma survivors often describe several cognitive difficulties that arise after the experience of abuse. They may have difficulties in remembering, making decisions, and in concentration and focusing. The ability to be attentive is easily impaired especially if the survivor is swamped by intrusive thoughts about the trauma. For some who also struggle with dissociation (a period of time when the individual drifts away from reality), completing tasks becomes a real problem.

Physically, trauma impacts sleep and appetite so that victims may experi ence unstable sleep patterns; night terrors or nightmares and night sweats; or they may eat too little or too much or have a poor diet. They sometimes may complain of having chest pains, headaches, back/neck pains, or stomach problems.

Survivors of childhood abuse especially struggle with the ghosts of their past when it comes to relationships—the ground on which they may expect the past violation to be reenacted. For a survivor who was controlled and coerced, an intimate relationship—especially one based on cooperation—may become too overwhelming, too outside the past pattern of abuse. It's not uncommon for a survivor to sabotage a healthy relationship.

Finally, trauma survivors tend to feel a deep disillusionment with their belief system (spiritually). They question their belief system, lose faith, and cannot believe that a higher power allowed such a transgression to happen to a vulnerable child. They may forever hold a violated sense of faith in the goodness of others.

So, we can see that the effects of child abuse not only carry well into adulthood, but can be completely devastating to a healthy adult life.

WHAT IS CHILD ABUSE?

Before we get into what constitutes child abuse, let's consider first the staggering statistics:

- Approximately six children are reported abused and neglected in America every minute—that's one child every ten seconds. (Prevent Child Abuse Data, 1998)
- Reported cases of suspected child abuse rose from 60,000 in 1974 to more than 2.4 million in 1989. (U.S. Department of Health and Human Services, 1990)
- In 1984, 2.8 million cases of suspected child abuse were reported. (U.S. Department of Health and Human services, 1996A)

The Child Abuse Prevention and Treatment Act was passed in 1974, and since then social service, mental health, and law enforcement agencies have tried to address the challenging issues of preventing child abuse and neglect. Our understanding of child abuse and neglect has also increased tremendously since then.

As a result of these new changes in the law, parents often ask themselves many questions that are at the core of child abuse and maltreatment, such as: At what age can a child be left alone? When does well-intentioned discipline become abuse? Is sleeping with your two-year-old appropriate? Is it abusive for children to witness their parents fighting? Is forcing a child to eat broccoli and beets abusive?

For an action to be seen as abusive, three important factors must be present: the act itself must be unacceptable (may differ by culture), the intent must be to cause harm, and the effect must be harmful. Any action against a child can be regarded as abusive if the physical, mental, or emotional health of a child is harmed or threatened by harm through any action of a parent/caregiver.

CAUSES OF CHILD ABUSE AND NEGLECT

There are as many causes of child abuse and neglect as there are cases of abuse. In general, women are prime caregivers of children, and there may be various reasons why they sometimes abuse children. Following are some causes of child abuse.

Women Who Experience Economic Stress Women who experience the stressor of poverty may also experience the ills of unemployment, homelessness, domestic violence, and poor education. Unfortunately, children born to such mothers also face an increased vulnerability to abuse and neglect. For many women, being handicapped by lack of financial resources leads them to be dependent on the wrong partner. For example:

Provencia fled a battering relationship in Florida and came to New Jersey to live in a Latino community where she thought she could safely raise her two girls, receive financial support, and resolve her immigration problems. As winter approached, that ideal soon faded. She became homeless before being befriended by someone whom she thought was a kind gentleman. Before long, she became involved with child protection authorities when her eight-year-old daughter was taken to the hospital with excessive vaginal bleeding. The child had been left in the care of the "kind gentleman."

Mothers Who Lack Social Support The information age has irrevocably changed the structure of society. Ironically, in spite of these advances, families seem to have become smaller and less connected to their extended families both emotionally and geographically, and, as such, this potential source of support is reduced. The startling divorce rate in the United States over the last three decades (now hovering at 50 percent of all marriages ending in divorce) has further eroded the close-knit family model that is important in a child's development.

Child care is a necessity, yet single parents without the means to properly support a household have to work, causing their children to become "latch-key" kids. Families with two parents have to decide between expensive child care or giving up additional income by having one parent stay at home. These choices can sometimes have damaging consequences. For example:

Wilma came to the United States from the West Indies several years ago, hoping to give her kids a better life. She was not well educated, and she depended on blue-collar wages that forced her to work long hours. She yearned for the support of her extended family at home

For an action to be seen as abusive, three important factors must be present:

+ The act itself must be unacceptable.

+ The intent must be to cause harm.

+ The effect must be harmful.

(in the West Indies) to raise her five children. The older kids began acting out as teenagers. In frustration, Wilma resorted to physically punishing her children, which was the way she was raised. Her problems multiplied when a younger son reported to a teacher that he was being "beaten" at home. "It worked for me," was Wilma's response to the social worker.

Women Who Abuse Substances A home in which a primary caregiver is substance abusing may also be a home that lacks the structure and discipline that a child needs. Sometimes a mother may resort to using drugs as a way to block out her own memories of childhood abuse, in the process neglecting her own children, and so history repeats itself. Not only are children faced with poor role models, but their basic needs may not be met. A significant number of children are maltreated in homes in which substance abuse is prevalent. For example:

Carmen is the mother of four children from three different fathers, none of whom are involved in helping her raise their children. Carmen, who grew up in a working-class area of Boston and who is herself a child from a broken home, has been substance abusing since the age of thirteen. She tries her best to be a good mother to her children, to turn things around for them, but there are days when her addiction to marijuana and alcohol take over.

At these times she is incapable of adequately caring for her kids. If there is food in the house, the children, who range in age from five to twelve years, are left to prepare their own meals and to take care of their own needs. Eating uncooked pasta out of a box and week-old food are common occurrences for these malnourished children. Indeed, the children sometimes go to bed uncertain whether their mother will be home for the night. One thing they are clear about is "telling on" their mother may result in removal from their home.

Women Who Have Psychological Difficulties The individual makeup of caregivers and their own upbringing play a role in child maltreatment. Mothers who lack self-esteem and have low frustration tolerance also have poor parenting skills. Depressed mothers or those who have other psychiatric disorders also struggle as caregivers. They usually don't have the emotional resources to parent adequately. For example:

Dina suffered with depression all her life, but it was after the birth of her third child that things seemed to "snap." Unkempt and lethargic, she began to look ten years older than she was. The "special room" in the basement where the children were sent as punishment became more frequently used. One afternoon her baby's screams led her down to the basement room. She found herself pressing "Tweedy," his special teddy bear, over his face; the more she pressed, the louder he screamed. Eventually, as if the child had no more fight left in him, he fell listlessly. Dina knew she had done something "really bad."

Mothers of Children with Special Needs Some children tax the resources of their parents because of their special needs. A child with disabilities, born prematurely or with other medical issues, or conceived during a stressful period in a parent's life is more likely to be abused or mistreated. For example:

Jenny was born "at a bad time." Her mother, Sandy, in the spring semester of her junior year, would drop out and become a wife and mom. Barry, Jenny's dad, would also do the right thing, completing college part-time and immediately finding work to support his family. Below the surface, Jenny's parents were miserable with themselves and their short-changed lives. To add to these problems, Jenny was born with a sleep apnea and required round-the-clock monitoring. Sandy, like most young mothers with special-needs babies, would often be short fused about Jenny's care. Barry was no help. He would come home after work only to run out again for evening classes. Jenny's crying and Sandy's complaints were the last thing he wanted to hear.

When Jenny was a year old, Sandy brought her for a checkup, only to be quizzed about a bruise on her cheek. "She fell a few days ago, trying to walk," was the excuse Sandy had prepared. After two more similar occurrences, the doctor felt pressed to call the local child protective services. The call was not in time, though, to save Jenny from her mother's latest violent outburst, during which she fractured Jenny's arm. When the police came to Sandy and Barry's apartment the following day, Barry insisted they were just going through "a bad time," a reflection of what Jenny's life had always been. Jenny was special—just not special enough.

Women Who Have Had Inadequate Parenting Models We are all expressions of our past. How we were nurtured as children influences the care we give our own children. For mothers whose own needs as children were unmet, parenting can be overwhelming. For women who were abused as children, mothering may bring up their own past issues. It is therefore important that women work through issues of a past trauma before they make a decision to have a baby. Unfortunately, for some who may have repressed painful traumatic memories, the birth of a child may be the thing to trigger recall of these past memories. For example:

Maiteh never knew her Vietnamese mother. Born to a prostitute, she was abandoned in the red light district and brought to the attention of child protective services. And so began a series of foster placements for Maiteh, while she awaited a permanent home with a family willing to adopt her. Maiteh was never adopted. She was left with the legacy of inconsistent mothering produced by too many part-time parents. Yearning for a sense of belonging, Maiteh became pregnant when she was barely sixteen. She planned to move out on her own and give her child the things she was not able to get herself. She did not count on the demands of an infant, the constant crying, the diaper changes. Alone and with no one to talk to, she resorted to what her mother had done to her. In fits of rage she would often shake her baby until one night she simply disappeared, leaving a sleeping baby to be found by the authorities.

We can all play an important role in identifying whether a child is being abused or neglected. Adults who take action make a positive difference and in some cases can save a child's life.

Women Who Have Abuse Histories Childhood abuse leaves deep scars on the psyche. Mothers who themselves were abused as children may parent in several different ways, fluctuating between being overprotective and hypervigilant with their own children, or sometimes abusing them. However, women who have been able to work through their own abuse history in therapy and reach a level of integration can become appropriate parents. For example:

Susan remembers being physically abused by her alcoholic father and spending many sleepless nights locked in her room without dinner. She vowed not to do the same with her own children. She left home after graduating high school, was at loose ends, and joined the wrong crowd for a time before becoming involved in a more stable relationship with a part-

ner she eventually married. In the comfort of this new relationship, her old fears came back. She began to see a therapist to work through these issues before making a decision to become a parent herself. Several years later, Susan is a loving mother to her two children. Now and then she notices the resentment and anger well up that life was not the same for her as a child, but she is able to discuss these feelings with her husband, who continues to be a source of strength and support.

HOW TO IDENTIFY WHETHER A CHILD IS BEING ABUSED, NEGLECTED, OR MALTREATED

As concerned citizens, we can all play an important role in identifying whether a child is being abused or neglected. Adults who take action make a positive difference and in some cases can save a child's life. The following sections describe some of the reactions that maltreated children usually exhibit.

Preschool (Two to Six Years)—Common Reactions to Abuse Children in this age group tend to display physical reactions of increased crying, lapses in toilet training, nightmares, and an unusual fear of darkness. They may have physical skin/bone injuries. Bruises and swelling are also usually telltale signs of abuse. Children that are neglected also have poor hygiene.

Some behavioral reactions to look for are an increase in whining, throwing tantrums, withdrawal, silence, and aggression. Children who engage in regressive behavior, such as thumb sucking or soiling underwear, after a period of competence in these areas may be conveying a message.

Emotionally abused children panic easily, get angry quickly, and have an increased irritability. Anxiety, especially separation anxiety, is prevalent among abused children.

Cognitively, a child who is being abused may show a sudden inattentiveness and distraction. The child may also have difficulty focusing and a poor memory. Oftentimes, the child may have a faraway look in her or his eyes, appearing to be daydreaming.

School Age (Seven to Fourteen Years)—Common Reactions to Abuse Children in this age group who have undergone some form of neglect or abuse generally complain of the following physical reactions: headaches, stomach-aches, nausea, vague aches and pains. They may suddenly wet their beds or have night terrors. Again, bruises or abrasions on the skin and severe injuries should be questioned.

Behavioral reactions are a withdrawn demeanor, lethargy or increased activity, clinging, irritability, disobedience, disruptiveness, resistance to authority, aggressive play, lying and stealing, and a marked drop in school attendance.

Emotionally, many abused children may be distrustful, subdued, have displaced fears, be self-blaming or describe a loss of interest, an increase in sadness/depression, and helplessness.

Cognitively, they may describe an inability to concentrate, exhibit a drop in school achievement, experience increased memory problems, or become judgmental of others and have fantasies with "savior" endings.

Adolescence (Fifteen to Eighteen Years)—Common Reactions to Abuse Of all age groups, adolescents may have the hardest time talking about their abuse, so vigilance around any physical and behavioral reactions they may exhibit becomes important.

Physical reactions of sleep disturbance, stealing/vandalism, substance abuse, eating disorders, increased physical activity, and vague physical complaints and painful menses are usually signs that something else may be going on. Behavioral signs are the exhibition of antisocial behavior, such as stealing/vandalism, accelerated entry into the adult world, an unusual increase in rebellion, and engaging in high-risk behaviors. Isolation, a decline in social interest and activities; running away; acting out sexually; and violence in dating relationships are also signs that an adolescent may be experiencing some form of abuse.

On an emotional level, adolescents who are abused may talk about revenge, express strong anger/rage, and may have suicidal thoughts or gestures. Other feelings they express are shame, hopelessness, helplessness, inadequacy, and depression.

> Adolescents may have the hardest time talking about their abuse, so vigilance around any physical and behavioral reactions they may exhibit becomes important.

Cognitively, adolescents who are abused have a foreshortened sense of the future, poor memory, and an inability to focus and be attentive. They may also express spiritual reactions of a loss of faith and a questioning of their faith and a higher power. If in the past the adolescent was a churchgoer, this activity becomes severely reduced. Although some of these reactions are the normal and natural behaviors of adolescents, if there is a sudden and unexplainable increase in these behaviors, it may be indicative of abuse.

CHILDREN WHO WITNESS DOMESTIC VIOLENCE

Children have always been affected by witnessing domestic violence, but only recently have authorities paid attention to the damage caused by this form of violence in the home. Social service and child protection agencies have designated social workers trained to deal with victims of domestic violence, and at most doctor's offices one can expect to be asked questions about domestic violence during regular medical check-ups.

In a home where domestic violence is occurring, children may themselves be abused physically, verbally, and emotionally while a parent is being abused. his complicates the child's ability to disclose the abuse and recover from the trauma since he or she may look to the abused parent to take the first action.

A child may also be the only witness to domestic violence in the home. This role can be quite stressful for a child who may feel allegiance to both parents but who may feel pressure from authorities to disclose pertinent information—a disclosure that can potentially affect the child's future with both parents. Some children may minimize the description of parental violence out of a sense of loyalty to parents they feel they have to protect.

In general, children who witness domestic violence may display the symptoms of Post-Traumatic Stress Disorder, and, in addition, they may take on some of the characteristics of the perpetrator partner. They may become physically abusive to family members, try to hurt pets in the home, hurt themselves, become fearful of leaving the victim parent alone, and exhibit physical, emotional, and behavioral problems at school or day care.

REPORTING ABUSE

Who Reports? State laws vary around who should be reporting abuse and neglect. In most states, educators are mandated to report abuse. Some states are more inclusive and specify

SOME TERMS COMMONLY USED IN CHILD MALTREATMENT

Bad touch: A term used by primary prevention programs for children to describe hitting, punching, biting, erotic touch, and other acts that hurt children.

Child protection agency: The designated social services agency in a state that investigates and provides rehabilitation services to children and families with problems of maltreatment.

False allegations: Sometimes a child's accusation of abuse against an adult may be false or ungrounded in truth. Knowing how a false allegation originated is most helpful in combating the negative effects. A child may falsely accuse to seek attention, seek revenge, or because he or she was coached by someone else (as sometimes happens in divorce cases).

Foster care: Out-of-home care provided for children who are placed outside of their families for protective purposes.

Good touch: A term used by child programs to describe appropriate forms of touch that are not erotic, such as hugs and pats.

Juvenile and family courts: These courts resolve conflicts and intervene in the lives of families in a manner that promotes the best interest of children.

Mandated reporter: A person who, in his or her professional capacity, is required by law to report suspected cases of child maltreatment to the authorities.

Neglect: Inattention to the basic needs (food, clothing, etc.) of a child by the caretaker.

Parent/Caretaker: Person responsible for the care of the child.

Physical abuse: The nonaccidental physical injury of a child by an adult, which may result from overdiscipline or punishment. Examples of physical abuse are kicking, punching, beating, and burning.

Sexual abuse: Any contact between a child and adult in which the child is used for the sexual stimulation of the adult. If the perpetrator is under eighteen years but significantly older than the child, it may also be deemed sexual abuse. When sexual abuse occurs within a family, it is called incest.

Substantiated: A finding made by a child protection agency after investigating a child abuse/neglect report that indicates that evidence exists to supports that abuse/neglect did occur.

Survivors: A term used to describe individuals who were abused/neglected and are coping adequately.

that all citizens are mandated to report. The reporting statute for child abuse in your state will indicate how to do the reporting. All states maintain a toll-free number to assist with the process.

What to Report? State statutes also define child maltreatment. Most state laws specify physical abuse, neglect, sexual abuse, and emotional and mental abuse by a child's caregiver as a transgression that should be reported.

When to Report State laws may vary, but most require reporting an incident of child abuse/neglect, within twenty-four hours. The onus does not fall on the reporter to produce evidence for making the report. In fact, waiting for proof may actually endanger a child's life.

Where to Report Each state designates agencies that are mandated to receive and investigate reports of suspected child abuse/neglect. For example, in Massachusetts, the Department of Social Services is the designated agency. The same agency may also be involved in the treatment and rehabilitation of affected families. It is important, for reasons of privacy and confidentiality for the families involved, to make reports only to authorized personnel.

How to Report Most states require both an oral and a written report in cases of suspected abuse. Having the following details helps when making a report:

- Child's name, age, and address
- Parent's name and address
- Nature of injury or condition observed
- Reporter's name and address (optional)

Reporting May Be Difficult One of the biggest obstacles to reporting child abuse/neglect may be the personal feelings of the reporter, who prefers not to get involved because of fear of personal harm from the abusive parent(s). Reporters may also not want to intervene in what might be considered a family issue. The person being reported might be an influential person in the community. These are normal and natural concerns, but remembering that one is protecting a child should help in overturning these concerns.

What Happens Next Once an official report of suspected child abuse/neglect is made, the onus is on the child protective agency to investigate whether abuse occurred. If the report is substantiated, the child will be assigned a caseworker whose task it will be to ascertain whether the child's safety is at risk in his or her current home environment.

In some cases, a child may be temporarily removed from the home while the parent(s) receives rehabilitative services or interventions in order to make the child's day-to-day life more secure. Once parents have demonstrated an ability to take care of their child, the child is returned home.

Abused and neglected children may need educational, psychological, and medical needs. The child protection agency that substantiates the abuse is responsible for ensuring the child receives these services.

SAFETY PLANNING

It is important that the child's therapy address the issue of safety and self-protection as a preventive strategy. This may entail educating a child about abuse (physical, emotional, and sexual), distinguishing between good and bad touch, and developing some skills in discriminating between adults that can be trusted and those that cannot. This psychoeducational aspect of therapy can empower a child to approach her or his future with confidence, armed with knowledge. The services a maltreated child receives can turn things around so that the child's resilient capacity is allowed to express itself.

—Priscilla Dass-Brailsford, Ed.D.

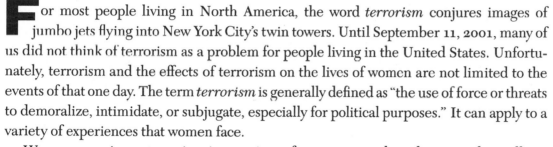

Terrorism

Another Form of Violence

For most people living in North America, the word *terrorism* conjures images of jumbo jets flying into New York City's twin towers. Until September 11, 2001, many of us did not think of terrorism as a problem for people living in the United States. Unfortunately, terrorism and the effects of terrorism on the lives of women are not limited to the events of that one day. The term *terrorism* is generally defined as "the use of force or threats to demoralize, intimidate, or subjugate, especially for political purposes." It can apply to a variety of experiences that women face.

Women experience terrorism in a variety of ways, some relatively rare, others all too common. Women living in or fleeing countries with political unrest experience bombings and the ongoing threat of violence. In the Middle East, suicide bombings have occurred frequently, leaving many in fear of ordinary life activities like using public transportation or shopping at the public market. For a number of years, terrorist bombings in London by those involved in the Northern Ireland conflict created uncertainty for public life. In the Middle East, London, and during the September 11 bombings, terrorists used fear and devastation of civilian populations as a means of achieving political goals.

In all too many instances, torture, including sexual violence against women, has been used as a means of demoralizing and intimidating women's family members and even entire ethnic groups. This was graphically demonstrated by the systematic raping of Muslim women by Christian Serbian men during that conflict. The stated goal was to subjugate and shame as well as to impregnate the women.

There are other forms of terrorism that don't involve wars and armies or even paramilitary groups. In the United States, the violence from gangs and drug dealers can be a form of terrorism. Gangs have historically used the threat of violence to prevent whole communities from reporting their crimes and identities; if the fear of violence prevents a citizen from reporting a drug dealer, that is terrorism. If the police are insensitive to the real dangers and risks that people are taking when they report such thugs, the situation becomes even more terrifying. Many children in inner city areas in this country know somebody who was killed in a drive-by shooting. In such communities, mothers become fearful of letting their children play outside; "hitting the floor" at the sound of gunshots becomes second nature.

In attempts to demoralize and intimidate—again, a form of terrorism—doctors and others working in clinics that provide abortions have been threatened, bombed, and killed by people opposed to abortions; if a woman has difficulty finding a doctor willing to perform an abortion because of fear or if a woman endures threats on the way in to a clinic where abortions are performed, that is terrorism. Burning of black churches, racist graffiti, and acts of hate violence are all terrorism against black Americans. Anti-Semitic graffiti, burning of synagogues, and shootings of Jews and immigrants are acts of terrorism.

> A person's response to acts of terrorism is affected by previous traumatic experiences. If you have had another traumatic experience, such as sexual assault, child abuse, or even a bad car accident, a terrorist act can bring back the feelings and symptoms you experienced before.

Women in abusive relationships often face terror on an individual level. Abusive partners may use violence and the threat of violence to prevent women from exercising their rights, associating with friends and family, engaging in normal activities, or even leaving the house let alone leave the relationship. Perhaps "terrorism" doesn't technically extend to this individual level, but certainly such experiences terrorize.

For women, the effects of terrorism are often not limited to their own injuries and fears about their own safety. Women are usually the practical and emotional caretakers of the entire family, especially the children and the frail. Women often feel and often are responsible for dealing with children's fears and injuries. These additional responsibilities can tax emotional resources when dealing with a terrorist event. Yet, because these responsibilities are generally an unacknowledged part of everyday life, women may not recognize the stress they create. They may wonder, "What's wrong with me?" when they see others without these additional responsibilities appearing to bounce back faster.

Psychologically speaking, terrorism is closely related to the concept of trauma. The goal of terrorist acts is to create fear, not only in the particular individuals directly harmed by the action but also in a broader group—to traumatize by disrupting the sense of the world as a safe place. This disruption of our sense of safety is one form or type of trauma or traumatic experience. The psychological effects, the consequences of those effects, and the methods for mitigating the various effects are similar to other forms of trauma.

At the same time, a person's response to acts of terrorism is affected by previous traumatic experiences. If you have had another traumatic experience, such as sexual assault, child abuse, or even a bad car accident, a terrorist act can bring back the feelings and symptoms you experienced before. In some cases, this may occur even if you have already made peace with the previous event.

> One of the keys to avoiding the negative effects of a vicarious traumatic experience is avoiding unnecessary exposure.

The effects of a trauma can also be experienced vicariously by anyone involved with the experience secondhand. After a terrorist incident, you can become emotionally connected to the event and experience fear even though you live far from the actual incident. When you consider yourself a part of a group under attack, you don't have to be there to feel attacked. If a person or community of your ethnic group, religion, or sexual orientation is attacked because of ethnicity, religion, or sexual orientation, it can feel threatening. Many Americans living far away from New York City, Washington,

D.C., and Pennsylvania were strongly affected by the September 11 bombings simply because it involved innocent citizens going about their everyday lives. Yet, the distance may lead us to downplay or ignore the psychological effects of an experience.

Psychologists working with trauma have learned that one of the keys to avoiding the negative effects of a vicarious traumatic experience is avoiding unnecessary exposure. That can be hard after a serious incident when we feel a strong desire to connect and stay in touch. We may find ourselves wanting to stay "glued to the tube," watching horrifying images over and over as many did in the days following September 11. However, once you have gotten the basic needed facts, it is a good idea to avoid endless repetition. Fulfill that desire to be in touch by connecting with family, neighbors, or a community or religious group rather than the TV. Limit children's exposure to these images as well and reassure them that they are safe, especially if they are far away from the event, or help them take the necessary steps to be safe if they are close to the danger.

A variety of physical symptoms can also be common after intense experiences of fear. These include intestinal upset, loss of appetite, increased appetite, shakiness or tremors, elevated blood pressure, and heart palpitations.

The fear created by a terrorist incident can lead to several common reactions. One immediate response to being made to be afraid is anger. We can also get angry in reaction to physical or emotional pain. In the aftermath of a trauma, however, don't let anger get in the way of good judgment. Avoid lashing out irrationally or reacting excessively. Stress can also increase a person's anger level, so monitor angry behavior carefully in the period following a terrorist incident to avoid acting in ways that will later be regretted. Implementing good anger-management tools, including things like taking a time-out if the situation is too stressful, can be helpful.

Another common reaction to fear is increased risk taking and aggressiveness. Some people are embarrassed by or uncomfortable with the experience of being afraid. There is an often unspoken desire to prove that one is not a coward. Although in Western culture this tendency is probably more common in men than women, women may experience it or need to deal with it in their sons, husbands, or friends.

Feeling violated is another common reaction. Our "safe zone" has been intruded upon, somebody we know or identify with has been harmed. This feeling can lead to a desire to "pull up the drawbridge" and reduce contact with anybody we consider an outsider. People who are "not us" are suspect.

A variety of physical symptoms can also be common after intense experiences of fear. These include intestinal upset, loss of appetite, increased appetite, shakiness or tremors, elevated blood pressure, and heart palpitations. Other symptoms may be more psychological, including anxiety, insomnia, nightmares, irritability, poor concentration, memory problems, hyper-alertness, and increased startle response.

Experiencing some or all of these symptoms in the period immediately following an experience of terrorism is normal and generally does not require professional attention unless there is some reason to be concerned about a heart attack or stroke (both of which can be triggered by intense fear). However, if any of these symptoms are severe, do not appear to be getting better, or last for more than a few weeks, it may be useful to seek professional attention.

In general, in the immediate period after a traumatic or terrorist incident, it is important to use all of the basic stress management tools: exercise, eat well, avoid excessive alcohol consumption, get adequate rest and sleep, spend time with loved ones, reconnect with the things that give your life meaning, and be kind to yourself and those around you. Remember that when we are under stress we are often not at our best.

Dealing with the long-term effects of terrorism is similar to the process of dealing with other traumatic experiences. Fear and an elevated sense of being unsafe are significant long-term psychological effects of any traumatic experience. After a sexual assault, women often feel unsafe in a variety of places where they previously felt quite comfortable. This increased fear can create real problems in daily life. This fear that results from a terrorist act is one of the goals of terrorism.

Adjusting in the aftermath of any trauma, including terrorism, is a matter of rationally assessing the real levels of danger. In some cases, that assessment will reveal unnecessary levels of vulnerability that must be corrected. The process is the same whether it is a young woman learning not to trust the safety of a drink handed to her by a stranger or a nation's people learning to be patient in airport lines while baggage is scrutinized. With that in mind, a person or a nation can balance behavior changes that appear reasonable with a resumption of previous activities that are not unreasonably dangerous.

That adjustment is, of course, easier to describe than to make. Part of the problem is that human minds aren't dispassionate computers. You may know that more people die each year from smoking cigarettes than from terrorist acts, but you may still be more worried about your children being killed by terrorists than about their taking up smoking. One way to help the process of emotional recovery after a terrorist act is to listen to your own fears and then actually get the facts about them. If an increased level of fearfulness is getting in the way of daily life or if other people suggest that a behavior seems excessive, seeing a professional can help.

—Nancy Lynn Baker, Ph.D., ABPP

The Impact of Chronic and Debilitating Illnesses on Women's Mental Health

One morning at age thirty-two, Olga stepped from her bed to the floor to discover severe discomfort in her left foot. "I literally couldn't take a step. It felt like I had a tennis ball under my foot." Now, twelve years later, she confides, "My feet are deformed. I can only wear tennis shoes." A joint in her left hand is also deformed and another joint in her right hand is swollen, red hot, and hurting.

Olga's particular form of arthritis is sometimes diagnosed as "unspecific" and sometimes as "psoriatic arthritis" because of the patches of severe psoriasis on her skin and scalp that are related to her particular form of arthritis. Whichever the technical diagnosis, Olga suffers from one of many chronic and debilitating illnesses that can strike a woman without warning.

Other illnesses present a slow compilation of symptoms that are often dismissed until the illness takes a sudden turn. Some can be specifically diagnosed and others remain elusive to a particular diagnosis and, sadly, a specific treatment. Two trademarks of most debilitating illnesses are chronic pain and extreme fatigue, two symptoms that, especially with no diagnosis, can be particularly frightening.

Debilitating illnesses that *are* diagnosed often promise little hope for a full recovery and can in an instant change a woman's life trajectory and that of her loved ones. Many of these debilitating illnesses are often progressive and sometimes fatal. The progression of these illnesses is nonspecific, unpredictable, and varies from person to person. The following information will help you understand a few specific chronic and debilitating illnesses commonly diagnosed in women. These illnesses come with an emotional cost, affecting a woman's mental health. However, there are also some things a woman can do to enhance her sense of resilience and hope in the face of chronic illness.

SOME COMMON CHRONIC AND DEBILITATING ILLNESSES

Chronic means "long duration or frequent recurrence," and *debilitating* means "to impair the strength of or make feeble." Many debilitating illnesses are related to autoimmune disorders, which challenge a woman's resilience both physically and emotionally because, in essence, her body begins to work against her.

Under normal conditions, the body's immune system kicks into action when it detects foreign bodies, usually bacteria or viruses, present in the system. For reasons that are unknown to the medical community, with an autoimmune disorder, the immune system attacks and destroys healthy cells and organ systems in the body.

Another fact, which also baffles the medical community, is that autoimmune disorders are more prevalent in women than in men. Some of the various autoimmune diseases include multiple sclerosis, scelroderma, arthritis, connective tissue disorders, lupus, fibromyalgia, chronic fatigue syndrome, and thyroid disorders. Other immune-related diseases (it is unclear whether immune system problems are a cause or a result of these diseases) include irritable bowel syndrome and Crohn's disease, which is reported to affect men and women at equal rates.

Women may also be debilitated by chronic pelvic pain, migraines, or severe premenstrual syndrome. Other women are periodically debilitated by illnesses such as chronic bronchitis or asthma, which are easily exacerbated by allergies or infections. Being diagnosed with any of these disorders is emotionally disorienting and causes feelings of uncertainty and fear.

> Autoimmune disorders are more prevalent in women than in men.

DIAGNOSIS AND THE STAGES OF ACCEPTANCE

For many illnesses, the exact time of onset can be difficult to identify. Some symptoms go unnoticed, fluctuate, get explained away, or are otherwise attributed to "overdoing it." Others are sudden, severe, and unmistakable. Because women are socialized to tend to the needs of others, they may not pay attention to their symptoms until they become unbearable and may even hide their difficulties to avoid feeling like a burden to others. Maureen Reid-Cunningham illuminated this dilemma in a paper on chronic illness by sharing what happened to her after she was diagnosed with chronic fatigue syndrome at age thirty-three:

At first, I tried to do everything I had been doing in my roles as mother, wife, professional, with extremely poor results. Although it seemed impossible to let go of any of my "duties," . . . I have had to learn to ask for help. This meant undoing the learning of generations of women on both sides of my family, which said, "Do your own work. Help others, but never ask for help."

Because women are taught to concern themselves with what their bodies *look* like, not how their bodies are working for them, symptoms may also be ignored until they are unmistakably "visible" on the body. The one exception to this is weight loss, which is, of course, immediately visible. Because our culture equates thinness with health, weight loss may not be considered a problem at all. No woman wants to think there may be anything seriously wrong with her physical health when she has finally lost those "last ten pounds!" Other women have a haunting sense that something is, indeed, very wrong. Either way, scheduling that doctor's appointment to find out can be quite unsettling.

Several things can happen as a result of that first visit. At best, a woman's concerns are met with compassion and taken seriously. At worst, her symptoms are dismissed, perhaps medicated temporarily. In reality, everything in between happens. Regardless, the diagnostic process is a scary time; feelings of uncertainty coincide with the frustrations of coordinating medical care.

It is important to remember that many chronic and debilitating illnesses are difficult to diagnose without the presence of a *combination* of symptoms that have culminated over a period of time. A single symptom, although significantly debilitating, may often be treated with a "wait-and-see" approach. Nevertheless, positives on some tests with negatives on others often indicate a need for more and more tests. Thus, this phase is usually filled with anxious waiting.

When the answers do come, a woman typically faces a heartbreaking reality of lifestyle changes that impact every facet of her life. While she may feel relieved that there is now a way to "name" the difficult experiences that have filled her life, a new set of emotional factors arises as she begins to learn about the nature of her illness and the course of its progression. Many women are not only concerned with the course of the illness itself, but they are equally concerned about how their illness will impact their relationships with others.

THE RELATIONAL IMPLICATIONS OF ADJUSTING TO LIFE WITH A CHRONIC ILLNESS

Maureen Reid-Cunningham, along with four other women who all suffer from chronic and debilitating illnesses, wrote a paper about their experiences. They concluded that "the quality of our relationships is central to our ability to live successfully with illness." They also identified three developmental stages of coping that include recognition, renegotiation, and regeneration. These stages are not linear; rather, they are cyclic in that the nature of chronic illnesses involves unpredictable periods of remission and recurrences.

The first stage described by Reid-Cunningham and her colleagues is termed "recognition." In this stage, women move through feelings of shock, and sometimes denial, into a "conscious awareness" that they will experience profound lifestyle changes as a result of their diagnosis. Supportive relationships help women move through this initial stage of adjustment, which is often filled with disbelief and shock.

Each woman gradually comes to accept her diagnosis much like women deal with the stages of grief—in her own way and her own time. As a part of this process, women can expect to move into a time of mourning over the loss of dreams and expectations they had for their lives, their lifestyles, and their relationships. Some of the possibilities may be quite frightening and difficult to face. Olga shared her feelings at the time she was diagnosed:

> Many women are not only concerned with the course of the illness itself, but they are equally concerned about how their illness will impact their relationships with others.

It was hard being told I had something that couldn't be cured. I had always figured you got sick and you just took something to make it go away. Now I was being told that not only was it not going to go away, but that I could expect to be in a wheelchair one day. It was very depressing. I'd go to see my doctor and there I was in my thirties sitting in the waiting room and everybody else was in their eighties. The thought of being in a wheelchair was something I just couldn't think about. It's my greatest fear. I just try to keep the thought out of my head.

And each time there is a shift in the illness, women reengage in a new process of recognition.

The second stage identified by the authors involves a process of "renegotiation" whereby a woman works to build room in her life for the management of her illness while working to see it as only a part of who she is and not as something that encompasses her whole identity. How a woman adjusts to lifestyle changes and renegotiates her identity in the context of her illness depends on many things, including her age at onset, the circumstances under which she is diagnosed, the quality of her relationships, the support she has in her life, as well as the amount of resources she has available to her to assist her in taking care of her responsibilities.

The age of onset and diagnosis has a great impact on a woman's ability to integrate her illness into her identity. Women diagnosed in early adulthood may be concerned about reproductive and fertility issues. During a woman's reproductive years, a diagnosis of lupus, for example, may evoke concerns regarding her fertility and her ability to carry a child full-term. Renegotiation around fertility issues can be particularly frightening as the image a woman has had of herself as a mother is suddenly uncertain.

For women with lupus and other autoimmune disorders, their immune systems can wreak havoc with the developing embryo just as it does with other organ systems in the body. The problem that this family of disorders causes in pregnancy is called "antiphospholipid syndrome." According to medical experts, most autoimmune disorders, even those whose effects on pregnancy are still not understood, are a cause of concern for pregnant women and for women who are considering conceiving.

> Caring for others while struggling with a chronic and debilitating illness takes a great deal of energy and can sometimes complicate efforts for the long-term management of these types of diseases.

Sadly, many of these disorders are not diagnosed until after a woman suffers a miscarriage or premature births. After a late-pregnancy loss, one woman shared this:

I never expected anything like this could happen to me, but there I was, pregnant in my mid-twenties with a perfect health history and then suddenly we discovered my baby was in distress and was severely underdeveloped. My daughter had to be delivered by emergency c-section at thirty-two weeks and because she was months behind in her development, she died shortly after birth. I am now being tested for a connective tissue disorder that wouldn't allow my body to properly nourish the baby. I am devastated with grief and guilt and on top of everything else, I don't know if I'll ever be able to have children of my own.

According to relational-cultural theorists Jean Baker Miller and Irene Stiver, caring for others and participating in growth-fostering relationships are important factors in a woman's physical and emotional health and are central to a woman's sense of worth. Paradoxically, caring for others while struggling with a chronic and debilitating illness takes a great deal of energy and can sometimes complicate efforts for the long-term management of these types of diseases.

For a woman to be unable to care for others is often a difficult adjustment and may evoke feelings of incompetence, frustration, disappointment, and fear. Sometimes it simply feels sad. Olga has felt this pain in one form or another throughout the course of her illness:

When I was first diagnosed my children were five and twelve years old. We were a very active family so I did what I could to keep up with my children. I had to just bear the pain and go with it. I was very irritable a lot of the time. Now I feel the saddest around my grandchildren. They have so much energy. I have a hard time just getting on the floor to play with them because I can't kneel. Then once I'm down I can't get back up without help. Those are the times when I ask, "Why me?"

Fortunately for Olga, physical activity is therapeutic for her particular diagnosis of psoriatic arthritis, and the joys of grandchildren serve to motivate her to continue to be active. The prescription for other women is rest, rest, and more rest. Regardless of the best course of action, a chronic debilitating illness can stop a woman in her tracks.

Maureen Reid-Cunningham and her colleagues suggest that the process of ongoing and cyclic renegotiation leads women to the process of "regeneration." Regeneration is described as a time of "meaning making," which is done through acts of giving intended to foster the adjustment of others who share their struggles. For women dealing with a chronic or debilitating illness, telling their stories, being heard, and hearing others are indicative of shifts in relationships and individual and collective growth from having adapted to the challenges of life with a chronic and debilitating illness.

MYTHS, STIGMAS, AND "WOMEN'S DISEASES"

Simply stated, myths and stigmas related to "women's diseases" clearly impact a woman's ability to advocate for her physical health. As women turn to the medical field for answers and understanding, they often find their caregivers struggling to identify the causes and cures of many of these diseases. Interestingly, the nature of "chronic" illnesses is problematic for patients and physicians in ways that leave both parties feeling frustrated and helpless.

In the worst-case scenario, medical professionals handle these feelings in ways that are oppressive and detrimental to women's mental health. Arthur Kleinman has written extensively on this issue and sums up this dilemma by stating: "Practitioners, trained to think of 'real' disease entities, with natural histories and precise outcomes, find chronic illness messy and threatening.... Predictably, the chronically ill become problem patients in care, and they reciprocally experience their care as a problem in the health care system."

In essence, women deal with the debilitating effects of their illness while struggling with the idea that they, themselves, are problem patients of sorts. To make matters worse, health care providers don't always agree that some of these diseases, like fibromyalgia and chronic fatigue syndrome, even exist. As a result, women are sometimes told: "It's all in your head." For women who struggle with debilitating symptoms, having their illness dismissed as something that is simply "made up" can be devastating.

> For women dealing with a chronic or debilitating illness, telling their stories, being heard, and hearing others are indicative of shifts in relationships and individual and collective growth from having adapted to the challenges of life with a chronic and debilitating illness.

One woman, whom I'll call Heather, was diagnosed with Crohn's disease after suffering through more than a year of tests. She shared the following about having had her symptoms repeatedly dismissed:

It was like I didn't exist as a person, or as a human being. It was thought I was making it up, or that I had a mental illness. I knew none of this was true, yet here was this doctor telling me I had brought this on myself. Quite honestly, at that point, it wasn't the illness that was so painful, it was that someone was telling me that it wasn't happening, that it wasn't real. It was the lowest point in my life and it changed me forever.

Sadly, Heather's dehumanizing experience speaks to the collective consciousness of all women who have experienced being ignored, ostracized, devalued, dismissed, oppressed, abused, or harassed in any number of contexts.

This phenomenon of "doubting" can feel like a modern-day version of the debate over the cause of hysteria in women, which actually began in the late 1800s. On April 21, 1896, Sigmund Freud, the "father of psychoanalysis," gave a paper on the etiology of hysteria to the Society for Psychiatry and Neurology in Vienna, Austria. Freud asserted that his female patients who presented with symptoms of hysteria all reported histories of early childhood sexual abuse perpetrated by male relatives, and most frequently by their own fathers.

Freud's thesis was highly criticized by his colleagues, thus leading him to doubt the validity of his patients' reports. In 1933, Freud denounced his earlier position and reported that he believed that his patients' accounts of sexual abuse came from their fantasies and wishes and were not based in reality. Joseph Carmen Smith, in his 1990 book entitled *The Psychoanalytic Roots of Patriarchy*, suggests that had Freud elaborated on his earlier position, his work may have shifted to understanding the makeup of the psyche of men who molest children, but instead, the focus shifted "onto the female, turning the analysand from victim to psyche-defective."

Irrespective of intent, "Freud's repression mirrors society's repression" of victims' experiences, whether they result from social *or* medical ills, according to Smith. This all follows the myth of meritocracy and our culture's victim-blaming mentality. In other words, if you work hard and are a good enough person, good things will come your way. If good things don't come your way, it is because you did something wrong, you brought your fate on yourself and are, in fact, deserving of the struggles in your life, whatever the context.

> For women who struggle with debilitating symptoms, having their illness dismissed as something that is simply "made up" can be devastating.

In a concrete sense, the myths and stigmas related to "women's diseases" are made visible when we look at Heather's experience, who, by all medical accounts, was diagnosed with a "valid" disease. The lifelong changes she described came from the fallout of this experience, which included the development of clinical depression. She now deals with the double stigma of having a chronic illness and a psychiatric diagnosis (which was *not* the cause of her illness) *and* the myth that she brought all of this on herself. The challenges to dealing with a chronic and debilitating illness are made even more complex by the paradoxical nature of treatment approaches, which often produce side effects that become, in and of themselves, the focus of treatment.

THE PARADOXICAL NATURE OF TREATMENT APPROACHES

At the time Olga received her diagnosis of psoriatic arthritis, she recalled having the illness explained to her in part as: "Your body has turned on you." Women are told that they need to "fight" their disease and, paradoxically, their own bodies. In my view, this perspective adds a new twist to the familiar experience of the "battle of the body." As women, we spend our lifetimes either battling the bulge or, if not, fearing the bulge. We put energy into fighting fat, defying age, and resisting urges. As if the illness wasn't enough, women are often faced with medication side effects that range from mere nuisances to life-threatening consequences.

Over the course of twelve years, Olga has taken seven different medications for her psoriatic arthritis that have caused hair thinning, facial hair growth, anemia, and weight gain, to name a few. She can track the course of her illness with the course of her weight, "Over the years I have gone from 118 to 125 to 140 and now I'm at 159. I'm short so every ounce shows on me." Medication side effects have also put her at risk for liver and kidney damage.

Sometimes the focus of treatment becomes managing the side effects of many of the more commonly used immune-suppressant drugs. Because of the nature of immune-suppressant drugs, infections develop that can cause problems with other areas in the body. Once again, women are advised to "fight back." The familiar term "fight or flight" has been used to describe human beings' response to stress. Most of us understand this term to mean that in times of life-threatening stress, human beings will aggressively defend themselves or they will run away from the threat. Until recently, no one had really questioned this response pattern that has been assigned as the "natural" response pattern of both women *and* men.

Shelley Taylor and her colleagues at UCLA recently discovered that women respond to stress very differently than men, both behaviorally and physiologically. These researchers have coined the term "tend and befriend" as a way of describing women's response to stress. To tend and befriend suggests that in times of adversity women work to mobilize support, cooperation, and collaboration instead of becoming aggressive or fleeing from the scene. As such, advising women to "fight" an illness, or anything for that matter, may feel foreign and alienating.

As an alternative, I would like to invite women to befriend the enemy or rather to develop a relationship with their bodies and their illness. This approach invites women to learn to listen to what their bodies are telling them and to respond empathically and compassionately to their physical and emotional needs. The goal then is to work with, not against, your body.

RECOMMENDATIONS

There are, as we've seen, many issues related to how a woman's mental health may be impacted by a chronic and debilitating illness. You may have experienced some of the issues raised, you may be just beginning your journey into life with a devastating diagnosis and simply feel overwhelmed. Here are some recommendations that could facilitate a sense of resilience and hope.

1. Be proactive and educate yourself, your loved ones, and your employer(s) about your illness. Ideally, this can be thought of as a *mutual* learning process that keeps everyone informed and educated. It will also serve to prepare the people in your life for the uncertainties that lie ahead and will reduce any "explaining" you would have to do during any flare-ups, which might require unpredictable changes in your level of activity.

2. Reduce the level of stress in your life. Personal, professional, and caregiving responsibilities are often unavoidable, but it's important to begin to ask for help when you need it. Women who hide or neglect their health ultimately increase their stress level, which, in turn, exacerbates the illness. This dynamic is part of a stress-related vicious cycle that is best dealt with by honest, straightforward communication.

3. Listen to your body. You, more than anyone else, know what your body needs and how it is responding to medication. Learn to love, nurture, and care for your own body in the same way you respond to the needs of others. Avoid a combative men-

1. *Be proactive and educate yourself, your loved ones, and your employer(s) about your illness.*

2. *Reduce the level of stress in your life.*

3. *Listen to your body.*

4. *Mobilize support and seek professional advice.*

5. *Discuss alternative treatment approaches with your doctor.*

tality with your body and, if you find yourself in a combative relationship with the medical community, seek support in advocating for your health.

4. Mobilize support and seek professional advice. The complexities of life with a chronic illness are disheartening and exhausting. It is unfair and unrealistic to expect yourself to be able to deal with the stigmas, the emotional fallout, the physical demands of the illness, and the treatment regimens on your own. Attend support groups and seek professional counseling. In addition to emotional support, support groups are also a good resource for getting information on new treatment approaches and research trends related to particular illnesses.

5. Discuss alternative treatment approaches with your doctor. Research alternative therapies, such as acupuncture, massage, and herbal remedies, and discuss them with your doctor. Learn how they might help your specific illness or the symptoms that your illness has presented you with. Be sure to understand how the proposed therapy may interact with other medications or treatments you are taking and be cautious of marketing techniques that exploit women's hopes in order to sell expensive remedies.

CONCLUSION

Researchers such as Jeffrey J. Sherman, Dennis C. Turk and Akiko Okifuji have suggested that a large proportion of women with fibromyalgia suffer from debilitating Post-Traumatic Stress Disorder from various traumas that exacerbates, not causes, the illness. In addition, researchers have begun to identify invasive bacterial infections as possible causes for a host of chronic illnesses including fibromyalgia, chronic fatigue syndrome, and Gulf War illness. As such, new and effective treatments for many of these diseases may be on the horizon. These discoveries serve to "legitimize" women's illness experiences and they also serve to legitimize and support further research into their etiologies and cures.

The dehumanizing quality of the myths and stigmas related to "women's diseases" may impact a woman's mental health more than any other aspect of her illness experience by evoking a deep and dangerous sense of shame, depression, and isolation. A woman can best foster her psychological resilience in mutually empowering relationships and in communities of support, which Jean Baker Miller and Irene Stiver suggest are critical to a woman's physical and emotional well-being. Establishing and maintaining mutually supportive relationships require honest and authentic communication, which is best accomplished when a woman feels free to be herself. Dealing with the uncertainties of a chronic and debilitating illness requires flexibility and patience with others, one's self, and one's body, as well as an openness to life and all of its possibilities.

—Dana L. Comstock, Ph.D.

Poverty and Women's Mental Health

Money can't buy happiness, so the saying goes. But perhaps only people who feel monetarily secure say this—those people who don't count pennies when buying something or who have money left at the end of the month. Who wishes to be poor, unable to meet basic survival needs for food, shelter, clothing, medical care, general expenses, and emergencies? Even members of religious communities who take a vow of poverty are protected because they are provided a lifetime of basic necessities. Unfortunately, there are those who experience a life of poverty. And because they are poor, they can experience negative mental health outcomes.

BELIEFS ABOUT THE CAUSES OF POVERTY

There are two major aspects of poverty. The first is people's beliefs and opinions about poverty. The second is the official government definition of poverty. Generally, people agree that *poverty* is the term used to describe the lowest rung of the socioeconomic ladder. Poverty can have subjective, personal, and evaluative meanings. People compare their financial situation to what they think is a poverty level. As a result, opinions differ regarding what poverty actually is in terms of an actual dollar amount.

WHO IS POOR? PUBLIC BELIEFS AND OPINIONS

In casual conversation, people who do not meet the federal government definition of poor will use the words *poor* or *poverty* to describe how they perceive their financial situation at any given time. When asked why they are feeling that they are "poor," it may be that they cannot afford a desired item rather than because they are without basic life necessities. This feeling can be different from people's view of their social class status, a subjective opinion that need not be tied to actual income. For example, in 1999 the *Monthly Labor Review* reported that the median family income was $50,046 (the point at which 50 percent of families are above and below this figure). Assume two families of the same size have this income. The first family lives in Mississippi, a state with a low cost of living. The second family lives in Hawaii, a state with a high cost of living. While both families are middle-class, their feeling about their financial situation is subjective, as their locations have a significant impact on their standard of living.

Furthermore, there are individualistic beliefs about why someone is poor that focus on personality attributes such as irresponsibility, lack of discipline and effort, or low ability and talent. Often these beliefs become stereotypes of who we view as poor people. There are other stereotypes of the poor. Are you more likely to feel sorry for a woman or a man, an ethnic minority individual or a white person, or an older versus a younger person? All of these situations tap our individualistic beliefs. Researchers who study stereotypes of poor versus middle-class women report that poor women are labeled negatively (e.g., irresponsible, dirty, hostile, impulsive) and middle-class women are given positive labels (e.g., intelligent, competent, happy, and self-competent). Many of these negative attitudes become linked to cultural groups that are thought to be guided collectively by "ghetto" norms because of the economic status of the neighborhood. The neighborhood is viewed as being a cultural umbrella wherein all members of that geographic location are viewed similarly, and all are assumed to hold norms that deviate from those of "nonghetto" America (e.g., values of achievement, intelligence, and family cohesion). The contradictions to this type of thinking are not contemplated. So, a single mother who is poor can be viewed more negatively than a single mother who is middle-class. The latter may gain more sympathy from those who hold these prejudices.

> Researchers who study stereotypes report that poor women are labeled negatively and middle-class women are given positive labels.

Structuralistic beliefs of the causes of poverty incorporate the larger socio-economic system such as low wages for some jobs, poor schools, prejudice, discrimination, and job availability. Fatalistic beliefs as to a person's poverty status focus on such things a bad luck, chance, or fate. In addition to people's personal perceptions of the poor, the media also shape opinions regarding poor people. My colleague Heather Bullock and I, while studying how newspapers report on poverty, found that while most articles were neutral in tone and sympathetically portrayed the difficulties facing the poor, they failed to contextualize poverty or illuminate its causes.

These beliefs regarding the causes of another person's poverty lead to value judgments regarding who are the deserving and the undeserving poor. We respond to poor women in these value-laden ways, such that our responses to them can shape these women's sense of self-worth. In this case, the experience of being poor becomes part of the self-concept, rather than a financial situation.

WHO IS POOR? GOVERNMENT DEFINITIONS

The federal government officially designates who is poor in any given year. There are many publications that report figures on poverty levels by racial or ethnic group, marital status, gender comparisons, and place of birth. As a result, it is difficult to compare women and men within any racial or ethnic group category. Also, economic data on special populations are presented for certain years and the 2000 Census publications become abstracted in the local media allowing general access to this information.

In 1999, a family of four was considered at the official poverty level if their income was at or below $17,029. This represented 11.8 percent of the U.S. population, about 6.6 million people. This figure improved slightly to 9.29 percent of families in poverty in 2000. Among these families, those with children under eighteen years of age with a female head of household were the poorest (34.3 percent). This figure is shocking, since an enormous economic boom occurred in the 1990s. For those at the official poverty level, both families with female heads of household and foreign-born populations are poorer than married couples and native-born people. Thus, the 1999 official poverty rate was almost 17 percent for foreign-born populations compared to about 11 percent for native-born populations.

Being married increases income. In 1998, 10 percent of married couples were below the poverty line in comparison to female heads of household at 51 percent for African American; 28.7 percent for American Indian/Alaska Native; 27 percent for Hispanic; 18 percent for white; 9.8 percent for Asian/Pacific Islander. Not only are female-headed households poorer than those of married households, but also they are larger with an average of 3.01 persons under eighteen years of age. Only families born in another country had more members (3.35) under eighteen years of age. While the number of families falling under the designation of poor and headed by fathers is few, these families have more income than female-headed families since men earn higher wages than women.

> Women who work, but are still poor, have very difficult lives. In 1999, there were 1 million women in this category.

The Working Poor The *working poor* is the term used by the federal government to describe those individuals who are working or looking for work and who have worked for at least twenty-seven weeks during the year but whose incomes fall below the official poverty threshold. Women who work, but are still poor, have very difficult lives. In 1999, there were 1 million women in this category. Of this group, African American women represent the highest percentage at 16 percent, followed by 10 percent Hispanic women, and 5 percent white women. Welfare reform regulations have resulted in more women working, but at the same time these women remain primarily in the working poor category. Multiple jobs, lost jobs, and looking for jobs are the realities for these women. While welfare reform in 1996 required women with children on governmental assistance to take a job or enroll in job training, there are many states that do not define the work requirement such that attending school or taking English lessons to further training skills is accepted.

Poor Women and Mental Health Poverty status clearly leads to a stressful life. Researchers have reported consistently that socially disadvantaged groups (e.g., women, racial minorities, the poor) can have mental health difficulties based on their disadvantaged status. Much of this research fails to examine how race, ethnicity, social class, gender, religion, sexual orientation, and other person- and group-specific factors intersect to produce certain mental health problems. Instead of examining these intersections, many studies use an additive approach and deal with the generic "woman" and poverty, or an ethnic-group woman and poverty, and ignore other contextual variables that influence behavior. Poor women are influenced by the sociopolitical, cultural, geographic, and situational factors that shape their lives despite our limitations for understanding how, given the lack of research on the topic.

> Women are overrepresented in psychiatric statistics. They are most frequently diagnosed with depression, neuroses, and eating disorders.

Women are overrepresented in psychiatric statistics. They are most frequently diagnosed with depression, neuroses (e.g., anxiety), and eating disorders (anorexia and bulimia). Other disorders occur alongside these psychological problems, such as substance abuse, chronic health problems (hypertension, HIV/AIDS, diabetes, cancer), and family dysfunction. In addition, we need to be aware that one outcome of poverty is powerlessness, a feeling of not being able to control one's life which is directly attributable to lack of money to cover basic necessities. I would argue that poor and working poor women feel this way. Poor women's powerlessness interacts with environmental factors such as neighborhood safety, job market forces that result in unemployment or fluctuating employment, and racism and discrimination for those who belong to devalued racial or ethnic groups. The interactive nature of these forces on the lives of poor women and how mental health is affected need to be factored in.

> One outcome of poverty is powerlessness, a feeling of not being able to control one's life which is directly attributable to lack of money.

Poverty is a negative life event. Unfortunately, the research on the negative life events has not focused on poor people. Instead, negative life events are studied primarily in psychiatric populations because the aversive nature of a negative life event is important to understand in order to provide appropriate therapeutic interventions. However, results from some of these studies can help the reader understand how the event of poverty as negative, chronic, and/or situational can have adverse consequences on the mental health of women. Researchers report that individuals who experience major negative life events have difficulty recovering from depressive illness. Poor women who have multiple negative life events become at risk for developing psychiatric conditions. Many go without mental health treatment because these persons may not come to the attention of the mental health professionals. Alternatively, they may enter another system as a result of the outcomes of psychological and psychiatric problems; for example, these women may end up in the child welfare system because the care of their children is being adversely affected by their mental health, and/or the legal system because of substance abuse or other factors.

The majority of poor women, as already mentioned, are mothers. Studies on coping and social support for poor mothers report that when they do not feel in control of their emotional functioning, they receive more social support than mothers who feel more emotional control. Researchers find that poor mothers' stress increases with age and number of children. But we can't be sure whether the number of children leads to the stress or whether the mother was stressed before the children were born. However, it is understandable that more emotional stress is related to these factors, especially since female-headed households averaged slightly over three children in 1999.

Caregiving roles also create stress. Women engage in more caregiving than men, and they provide care for their own children as well as for other family members and friends.

> Researchers find that poor mothers' stress increases with age and number of children. But we can't be sure whether the number of children leads to the stress or whether the mother was stressed before the children were born.

The result can be multiple-role strain, placing women at a disadvantage for mental health problems. Caregiver stress can last a long time and result in feelings of depression, stress, frustration, and helplessness.

Domestic violence is a mental health issue that affects all women. For poor women, domestic violence represents further victimization. Women who are poor and racial minorities are more likely to be studied by researchers than middle-class and white women. Interestingly, studies of racial minority (primarily African American) and white women who are experiencing domestic partner violence indicate mainly similarities between these groups of women. Differences that are found often indicate that racial minority women have different supportive social networks aimed at trying to decrease partner violence than do white women. White and African American women use different professional help services, with African American women more likely to use emergency medical services, while white women are more likely to use social services or law enforcement to access help in a domestic violence situation. Surveys of shelters for battered women find that African American women tend to have more children and are poorer than white women in the shelter. When a woman and her children go to a shelter for battered women, we know that her children have been exposed, and at times, are also victims of violence. Youth who are exposed to violence experience negative psychological influences that further place a family in peril for psychological problems.

The work of Nadine Kaslow helps us to understand the interactive effects of poverty on women's lives. She studies domestic violence in low-income women who attempt suicide. Her research indicates that abused women are more likely to attempt suicide than non-abused women based on their lack of powerlessness, depression, and as a way to escape an intolerable living situation where every aspect of their environment is controlled by their partners. Kaslow found that women who attempted suicide compared to women who did not have higher rates of stressful negative life events, hopelessness, childhood trauma, psychological problems such as depression, and substance use and abuse.

—*Karen Fraser Wyche, Ph.D.*

RELATED ENTRIES

Adjusting to Divorce

Domestic Violence

Stress Management for Women

Racism and Mental Health

The *Oxford English Dictionary* defines *racism* as discrimination against or antagonism toward other races coupled with the belief that there are characteristics, abilities, or qualities specific to each race. Racism may assume personal as well as institutional forms.

Personal racism may be expressed by one person's hostility or aggression toward another person or group based on race or ethnicity. Racism is generally a learned behavior based on distorted information about other ethnic groups devaluing those groups and idealizing information about one's own group.

This information about others can be passed along directly by family members and peers or indirectly from our environment from the time we are very young. Even if we have never personally met an individual from a disparaged ethnic group, we have indirectly absorbed information about him or her via movies, television programs, newspaper articles, and other media outlets. Such outlets state or insinuate which people or groups are considered good, smart, safe to be around, and at-risk and which are considered bad, stupid, and dangerous. The media may simply exclude members of socially marginalized groups in depictions of American life except when focusing on some socially unacceptable behavior deemed characteristic of the marginalized group—depicting marginalized group members as if they are represented by their worst exceptions while members of the majority group are represented by their idealized exceptions.

These negative perceptions of stigmatized groups and idealized depictions of majority groups are reinforced over time and become less likely to be questioned or challenged by the people who hold them. Persons who hold racist beliefs would have to challenge the idealized beliefs that they hold about their own race if they were to challenge the validity of their racism against others.

When access to social opportunities is selectively denied to members of certain ethnic and racial groups, their position in the social hierarchy is diminished—and then used to defend the practices that serve as barriers to the very opportunities needed to transform their status. For example, a racist stereotype of African Americans was that they were of inferior intellectual ability compared to white Americans. Based on this mythic assumption alone, African Americans were then denied training and education. Then their subsequent inability to get jobs because they were denied the opportunities to acquire skills and training was used to further the "inferior intellect" argument, even though their failure was a function of absence of opportunity, not a function of ability at all. In this context, behaving toward the negatively stigmatized group members in ways that would be totally unacceptable if they were members of the majority is easier to do without question. This brings us to institutional forms of racism.

Institutional racism is more complex than personal racism. When personal bigotries are embedded in the very rules that govern our social institutions, racism becomes institutionalized. For example, laws that permitted states and other municipalities to deny African Americans the right to vote, to live in particular neighborhoods, to attend schools, and enjoy other public services and social opportunities accorded white Americans—even though both groups' tax dollars supported these things—are forms of institutional racism. They are not the result of an individual who simply dislikes African Americans and chooses to not associate with them or even behaves in a hostile manner toward them. They also are not the result of a fair assessment of an individual's ability or talents. When the rules are arranged to facilitate opportunities for white Americans and deny them to African Americans, Latinos, Asian Americans, and other persons of color in ways that make those rules a part of the institution, the discrimination is institutionalized: One need do nothing for racism and discrimination to occur.

> When the rules are arranged to facilitate opportunities for white Americans and deny them to persons of color in ways that make those rules a part of the institution, the discrimination is institutionalized: One need do nothing for racism and discrimination to occur.

In institutional racism, racial discrimination can be accomplished even if the parties involved have no particular animosity toward one another or toward people of color in general. Racist outcomes are assured because they are embedded in the rules that govern the way the system works. If the rules of the game are rigged against you, you can be good and lose or bad and lose; your realistic efforts don't alter the outcome of the game.

Institutional racism is much more difficult to challenge and address by individuals who are victimized by it because there is no one person to "blame"; it is embedded in and concealed by the way the system works. As such, it can be less visible and harder to identify by individuals who are victimized by it. This is relevant to the effect of racism on mental health. Being able to identify the location of social barriers is crucial to developing skills needed to negotiate them as well as to avoid inappropriate self-blame. Because institutional social discrimination is hard to see, it creates a condition in which its victims can come to see themselves as defective or deficient and come to believe the very rationales that are used to justify discrimination in the first place.

In the United States, racism is commonly viewed as a form of social discrimination and negative stigmatization that have historically been and continue to be directed toward people of color, referred to as racial minority groups. Racism in the United States has been a ubiquitous social reality and may be seen to contribute to the mental health vulnerability of its victims.

Racism has the potential to make mundane life events more difficult and extreme life difficulties catastrophic. Negotiating racial barriers as an everyday part of life drains people of the energy required to manage other routine life stressors that have little to do with race. This additional burden requires additional tangible and psychological resources.

Negotiating an everyday climate of social hostility, patterned injustice, or protracted hardship exposes people to chronic levels of stress. Over time, this stress, particularly when coupled with other normal life stressors, can have negative effects on the psychological equilibrium needed to maintain good mental health.

Invisibility—the ways that people who are targets of racism are not seen and their performance or ability is not judged on the basis of who they are as individuals—may be deemed a negative consequence of racism. Rather than being judged by individual merit, they are seen as if they were the sum of the negative stereotypes. This experience of being chronically disrespected, of having one's feelings treated as if they are unimportant, having one's talents and abilities disregarded or impugned has negative effects on the mental health of an individual in a variety of ways.

> Negotiating an everyday climate of social hostility, patterned injustice, or protracted hardship exposes people to chronic levels of stress.

One's family and community can mitigate the negative characterizations that are a part of racial stigma and facilitate coping. An individual may internalize the negative stereotypes and come to believe that they are in whole or in part valid depictions of him- or herself. This is referred to as internalized racism.

Social scientists who study the consequences of prejudice observe that when people are forced to experience social injustices like racism they develop feelings and conflicts about their unfair negative treatment. When there are no safe, socially acceptable outlets for the resulting expressions of anger, rage, sadness, and frustration that naturally and appropriately develop, they may turn those feelings against themselves and others who are like them. The individual faces a double bind when any of the characteristics associated with negative stereotypes are synonymous with appropriate responses to being discriminated against.

For example, anger is a common response to unjust treatment, but exaggerated depictions of anger have also been a way of negatively stereotyping some ethnic minority groups, such as African Americans. An individual may avoid displaying anger at discrimination in order to avoid exhibiting the behavior of the stereotype. The options such individuals face are to suppress their anger, direct it inward, redirect it in creative ways, or express it overtly in appropriate ways. Suppressing anger uses a lot of psychic energy and is not a good long-term solution. Directing the anger inward, toward the self, often results in self-destructive behavior. Redirecting anger in creative ways requires sufficient skill as well as a minimal level of emotional, tangible, and psychological resources. Expressing anger overtly, however, gets us back to the reinforcement of the negative stereotype of the group. Individuals in this situation are damned if they do and damned if they don't, the essence of a double bind.

> Anger is a common response to unjust treatment, but exaggerated depictions of anger have also been a way of negatively stereotyping some ethnic minority groups, such as African Americans.

When people are constantly forced to endure no-win situations, they can become frustrated, demoralized, and hopeless. What began as appropriate anger can fester into rage as well as depression, which when expressed can be destructive to both oneself and to others—substance abuse, domestic violence, major depressive symptoms, cardiovascular diseases, and other health as well as mental health problems that compromise an individual's capacity to function in healthy ways.

Not all ways of responding to or coping with racism are problematic or maladaptive. Indeed, throughout history, many individuals have forged creative individual and group strategies for coping with and successfully negotiating racial barriers and hostility. However, having to do so drains them of resources they may need for other life tasks. For example, many African American parents have long understood the need to prepare their children to negotiate the racism that they will inevitably face. This process of racial socialization is an additional task required of parents that is not required by their white counterparts. As such, it becomes an additional dimension to the already difficult task of parenting. This process requires parents to accept that they cannot protect their child from racist slights or barriers, nor can they protect them from the feelings that both they and their children will have as a result. A major part of the parental role is to protect children. Parents who are not allowed to do this are left with feelings of hopelessness, frustration, and inadequacy. How extreme these feelings are depends on other racial barriers the parents must address, their own family history, and the adequacy of their coping styles as individuals. While they must support their child's feelings, they are also obliged to teach them concrete problem-solving skills that would facilitate their ability to address racial barriers as well as other life tasks that racism complicates.

Just as it would be inaccurate to depict all responses to racism as problematic, it would be just as inaccurate to assume that all individuals who experience racism are inevitably debilitated by it. We know that just as adversity can contribute to psychological vulnerability, it can also contribute to psychological resilience. Many individuals who are forced to negotiate societal barriers like racism can, with appropriate support during development, become highly resilient individuals. Such individuals seem to have the ability to keep toxic and malevolent forces around them at bay. They may have learned an ability to adopt a psychological detachment to social injustice and other forms of malevolence. Hence, they may be far less likely than other individuals to internalize its toxic effects.

Resilience requires the presence of a complementary balance among adversity, social and emotional support, basic resources, the presence of social and other skills that enhance the ability to negotiate social difficulty, and periods of respite or safety from adversity—no amount of support is sufficient to counteract unremitting bouts of social adversity with little respite. Resilience also refers to a difficult-to-define quality found in some individuals who are able to take adverse circumstances and not only manage them but enhance their sense of self-adequacy and competence in the process. This greater sense of competence and confidence, in turn, allows them to approach negotiating barriers with more confidence as well, maximizing the potential for positive outcomes. This may explain why throughout history many individuals have transcended egregious social barriers and traumas without experiencing distortions in themselves as a result. People who are accustomed to negotiating the social world from a point of advantage may be less well equipped to manage that world when they are at a disadvantage, having fewer strategies than individuals who have had to learn to do so in order to survive.

Despite the fact that many people have not been psychologically crippled by racism, and despite examples of many individuals who thrive despite great social adversity, there is always a price to be paid for racism. The energy that is utilized anticipating and negotiating racial barriers, neutralizing racial slights, and recovering from the injuries of racism is not available for other aspects of life. The fact that many people manage to survive and perhaps even overcome racism does not in any way mitigate its potentially toxic and debilitating effects on any individual's mental health.

—*Beverly Greene, Ph.D., ABPP*

RELATED ENTRIES

Anger: That Most Unfeminine Emotion

Depressive Disorders

Stress Management for Women

Women and Addictions

Women of Color and Relationships

PART TWO

Mental Disorders

Anxiety Disorders

INTRODUCTION

A woman sits at an oak desk, her loose-leafed papers spread before her in disarray. She wears a long nightdress and an anxious, distressed expression. She fidgets, sighs, bites her cuticle, gnaws her pencil. She is trying, failing, to fight off the attack of "nervous depression—a slight hysterical tendency" to which she is increasingly prone.

The woman in question is the nameless narrator in Charlotte Perkins Gilman's classic Victorian tale of female subordination, *The Yellow Wallpaper*. She might as well, though, be any one of us—the woman who appears in the glossy drug ad pages of the *American Journal of Psychiatry*, or the one in the television commercial, sitting with furrowed brow while a disembodied voice expounds on the curative properties of a certain medication.

For over a century, anxiety in various guises has been associated with women; not only is the psychological canon replete with anxious women, there is also a lengthy history of locating the cause in women's biology. *Hysteria* means, literally, "wandering uterus," and to this organ's intransigence the ancient Greeks ascribed a host of physical and mental symptoms. According to Hippocrates: "And if you then palpate the uterus, it is not in its proper place; her heart palpitates, she gnashes her teeth, there is copious sweat, and . . . they do all sorts of unheard-of things."

This anatomical view of hysteria persisted, with some variations, for over two millennia. With Freud, however, hysteria migrated from the physiological to the psychic realm. In *Dora: Analysis of a Case of Hysteria,* he posited that hysterical symptoms were caused by unconscious conflicts, that the symptoms themselves expressed those conflicts symbolically, and that treatment would entail making the unconscious conscious through analysis.

For Freud, the unconscious conflict in question was invariably a sexual one. Feminist revisionists, alternatively, have suggested that the manifestations of hysteria—the shortness of breath, palpitations, throat tightness, and weakness—were actually a vivid and accurate rendering of women's voicelessness and powerlessness.

Far apart though they may seem, Freud and his critics agree on one thing: that anxious symptoms originate in the unconscious but are experienced all too consciously by both mind and body. This view of anxiety provides a framework for understanding a wide range of symptoms, from the heart-thumping intensity of a panic attack, to compulsive hand washing, to the fearful isolation of the agoraphobic. A century after Freud, neurobiologists are finding evidence that supports the role of the unconscious in producing anxiety. For instance, stimulation of the amygdala, a brain region associated with emotion and memory, produces a physiological response akin to panic without being precipitated by anything conscious.

The classification of anxiety disorders, as well, began with Freud, who characterized four major clinical syndromes: (1) general irritability; (2) chronic apprehension; (3) anxiety attacks; and (4) phobic avoidance. Still, the tome of psychiatric illness, the *Diagnostic and Statistical Manual* (*DSM*), retained a very diffuse concept of anxiety for most of the nineteenth century. In 1980, the *DSM-III* was published, setting down for the first time the modern classes of anxiety disorders: Panic Disorder, Generalized Anxiety Disorder, Post-Traumatic Stress Disorder, Social Phobia, Obsessive-Compulsive Disorder. Four of these disorders are discussed in this chapter; Post-Traumatic Stress Disorder (PTSD) is covered elsewhere in this text.

> ✦
>
> The classification of anxiety disorders began with Freud, who characterized four major clinical syndromes: (1) general irritability; (2) chronic apprehension; (3) anxiety attacks; and (4) phobic avoidance.

Interestingly, women remain two to three times more likely than men to develop anxiety disorders. What, if we dispense with the theory of uterine intransigence, can account for this difference? The theories set forth to explain the gender imbalance reflect the age-old debate between nature and nurture, between innate and acquired susceptibility to illness. According to the biological determinists, fluctuations in the level of estrogen at various times during a woman's life (menses, pregnancy, menopause), via effects on serotonin and other neurotransmitters, confer a predisposition to both mood and anxiety disorders. Evidence for this theory derives from epidemiological findings that symptoms of anxiety worsen premenstrually as well as postpartum (both periods associated with a rapid decline in estrogen levels). However, estrogen treatment of mood and anxiety disorders has not been conclusively shown to ameliorate symptoms, suggesting a more complex interaction between hormonal shifts and psychological illness.

Those in the biological camp also propose an evolutionary explanation for women's higher level of anxiety. Historically, women who were more vigilant, more closely attuned to their environments were more likely to protect themselves and their children. In this model, fear of certain environments (as in agoraphobia and Social Phobia) might have conferred survival value.

Nonsense, say those in the nurture camp. One need not look beyond women's life experience to explain their increased risk. They point to the increased risk of sexual abuse among women. In fact, women with a history of childhood physical or sexual abuse have a higher risk of both depression and anxiety and have a heightened adrenaline response—in other words, they are more physiologically "primed"—to mild stress.

> ✦
>
> Women remain two to three times more likely than men to develop anxiety disorders.

These critics also note that anxiety is a more acceptable condition in women than it is in men. Women are likely to absorb the anxiety and fearfulness of their partners, becoming the family bearer of worry and tension.

Finally, say the environmentalists, women's entry into the workplace spawned new anxieties about how to negotiate the balance between the personal and the professional. Two decades of feminist revisions to psychological theories have taught us that women develop in relation to others, and that for them, the work-world issues of success and competitiveness, self-esteem and competency can be fraught with difficulty. Surely, this transition alone could account for increased levels of psychological distress.

It is likely the case that all of these elements play a role in heightening women's risk of depression and anxiety, just as likely that we will never ferret out the precise contribution of each. Perhaps the best we can hope for is an awareness that anxiety disorders are complex, multifactorial conditions requiring an integrated approach to treatment.

GENERALIZED ANXIETY DISORDER

Mrs. P., a forty-five-year-old court stenographer, presents to her primary care doctor for complaints of chronic muscle tension, difficulty sleeping, fatigue, and irritability. She has had difficulty concentrating at work and is short-tempered with her family. Her husband adds that she has "always been a worrier" and that she often seems overly distressed about things of minor importance.

The preceding case could describe a woman with depression, or one with any number of medical conditions. Most likely, however, is a diagnosis of Generalized Anxiety Disorder (GAD), a condition characterized by excessive anxiety and worry about a number of life events or circumstances. The subjective feeling of anxiety is accompanied by signs of physical distress; for this reason, many people first go to their family physicians for treatment.

Now, some of us are worriers. When I was born, my mother worried that I would not learn to spell my name, prompting her to switch from a three-syllable to a two-syllable appellation. My great-grandmother in Russia probably worried that rain would fall on her clothesline, or that the house would burn down during the night. It's in our blood.

What sets GAD apart from run-of-the-mill worrying is that the degree of concern is excessive—out of proportion to the context—so that it causes the person distress and interferes with her day-to-day functioning. In fact, according to one study, GAD was associated with more lost workdays than any other condition, including asthma, hypertension, diabetes, arthritis, and Major Depression.

Female gender is a risk factor for GAD; the lifetime risk is 3.6 percent in men, 6.6 percent in women. This difference holds true across cultures as diverse as Brazil and Turkey. The difference emerges early in life; at age six, girls already have a twofold risk compared with boys.

One wonders whether various psychosocial aspects of girls' development might account for this disparity. And indeed, several factors have been shown to increase girls' risk of developing GAD: self-consciousness, lower self-esteem, physical illness, to name a few. But even controlling for these variables, girls remain at higher risk, suggesting a biologic basis.

Data from epidemiological studies show that, in addition to gender, several psychosocial factors are associated with GAD. In particular, ethnic-minority status and low socioeconomic status are correlated with high rates of GAD. Among African American women, the incidence may be as high as 10 percent.

PANIC DISORDER

Mrs. D. is a woman in her forties, married, a secretary in the insurance office of a local hospital. She is brought by her husband to the emergency room because of the abrupt onset of

MODERN CLASSES OF
ANXIETY DISORDERS

Generalized Anxiety Disorder

Panic Disorder

Social Phobia

Obsessive-Compulsive Disorder

Post-Traumatic Stress Disorder

The subjective feeling of anxiety is accompanied by signs of physical distress; for this reason, many people first go to their family physicians for treatment.

difficulty breathing, palpitations, chest pain, and a panicky feeling that she is "going to die." Her husband says that these symptoms came on "out of the blue," just as the family was sitting down to dinner. She has not been sick, nor has she lately seemed anxious or depressed. On examination, her heart rate is rapid, her blood pressure slightly elevated, but otherwise her exam and electrocardiogram are normal.

The hallmark of Panic Disorder is the panic attack. As in the case described here, panic attacks are defined as the abrupt onset of an acutely distressing physical state: palpitations or racing heartbeat, shortness of breath, dizziness, tingling sensations in the hands, nausea, or dizziness. This very physical experience is accompanied by an intense subjective feeling of anxiety or fear; usually, a fear of dying, losing control, or "going crazy." Panic attacks are very discrete events, occurring over several minutes; they may be preceded by a fear-provoking stimulus, such as an exam or job interview, or they may seem to arise spontaneously. Spontaneous panic attacks are perceived as "coming out of the blue," under entirely normal, nonstressful circumstances. To constitute full-blown Panic Disorder, two or more spontaneous panic attacks must have occurred.

> Spontaneous panic attacks are perceived as "coming out of the blue," under entirely normal, nonstressful circumstances. To constitute full-blown Panic Disorder, two or more spontaneous panic attacks must have occurred.

Panic Disorder is often, though not inevitably, accompanied by agoraphobia; this likelihood is higher in women than in men. *Agoraphobia* means, literally, fear of the marketplace. The moniker is interesting in itself, suggesting on the one hand, a phobic avoidance of the public places in which women have traditionally been found; and, on the other, a reluctance to enter the more modern "markets"—for instance, businesses, professional institutions—inhabited by men. In the most extreme cases, agoraphobics are confined to their homes for months or even years; those less severely afflicted leave the home but tend to avoid public places, such as buses, trains, and bridges, from which rapid escape would be impossible.

Panic Disorder, like GAD, is twice as common among women than men (2.3 percent versus 1.0 percent incidence). As with GAD, too, this difference holds true across cultures. In a recent study, rates of Panic Disorder were similar in African American, Hispanic, and white groups, although the rate of agoraphobia was higher among African Americans.

Perhaps because panic attacks are defined by relatively discrete, reproducible physiologic symptoms, they have been extensively studied from a biological perspective. Multiple neurotransmitter systems have been implicated, including serotonin, norepinephrine, and gamma-aminobutyric acid (GABA), the neurotransmitter that induces relaxation and sleep. These neurotransmitters may exert their effects by interfering with the body's internal stress-regulation system. This might explain the effectiveness of a variety of medications in Panic Disorder, as discussed later.

More recently, researchers have postulated a link between biologic and psychosocial precipitants of Panic Disorder. They suggest that a propensity to anxiety may be linked to early parental loss or separation, leading to subsequent problems with attachment. In this model, children with an underlying predisposition to anxiety might suffer a disruption in the parental relationship, leading to a heightened response to future separations or losses.

SOCIAL PHOBIA

Ms. M. is a twenty-five-year-old graduate student in music who presents to her school clinic for help with longstanding social fears. She does well in her assignments, but is so anxious in class that she cannot ask or answer a question. She avoids socializing at school and spends most of her time at home reading or studying. As a child, she was extremely shy and had difficulty transitioning to school. She would like to have friends, but each time she approaches someone to talk, she panics.

The fear of humiliating oneself in public is so ubiquitous that labeling it a disorder might seem inapt. Like a propensity to worry, shyness and self-consciousness are character traits that afflict many, if not most, of us at one time or another. In fact, community studies show that roughly one-third of all people consider themselves to be more anxious than other people in social situations. Such anxiety only crosses the threshold for Social Phobia when it becomes persistent, irrational, and interferes with daily functioning.

The defining feature of Social Phobia is an intense fear of social situations in which a person might act in a humiliating manner. People with Social Phobia tend to avoid public encounters, such as parties, interviews, and restaurants, or to endure them only with great difficulty. They also recognize that their anxiety is out of proportion to the actual situation. Common themes in Social Phobia include fears about meeting new people, making oral presentations, using a public restroom, writing, talking or eating in public.

Social Phobia is often complicated by other conditions, such as depression, Panic Disorder, and agoraphobia. Because these conditions also contribute to social withdrawal (and because sufferers are loathe to come to treatment), Social Phobia can be difficult to diagnose. A key factor is that people with Social Phobia are afraid to interact with *people,* whereas those with agoraphobia are afraid of *environments* or situations from which they cannot easily escape.

The rate of Social Phobia has been variably reported. More recent estimates have placed the lifetime prevalence at 13.3 percent, making it the third most common psychological disorder, after Major Depression (17.1 percent) and alcohol dependence (14.1 percent). Women are more often affected than men, with a ratio of 3:2. Interestingly, al-

> The defining feature of Social Phobia is an intense fear of social situations in which a person might act in a humiliating manner. People with Social Phobia tend to avoid public encounters, such as parties, interviews, and restaurants, or to endure them only with great difficulty.

though women are more likely to have Social Phobia, men are more likely to seek treatment. Some researchers have attributed this discrepancy to gender role typing; they argue that men have traditionally been expected to be more confident and outgoing in social situations than women, therefore reticence would for them cause more impairment and, possibly, more subjective distress. Data from some studies of natural shyness support this theory; shy boys are more likely to suffer social and occupational dysfunction as adults than are shy girls.

OBSESSIVE-COMPULSIVE DISORDER

Mr. B. is a thirty-three-year-old accountant who presents for psychological evaluation because of intrusive, unpleasant thoughts. With great difficulty he reveals to the interviewer that he cannot get the phrase "My hands are dirty" out of his head. He washes his hands thirty times a day; as a result, they are chapped and red. Between the time spent washing and the effort he exerts to resist the compulsion, he estimates that he loses several work hours per day.

By way of the media and popular books, the term *obsessive-compulsive disorder* has acquired a level of public recognition; it elicits a knowing half-smile. Obsessions and compulsions are the sine qua non of neurosis; they are normal behaviors and preoccupations taken to extremes. OCD is defined, in the *DSM-IV*, by the presence of either obsessions (recurrent, persistent thoughts, images, or impulses) or compulsions (repetitive, ritualized behaviors) that are time-consuming, distressing, and that interfere with a person's functioning and relationships.

> OCD is a relatively common disorder, with an incidence of 2 to 3 percent in the United States. Unlike other anxiety disorders, OCD has a gender ratio of nearly 1:1.

Obsessions may include repetitive, negative thoughts, such as "My hands are dirty" or "I didn't lock the door," or they may comprise intrusive, unwelcome images, for example, of sexual assaults or aggressive acts. Common themes for obsessions include cleaning and contamination fears, order and symmetry, counting, sex and aggression, and specific phobias.

Compulsions are defined as behaviors that an individual feels driven to perform and which are aimed at alleviating anxiety. Common compulsions include hand washing or repetitive checking (e.g., to be sure the door is locked, the stove is off). However, compulsions can also be internal: for example, a person who believes he has sinned may compulsively pray. Compulsions can also include complex behaviors. A woman driving a car might be plagued by the thought that she has run someone over. She will stop, retrace her path, anxiously looking for evidence of an accident.

OCD is a relatively common disorder, with an incidence of 2 to 3 percent in the United States. Unlike other anxiety disorders, OCD has a gender ratio of nearly 1:1. In men, the disorder may present earlier, and be associated with greater social and occupational difficulty. Women and men also differ somewhat in symptomatology: Although contamination fears and checking predominate for both sexes, men are more likely to suffer from sexual, symmetry, and exactness obsessions, whereas aggressive obsessions and cleaning compulsions predominate among women.

COMORBIDITY AND OUTCOME

Most anxiety disorders have a persistent, chronic course. Without treatment roughly two-thirds of affected persons will remain symptomatic at five-year follow-up. Additionally, anxiety disorders tend to coexist, both with one another and with a host of other conditions. Major Depression, substance abuse, and eating disorders are often comorbid with anxiety.

TREATMENT

The treatment options for anxiety disorders include psychotherapy, cognitive behavioral therapy (CBT), and pharmacologic options. As therapy options are covered elsewhere in this text, I confine this discussion to pharmacologic treatments.

Benzodiazepines have long been the mainstay of anxiety treatment and are still considered by some to be the treatment of choice for GAD and Panic Disorder. Also called "minor tranquilizers," this class of drugs includes Valium, Xanax, and Klonopin. About three-fourths of patients are effectively treated with these agents. However, the benzodiazepines are more helpful for the physical than the psychic manifestations of anxiety, such as feelings of worry, irritability, and oversensitivity. Also, these drugs have significant side effects, such as sedation, memory problems, and incoordination. Unlike most drugs used in psychiatry, these agents also have the potential for addiction. Because of these risks, clinicians have sought other drugs to manage anxiety.

The SSRIs, or serotonin reuptake inhibitors, were initially developed to treat depression, but their efficacy in treating anxiety disorders was quickly recognized. A number of these drugs are now approved for various anxiety disorders, including Luvox, Zoloft, Prozac, Paxil, and Celexa. For OCD, high doses of SSRIs are now the standard of care. These newer agents lack the addictive potential of the benzodiazepines; they also compare favorably in the area of side effects. The SSRIs are roughly equivalent to the benzodiazepines in their effectiveness for anxiety; unlike these older agents, though, the SSRIs are better at treating psychic than physiologic symptoms.

A number of other drugs have been used as alternatives for those who can't tolerate or don't improve on the benzodiazepines or SSRIs. These drugs include, but are not limited to, Effexor, Buspar, Serzone, and Remeron. Most of these agents are antidepressants with a different method of action than the SSRIs. Older antidepressants, including the tricyclics and MAOIs, have also shown efficacy.

—*Susan Mahler, M.D.*

RELATED ENTRIES

Post-Traumatic Stress Disorder

Eating Disorders and Disconnections

How to Find and Choose a Therapist

Questions to Ask a Psychiatrist

Cognitive Behavioral Therapy

Dialectical Behavioral Therapy

Insight-Oriented Psychotherapy

Depressive Disorders

Depression. The word has become a part of our cultural lexicon, the buzz-word of the late twentieth century. Books on Prozac and its kin proliferate; the media, it seems, cannot get their fill. Even Tony Soprano, television's quintessential tough guy, takes anti-depressant medication. We have become a society both addicted to, and inured to, the illness that is depression.

Maybe this is a problem of terminology. Surely, all of us have felt blue, dejected, down-in-the-dumps. *Depressed* connotes hardly more than that; as William Styron, whose depression nearly cost him his life, put it, this is "a true wimp of a word for such a major illness."

Given these difficulties, how do we tease apart the popular from the pathological, the familiar, rueful experience of sadness from the more fulminant collapse of Major Depression? As clinicians, we rely on specific guidelines in discerning when a deviation from normal emotion becomes a clinical event. But for those who have suffered from Major Depression, for those for whom a certain light oppresses, the experience is less a collection of symptoms than it is a journey into a most inhospitable land.

HISTORICAL OVERVIEW

Depression has been with us for as long as we humans have been sentient. *Melancholia,* as the illness was formerly, and more aptly, called, derives from the Greek for "black bile" and reflects a long-held belief that gloomy temperament predisposed a person to the illness. In fact, introspection and shyness are associated with a somewhat increased risk of depression, but these temperamental features are actually better correlated with a less severe, more protracted mood disorder, Dysthymia.

Still, temperamental issues are relevant. For centuries it has been noted that disorders of mood are frequently associated with an artistic bent. An abbreviated list of writers and artists believed to have suffered from Major Depression includes T. S. Eliot, Emily Dickinson, Virginia Woolf, Sylvia Plath, Edgar Allan Poe, Robert Lowell, William Faulkner, Henry James, Herman Melville, Ernest Hemingway, William Styron, and Georgia O'Keeffe.

What is the link between artistry and depression? It has been suggested that a tendency for introspection, for immersion in the internal landscape of the imagination, is a natural companion to the reticent, if not antisocial, depressive temperament. Perhaps, too, a predisposition toward intense feeling states is a precursor to depression. Also possible is the theory that art, poetry, and music emerge as the creative outlet for the pain of depression, allowing the sufferer not only self-expression, but also a form of triumph over her private demons.

ETIOLOGY

Temperament aside, where do we look for the origins of depression? Freud disapproved of the black bile theory; instead, he postulated the origins of depression in loss, an idea that retains a certain amount of currency. In *Mourning and Melancholia,* Freud drew a parallel between the ordinary process of mourning and the pathological state of clinical depression. In both states, he suggested, an individual suffers the (real or imagined) loss of a loved one. However, the melancholic, unlike the bereaved person, is unable to tolerate this loss. He feels rejected and abandoned, as well as grief-stricken. The feelings of rejection and abandonment, which cannot be ascribed to the lost person, are instead internalized, or "introjected." The individual is subsequently plagued by guilt and self-reproach, the hallmarks of depressive illness.

Freud's version of events correlates well with modern studies of depression. Construing Freud's notion of *loss* to mean early *trauma*—such as abuse, parental illness, the presence of substance abuse, and so forth—we find extensive evidence for a link to depression. The presence of childhood sexual abuse is a clear risk factor for depression in adult life. This increased risk may be a result of lasting changes in brain chemistry, particularly in the system of stress regulation, known as the hypothalamic-pituitary axis (HPA). Not only do depressed people have elevated levels of cortisol, a stress hormone, they also may exhibit a greater response to milder forms of stress in adulthood. Moreover, there is some evidence to suggest that the HPA axis is more reactive to stress in women than in men.

Despite such studies, the precise neurobiology of depression remains elusive. In the 1960s, scientists proposed the first neurochemical model to account for depressive illness. They observed that medications that tended to raise the brain concentration of three neurotransmitters, norepinephrine, serotonin, and dopamine, had a mood-elevating effect; whereas medications that lowered levels of those same substances caused mood depression. They therefore theorized that deficiencies of these neurotransmitters were implicated in the pathophysiology of depression, a theory that came to be known as the *biogenic amine hypothesis.* The tricyclic antidepressants, including Tofranil, Elavil, Norpramin, and Pamelor, were the first drugs marketed for the biological treatment of depression.

The tricyclics act by inhibiting the neurons in the brain from breaking down or reabsorbing neurotransmitters at the receptor sites, allowing these chemicals to exert a more prolonged effect. In particular, the tricylics acted on norepinephrine receptors and, to a lesser degree, serotonin receptors. More recent agents, including Prozac, Paxil, Zoloft, and Celexa, act predominantly on the serotonin system.

The problem with the biogenic amine theory, however, was that, while the neurochemical changes occurred within minutes, the clinical evidence of recovery from depression could take weeks. It is now thought that clinical improvement is correlated not with absolute levels of neurotransmitters, but with a decrease in the numbers of receptors for serotonin and norepinephrine, a change that occurs over a period of several weeks.

What, however, accounts for the biochemical derangement to begin with? Returning to our discussion of the role of trauma and elevated levels of cortisol, we can add to this picture the fact that sustained secretion of cortisol causes long-term changes in the brain, including death or inhibition of existing neurons and suppression of neurogenesis, the production of new nerve cells.

Several novel studies have shown that antidepressants, as well as electroconvulsive therapy (ECT), may prevent or reverse some of these changes. If these studies are confirmed, they may redefine our understanding of the etiology of depression, with important implications for the development of new treatments.

CLINICAL FEATURES

Perhaps the most compelling evidence that depression is a physical illness comes from observing affected persons. Hippocrates (A.D. 460–370 B.C.) described the state of melancholia as "an aversion to food, despondency, sleeplessness, irritability and restlessness." He might as well have been reading from the *DSM-IV*, as he cited four of the modern diagnostic criteria for Major Depression: sad or depressed mood, insomnia, loss of energy, and loss of appetite. In addition to these symptoms, the checklist also includes poor concentration, anhedonia, feelings of worthlessness or guilt, and thoughts of suicide. Five of these criteria must be fulfilled, over a period of at least two weeks, for a diagnosis of Major Depression to be made. These conditions are elaborated in the following sections.

Depressed Mood Unlike normal sadness, the melancholy of depression is often unprovoked by external events. The sadness is persistent, unremitting, unresponsive to changes in the environment. Similarly, happy circumstances have little effect on the depressed person. A peculiar, somatic quality has been ascribed to the pain of depression. Styron has written, "The gray drizzle of horror induced by depression takes on the quality of physical pain." Alternatively, some individuals describe feeling numb rather than sad.

Insomnia The sleep disturbance in Major Depression has many manifestations. There may be early morning awakening, or frequent awakenings throughout the night. Sleep is experienced as fragmented and unrefreshing. In other cases, depressed persons report excessive sleep, called hypersomnia.

Changes in Energy Depressed people may report both a decrease in energy (anergia) and a simultaneous increase in agitation, restlessness, or irritability. The anergia of depression is often experienced as a "leaden paralysis," which makes the smallest activities (taking a shower, talking on the phone) onerous and exhausting. Mental activity is also experienced as being torpid and ineffectual. Often these people appear physically slowed down, with slumping shoulders, inexpressiveness, and slowed speech.

Appetite Changes Classically, depression is associated with a failure to eat, also called anorexia. This may be related to decreased appetite, blunted taste sensations, or inadequate energy to prepare food. Some people eat normally but describe an inability to enjoy food. Appetite may also be increased, particularly in younger people and women, sometimes accompanied by carbohydrate cravings. Both weight loss and weight gain are common in depression.

Concentration Along with slowed thought processes, poor concentration is a hallmark of a depressive episode. Individuals report that they are no longer able to read a book, study, or work effectively, or even to watch television. Not only impaired thinking but also ideas of guilt or self-reproach may interfere with concentration.

Anhedonia *Anhedonia* means "loss of pleasure," and this, perhaps more than anything else, describes the experience of Major Depression. Concurrent with an enhanced ability to feel pain is a complete inability to access pleasurable feelings. People report that they are unable to enjoy the very things that used to give them the most pleasure, such as their children, hobbies, music, books. They see in the world around them only further evidence of their own pain and feel cut off from people who seem to be engaged and vital. Perhaps Shakespeare's Hamlet put it best: "How weary, stale, flat and unprofitable seem to me all the uses of the world" (Act I, Scene II).

Feelings of Inappropriate Guilt People in the throes of depression may not report feeling guilty *per se*, but on questioning it is clear that they spend much of their time ruminating on mistakes they have made, inadequacies, lost opportunities, and perceived failures. In some cases they describe feeling as though they are being punished for past wrongs.

Suicidal Thoughts Thoughts of suicide, called suicidal ideation, occur in up to two-thirds of people with severe depression. Fortunately, only a fraction of these attempt suicide, and of these, fewer still succeed. Risk factors associated with suicide are covered in further detail subsequently. It is imperative, however, to ask depressed people specifically about thoughts of and plans for suicide. There is no evidence that asking about suicide precipitates an attempt; in contrast, there is considerable evidence that concerned questioning saves lives.

The preceding are the clinical features of both typical and atypical Major Depression. Typical depression usually results in loss of appetite and decreased sleep; whereas atypical depression is oftentimes accompanied by weight gain and excessive sleep. Both typical and atypical major depressions are thought to be different facets of the same prismatic picture, and both respond to treatment. It is thought that women suffer more frequently from atypical depressions.

EPIDEMIOLOGY

Major Depression is the most common of all mental disorders in Western populations. The lifetime prevalence in the United States is 21.3 percent for women, 12.7 percent for men. This striking difference in risk emerges in adolescence and persists through midlife. A number of theories have been put forward to explain the gender imbalance, including hormonal factors, differences in reporting of symptoms, victimization, gender role, and life stress. While the gender imbalance holds true across cultures, the difference is less pronounced in some non-U.S. populations. Although ethnicity does not seem to be implicated, lower socioeconomic status is a risk factor for depression. It is important to note, however, that differences in diagnosis—for instance, a bias toward a diagnosis of schizophrenia, rather than mood disorders, among African Americans—may delay treatment for Major Depression among minorities. Urban residence is also a risk factor, as is unemployment.

Marital status has clearly emerged as a risk factor for depression. Rates of Major Depression are highest among people of both sexes who are separated or divorced. However, single women have a lower rate of depression than do single men. In addition, persons living alone have double the rate of depression of those living with others. Taken together,

CRITERIA FOR A DIAGNOSIS OF MAJOR DEPRESSION

Five of the following criteria must be fulfilled over a period of at least two weeks:

+ *Sad or depressed mood*
+ *Insomnia*
+ *Loss of energy*
+ *Loss of appetite*
+ *Poor concentration*
+ *Anhedonia (the inability to feel pleasure)*
+ *Feelings of worthlessness or guilt*
+ *Thoughts of suicide*

these findings suggest that it may not be marital status *per se* that predisposes to Major Depression, but rather the availability of supports and adequacy of relationships.

Despite a good deal of overlap, depression may present somewhat differently in women than in men. Women tend to become ill earlier than men, with an average age of onset in the late twenties. They may be more apt to develop a seasonal pattern to their symptoms. They also present with more "atypical" symptoms, namely, increased (rather than decreased) appetite and sleep. They may show more variability in mood in response to social situations, a phenomenon called "mood reactivity."

Hormonal factors seem to be implicated to some extent in Major Depression. Depressive episodes are more likely to occur during the premenstrual period, and preexisting depressive symptoms may worsen during this time. About 20 percent of women experience depressive symptoms during pregnancy and 10 to 15 percent experience postpartum depression. However, the rate of depression does not increase after menopause, suggesting that it is not estrogen deficiency but rather hormonal shifts that contribute to higher rates of depression.

Genetics clearly play a role. Major Depression is two to three times more common in the first-degree biological relatives of affected people than in the general population. Twin studies show that there is a 50 percent concordance rate in identical twins, compared with a 20 percent concordance rate in fraternal twins. However, no single gene has been associated with depression, and it is likely that the genetics of depression are complex.

Although some people experience a single major depressive episode, more commonly the illness recurs. On average, the number of episodes in an individual's lifetime is five to six. Given that these episodes last roughly six months, it becomes rapidly clear that this is a disabling condition that can claim years of a person's life. Add to this the fact that some individuals remain depressed for years, and that many others recover incompletely, and the picture becomes even more dire. Most people with Major Depression never get appropriate treatment, a tragic situation given the wide availability and efficacy of treatments.

Management of Major Depression usually includes medications, sometimes combined with psychotherapy. Medications, which include the SSRIs, tricyclic antidepressants, and newer "hybrid" agents, are effective for 45 to 60 percent of patients. People who fail to improve on one drug have a 50 percent chance of recovery when switched to a different class of drugs.

In general, the SSRIs are used first, because of a lower incidence of side effects and relative safety from overdose. Women in particular may respond better to SSRIs, while men may respond better to tricyclic antidepressants. Those with atypical symptoms also respond preferentially to the SSRIs. A third class of medications, called monoamine oxidase inhibitors, is usually considered a third-tier choice, because of the need for dietary restrictions and the potential for dangerous interactions. However, these drugs are often effective when other medications have failed.

Psychotherapy has been shown to be effective in treating depression, particularly in combination with medications. Both cognitive behavioral and dynamic (interpersonal) therapies have been used, with equal efficacy. However, for severe cases of depression, medication is clearly indicated. Many people who are profoundly depressed are unable to use therapy effectively; once treated with medication, these same people become actively engaged in therapy.

Electroconvulsive therapy, or ECT, is a treatment that has understandably acquired an ominous, if not downright grisly, reputation. Dating to 1934, before the use of effective medications, the treatment was originally used to treat psychosis. However, as the technique was refined, it became clear that ECT was highly effective for both depression and mania. Currently, the treatment is used in a number of circumstances: when medications have failed, when medications are contraindicated (e.g., in the medically ill), when there has been a prior response to ECT, or when there is an acute risk of suicide. The response rate to ECT is 70 percent, making it the most effective treatment available for depression. Just how it works is unclear; current belief is that the administration of electrical current causes lasting changes in brain chemistry. As it is used today, the procedure is extremely safe, the most common side effect being memory loss, which is usually short-lived.

RELATED DISORDERS

Dysthymia Dysthymia can be difficult to distinguish from Major Depression. Like depression, it is associated with a low mood, despondency, fatigue, and disinterest. Unlike those with Major Depression, however, people with Dysthymic Disorder tend to complain of long-standing, chronic depression. They are unable to recall a distinct shift in mood symptoms; instead, such individuals report that they have felt this way "my whole life."

The criteria for Dysthymic Disorder reflect this emphasis on chronicity; the symptoms must have been present for a minimum of two years. Key features include changes in appetite and sleep, low energy, low self-esteem, poor concentration, and feelings of hopelessness. Note here the overlap with Major Depression, with less emphasis on physical symptoms and the absence of suicidal thoughts. The illness is possibly best characterized as a long-standing, low-grade depression, with fluctuations in symptoms. However, about 20 percent of those with Dysthymia go on to develop Major Depression, a condition that is sometimes called "double depression." Dysthymia affects about 3 percent of the population, women twice as often as men.

People with Dysthymia most often are able to function adequately. However, they are often perceived to be gloomy and brooding characters, those for whom "the glass is always half empty." To this extent, Dysthymia seems to be, at least partially, a matter of personality style or temperament. Unlike Major Depression, it does not respond robustly to medication, although antidepressants are sometimes helpful.

Cyclothymia Cyclothymia is generally considered to be a mild form of Bipolar Disorder. Essentially, these individuals suffer from mild depressions and mild elevations in mood, over a long period of time, which do not meet full criteria for either Major Depression or mania. The changes in mood may occur abruptly and often, sometimes within hours, causing considerable disruption and distress. People with cyclothymia often feel out of control of their moods, and those around them find them argumentative and unpredictable.

The treatment of cyclothymia is challenging; as many as half of those treated with antidepressants develop manic or hypomanic symptoms. The best-documented treatment for cyclothymia is lithium, a mood stabilizer.

SUICIDE

Suicide is now the eighth leading cause of death in the United States; about 15 percent of all those with Major Depression eventually commit suicide. Fully half of all suicides occur among those with a primary depressive disorder; other high-risk conditions include alcoholism, anxiety disorders, schizophrenia, and bipolar disorder. Demographically, the risk of suicide increases with age; the elderly comprise 25 percent of suicide victims, though they account for only 10 percent of the population. This fact notwithstanding, among individuals age fifteen to twenty-four, suicide is the third leading cause of death.

There is a complicated relationship between ethnicity and suicide rates. Historically, rates have been lower among minority groups, possibly because of greater cohesiveness and social prohibitions against suicide. However, the rate among African Americans is increasing, and among inner-city youth, the risk of suicide far surpasses the national rate.

Women attempt suicide at roughly twice the rate of men. However, men are more lethal in their attempts; twice as many men as women will succeed in killing themselves. In the past, it was theorized that men's higher death rate was attributable to the use of more lethal, "all-or-nothing" means, such as shooting, hanging, and carbon monoxide. However, the most common means of suicide for both sexes is drug overdose. Moreover, the use of firearms among female suicide victims is increasing. More recently, it has been suggested that women's cognitive style might be protective against suicide. That is, women are more apt to be embedded in relationships and to make decisions based on a wide range of concerns than are men. For them, the decision to commit suicide may be more ambivalent, less impulsive. On the other hand, this very same style of functioning might account for women's higher risk of depressive illness. For women (but not men) the risk of developing depression is increased by the presence of stressful events among those around them.

About 10 percent of those who attempt suicide will make a repeat attempt in the next two years. And about one in eighteen attempters will ultimately complete suicide. Two-thirds of suicide victims have had psychiatric treatment during the past year, a figure that is humbling, if not downright embarrassing, to health professionals. However, the majority of those who complete suicide are not in treatment at the time of death. It has often been noted that suicide among depressed people occurs, not at the nadir of illness, but in the early days of recovery. At this time, it is thought, the person has enough energy to take action, while not yet feeling well enough to want to live.

—*Susan Mahler, M.D.*

Bipolar Disorder

It is easy for me to understand why there is a tendency to romanticize manic-depression. The people I know who struggle with bipolar disorder, as the illness is now more officially known, are those that have most captured my imagination and attention in life.

This is not to say that bipolar disorder *should* be romanticized. Many painful misunderstandings about the disastrous consequences of this illness have occurred as a result of our tendency to put a high gloss on the suffering wrought by mental illness. Bipolar disorder is especially vulnerable to that gloss because it is characterized by both vibrant expressiveness as well as black despair, and both moods can be captivating—as well as devastating. This cycle can make the illness an addictive torture for the person who suffers from it. Bipolar disorder catapults a person between the two "poles," or extremes, of his or her personality —the highs and the lows.

During the highs, a person can range from feeling energized (often referred to as "hypomania")—productive at work or fiery and charming at a dinner party—to losing touch almost completely with reality. On the extreme end, mania can lead to hallucinating or bingeing (on sleeplessness, shopping, or sex), or becoming fearful enough to believe, as a friend of mine in the grips of this illness did, that one's own family is secretly made up of actors hired to play the roles of loved ones. Mania can offer a departure from earthbound daily life and is often recalled by sufferers as rapturous, magical, intoxicating. The psychosis brought on by extreme mania, however, is not considered enjoyable as it pushes a person one step beyond elation into a darker, more frightened state.

Mania almost always swings back on itself, like a mood pendulum, into depression. The low of bipolar disorder is not unlike the despair of unipolar major depressive disorder. Both are indicated by the same checklist of symptoms: persistent sadness; loss of interest or pleasure in activities that were once enjoyed; significant changes in appetite or body weight; difficulty sleeping or sleeping too much; loss of energy; feelings of worthlessness or inappropriate guilt; difficulty thinking or concentrating; and recurrent thoughts of death or suicide. The sadness brought on by major depressive disorder, however, does not have a partner emotion, like mania. Bipolar disorder also presents particular feelings of guilt and shame experienced by the sufferer who recalls—sometimes only in fragments—his or her past manic behavior.

The patterns and severity of the high and low episodes determine different types of bipolar disorder. Bipolar I, the most severe form of this illness, is indicated, in an outline set forth by the *Diagnostic and Statistical Manual of Mental Disorders, Fourth Edition* (*DSM-IV*), by the occurrence of one or more manic episodes (which frequently include hallucinations and extreme paranoia) or mixed episodes (rapidly alternating feelings of mania and depression that last for at least a week). In addition, the person also experiences one or more major depressions. Bipolar II disorder is similarly expressed by one or more depressive episodes, but the "high" cycle presents itself as hypomania, a version that results in agitation but rarely in delusions or hallucinations. Bipolar disorder with "rapid cycling" is defined as four or more mood episodes, in any combination or order within a year.

Patients struggling with bipolar are often misdiagnosed. According to the *DSM-IV*, some clinicians may misdiagnose bipolar disorder as schizophrenia in varying ethnic groups and in younger people. In fact, the manic behavior of Bipolar I—hallucinations, paranoia, delusions, believing one is divinely inspired—is nearly indistinguishable from the manner of schizophrenia. Clinicians rely on varying methods to tell the difference.

First, if the patient responds to lithium, the illness is determined to be bipolar. In this sense, lithium, which is the medication most frequently used to treat bipolar disorder, also acts as an interpreter for clinicians. Secondly, bipolar and schizophrenia are differentiated by the emotion, or lack thereof, that informs the mania. If the patient's hallucinations and delusions are expressed with expansive emotions such as happiness or even fear, then the mania is considered "mood congruent" and the diagnosis is likely to be bipolar disorder. If the psychotic symptoms are devoid of mood—if the patient seems flat or emotionless—the patient is considered "mood incongruent" and the diagnosis is likely to be schizophrenia.

Interestingly, bipolar disorder also gives a certain feeling of contagiousness; people close to the patient speak of feeling a similar edginess and raciness to that of the mania of the patient. Clinicians sometimes rely on this instinct to guide them toward a diagnosis of bipolar disorder. Since the diagnosis for these mood disorders cannot be made physiologically— for example, by a blood test—the assessment must be made by this rather old-fashioned system using intuition and judgment. In order to define the problem, clinicians must study the patient's response to medications, symptoms, and family history. Studies have shown that people with first-degree biological relatives with Bipolar I or II have elevated rates of both bipolar disorder and depression as compared to the general population. In addition, findings from family, twin, and adoption studies have strongly demonstrated that genetic factors create a vulnerability to the illness.

> The major clinical problem in treating bipolar disorder is not that medications are ineffective but rather that patients often resist taking them.

Although bipolar disorder seems utterly unique in the midst of its expression, more than 2.3 million adult Americans struggle with the illness. Its onset most commonly occurs in late adolescence (some experts more specifically cite the average age as eighteen), but it is possible for the illness to manifest itself at any time. Men and women suffer at the same rate: unlike major depression, which affects twice as many women as men, bipolar is evenly distributed between the sexes. Men, however, usually begin with a manic episode whereas women tend toward depression initially. The disorder also exists indiscriminately among all races, ethnic groups, and social classes.

Research on the cause of bipolar disorder continues to deepen. More answers are expected in the near future from scientists studying the genes and neural circuits in the brain that may determine the illness. There are also researchers studying the nongenetic environmental factors, such as stress and environment, that contribute to the disorder. In the meantime, the best explanation is that brain abnormalities as well as the structure and function of certain brain circuits are the underlying cause of this mood disorder.

While it has not been found that the illness ever actually goes away once discovered, it can be successfully treated with medication in the majority of cases. Bipolar disorder with rapid cycling, however, is often more resistant to treatment than non-rapid-cyling bipolar disorder. Lithium, as mentioned earlier, is generally considered the most effective pharmacological method for controlling mania and depression and reducing the likelihood of recurrence. But lithium doesn't work for everyone and can cause uncomfortable side effects, such as weight gain, tremor, frequent urination, and nausea. Other mood-stabilizing medications (covered elsewhere in this book) have been used to treat this illness effectively.

The major clinical problem in treating bipolar disorder, however, is not that medications are ineffective but rather that patients often resist taking them. One of the great ironies of bipolar disorder is that it offers such intense emotion, it distracts the sufferer from the realization that these feelings come at a steep price. The price, indeed, is sometimes life itself: it has been found that, without treatment, the illness can lead to suicide in nearly 10 to 15 percent of cases in both Bipolar I and II. (Sadly, the illness can hold a person in its sway until enough havoc has been wreaked to sufficiently persuade the sufferer that it's worth balancing one's moods.)

Studies have recently shown that the combination of psychotherapy and medication results in greater improvement than either treatment alone. The rate of response is approximately 60 versus 40 percent. Family members also play an important role in controlling the illness. Many people with bipolar disorder have spoken and written about being helped immensely by the unyielding support of their intimates. "Trapped in the dead body of depression, I was able to find relief in touch—the touch of friends and family who wanted to keep me from hurting myself," my own sister, Maud Casey, once wrote about her struggle with bipolar disorder. "[A childhood friend's] touch reminded me of the power of wordless physical connection, of what I would lose if I died." Beyond providing this vital glimpse of comfort and safety, family members can also help in practical ways. It is important to learn about the illness so as to recognize the symptoms when they appear. Often sufferers cannot discern symptoms for themselves when they are caught in the cycle of this mood disorder. Studies have in fact shown that approximately 50 percent of patients with acute mania do not realize they are experiencing manic symptoms. Families should involve themselves, when possible, in helping their relative receive and understand the appropriate diagnosis and treatment, which includes securing a good therapist and psychopharmacologist. In addition, a person struggling with bipolar disorder might want to set an emergency plan, while in good health, with a close friend or family member detailing what should be done if a manic or depressive episode descends. This plan should include such information as how to contact the person's doctor and when and if, as well as where, the person would like to be hospitalized.

In my own life, I have seen friends and family members through the racing terror of mania, the subsequent grind of depression, and finally the resolution that they must find a way to live with bipolar disorder. I have also seen these people achieve health and vitality again through the varying resources that are available to them—therapy, medication, and human connection. Bipolar disorder is an undoubtedly dramatic and terrifying illness, but the hope for recovery grows consistently stronger than the pull toward darkness.

—*Nell Casey*

RELATED ENTRIES

Mood Stabilizers

Antidepressants

Depressive Disorders

Polypharmacy

Post-Traumatic Stress Disorder

The image of the typical Vietnam veteran is familiar—a promising young man is shipped abroad to fight in a questionable war. After his tour of duty, he returns home to the United States, but instead of the homecoming celebration that most young men expected when they enrolled or were drafted, he endures the humiliation of defeat, criticism from peers, and a feeling that he doesn't belong. Broken by this negative reception and by the images of war, he withdraws from his community and his family. He does not believe others can understand his experience; he appears jumpy and startles easily; he cannot sleep at night, awakening repeatedly with recurring nightmares. His life is a daily battle; he becomes depressed, and often he escapes into drugs or alcohol. He has Post-Traumatic Stress Disorder, or PTSD.

Post-Traumatic Stress Disorder has been part of the human experience for generations. During much of the twentieth century, PTSD was known as shell shock or war neurosis and was seen frequently in men returning from battle. Shell shock and war neuroses happened to men, not to women—until approximately twenty-five years ago.

The feminist moment of the late 1960s and 1970s allowed women to talk about their traumatic experiences in a real way. They talked of sexual abuse as children, they talked about rape as adult women, they talked about domestic violence—beatings from husbands and boyfriends, fathers and stepfathers. Many had spent a lifetime in battle. The traumas they shared with each other were often at least as enduring as those experienced by men in war times, but they were hidden secrets of a patriarchal society.

Prior to the seventies, these women who were betrayed by their most intimate family members were labeled as hysterical and the mental health community often dismissed their stories of abuse as fantasy. Instead of being treated for PTSD symptoms, these women were silenced and condemned to isolation.

Today, the research into Post-Traumatic Stress Disorder is extensive and includes human responses to a wide array of traumas, including childhood abuse (physical and sexual abuse and emotional neglect), domestic violence, natural disasters, war experiences, sexual and physical assault, terrorism, and motor vehicle accidents. Essentially, the diagnosis can be made if a person has been exposed to a life-threatening experience or has witnessed another person in a life-threatening situation (see table 1) and has symptoms of hyperarousal, numbness, and intrusive memories of the event. While the extent of trauma to any individual is a highly subjective experience, the diagnosis is reserved for those who have had an overwhelming experience and who chronically relive this experience.

While PTSD affects an individual in many areas of her life, the most debilitating effects can be the destruction of relationships. Many survivors of violence feel intense longings for safe connections with others, but the longings are often accompanied by other extreme feelings, such as the terror of being violated again, rage at past perpetrators or violations, or despair at feeling alone and overwhelmed.

SYMPTOMS AND EFFECTS OF PTSD

The chronic symptoms of PTSD are reexperiencing the violation through nightmares, flashbacks, or intrusive memories. These reexperiences can be triggered by the emotional vulnerability needed to form more intimate relationships. Closeness with another person can feel violating even when the person understands intellectually that little threat exists.

These contradictory messages make relationships very confusing for the person suffering with PTSD. The response to the perceived threat may be to become afraid and to flee relationships, to feel anger, to feel the need to fight continually to protect yourself, or to feel over-

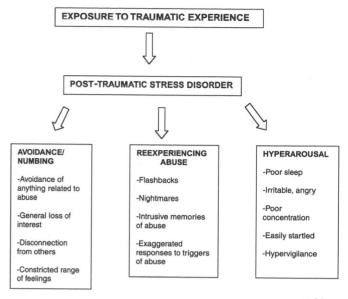

Table 1

whelmed, frozen, and powerless in relationships. Survivors who were violated in childhood often had little chance to experience healthy relationships as a child, and they therefore may find it difficult as an adult to identify safe people—some survivors find themselves in disrespectful, even violent relationships again and again.

This chaotic relational pattern is difficult for both the traumatized individual and the person with whom he or she is trying to relate. Many women with this pattern of relationships have been diagnosed with borderline personality disorder. The vast majority of individuals who have been labeled "borderline" have had significant relational disconnections throughout their lives; many have suffered childhood abuse. There is a stigma attached to this diagnosis. Women with it are seen as too needy, out of control, difficult to manage. In fact, researchers have documented that when individuals carry this diagnosis, clinicians respond to them in a more angry, punitive way. For all of these reasons, borderline personality disorder is a diagnosis I do not use. I have found it more helpful to understand the erratic behaviors as resulting from the dysregulated brain chemistry that seems to coincide with early childhood traumas.

Many people exposed to violence develop coping strategies such as eating disorders, drug or alcohol abuse, or self-mutilation to manage the symptoms of PTSD. Though these strategies feel protective, they also make it even more difficult for the individuals to reach out to others for help or comfort and instead keep survivors locked in "condemned isolation."

UNDERSTANDING PTSD

On September 11, 2001, Pam was in the south tower of the World Trade Center when the north tower was struck. There was a period of confusion before the second plane hit her building: People inside the building learned that there had been a plane crash, and first they were told that they needed to evacuate their building. Then a second message came, saying things were okay and they could stay where they were. Then the final panic hit when the sec-

ond plane crashed into their building. Some people were leaving, some people were return-ing, and everyone was fearful and confused. Pam made it out safely, but many, many of her friends died that day.

She was back to work within a week at a makeshift office in New Jersey; most of her col-leagues admired this, but she felt disconnected from them. She did not know what else to do. She was sleeping poorly and using alcohol to overcome tenseness; she increased her dosage of antidepressant, hoping that would ease the overwhelming desire to stay in bed, to retreat from everything. She felt distant and remote from even her closest friends.

It had been a long year since that traumatic day. Pam was looking forward to going to Maine, where she would join a few of her close friends from New York City for some rest and relaxation for a couple of weeks at the end of the summer. They would be in Rockland during the annual Lobster Festival. Pam envisioned eating many lobster rolls, taking quiet walks on the beach, listening to music.

As she approached the gate to the festival, she began to feel slightly lightheaded and a fa-miliar anxiety began to grow in her chest. The chaos, all the people, loud noises—chaotic places always brought the experience of September 11 back to her again and again; it never went away.

Human-sized lobsters, each decorated by a local artist, were scattered throughout the city, with a large concentration at the community green in the center of town. Pam walked to the green to get away from the crowd, from the confusion. She admired the artwork—there was the New England Patriot football player lobster, the Spiderman lobster, and even a lobster paying tribute to September 11 and the terrorist attacks. It was decorated with burning twin towers. She stared at it and felt nothing.

Pam suffers from PTSD.

Our society struggles to understand why bad things happen to good people, and we struggle even more to understand what effect traumas have on an individual's brain and body. It used to be that the person who developed shell shock was considered damaged or at fault in some way.

The feminist movement in the seventies with its focus on exposing and ending violence against women offered an alternative way of looking at trauma symptoms. The theory from the rape crisis movement was that it was not the reaction but rather the trauma that was ab-normal. This shifted the blame away from the traumatized person back to the perpetrator, where it belonged. While this was an important step in decreasing the amount of shame and stigma attached to the victim of the trauma, it may not be accurate.

Today's definition of PTSD remains empathic with the victims of trauma but also tries to understand the reactions of people who have been traumatized. And it is clear that not everyone who has had a life-threatening event develops chronic PTSD. Most people (75 percent) exposed to trauma will have an acute stress response that resolves within six months. Those people who do develop chronic PTSD are having a unique reaction to an ab-normal event.

Researchers are trying to understand this incredibly complex illness, and the body of re-search results is growing. There are certain situations that tend to be predictive of a person developing PTSD. These include (1) trauma at an early age, (2) chronic trauma, (3) violence from family or known individuals, and (4) severe trauma. Adults who have had a history of trauma earlier in their lives have a higher chance of developing PTSD if they are retraumatized as adults, even if they did not develop PTSD from the first trauma event. One intriguing research finding is that an appropriate, compassionate response to a trauma in childhood can have a dramatic positive impact on a child's ability to heal from a trauma and to avoid chronic PTSD.

THE NEUROBIOLOGY OF PTSD

So far, there have been many interesting findings about the neurobiology of PTSD. Nothing has yet to answer the classic "which came first, the chicken or the egg?" question: Are the differences seen in patients with PTSD the result of the trauma or do they predate the trauma? Not surprisingly, there are, however, clear findings of a disrupted stress response system.

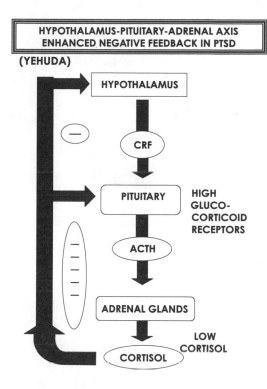

The stress response has two arms: One arm is the sympathetic nervous system, part of the central nervous system; and the other arm is the hypothalamic-pituitary-adrenal (HPA) axis. Rachel Yehuda is one of the foremost researchers in the field of PTSD studies. Her research has focused on dysregulation of the HPA axis. Humans have sympathetic nerves running throughout their bodies and brains. These nerves are stimulated in times of stress to release norepinephrine (adrenaline), which travels to many organs, preparing a person for flight or to fight during an acute stress situation. The norepinephrine helps to divert blood away from nonessential flight-or-fight organs, such as the stomach, and to divert it to large muscles and the heart to help the body prepare to confront the immediate challenge.

Figure 1

Most essential systems in the human body are balanced by another system that helps to modulate response. The stress response is balanced by the HPA axis. Though the hypothalamus and pituitary (both located in the brain) excrete many hormones and chemicals, it is the hormones and chemicals that lead to the production of the antistress hormone cortisol that is most important to the stress response system.

This antistress system starts with the release of cortisol-releasing factor (CRF) from the hypothalamus. CRF travels to the pituitary gland, stimulating the release of adrenocorticotropin hormone, which travels to the adrenal glands, causing the production and release of cortisol. Cortisol then feeds back on the sympathetic nervous system and turns off the release of norepinephrine. With this loop, the stress response is self-regulated.

Based on this model, one would expect that both norepinephrine and cortisol levels would increase during a time of acute stress. Interestingly, Yehuda and others have found, cortisol levels in people who suffer with PTSD are actually low at the time of the trauma rather than high (see figure 1). This results in a lower ability to buffer stress, meaning that for those individuals with PTSD, even small traumas have a rather large effect.

The research model of "inescapable shock" can be helpful in understanding what this dysregulated chemistry looks like. Though this is a model based on research on animals, many feel that it may closely replicate what is happening in the human body under chronic stress. In this model, a rat is repeatedly exposed to a mild shock without the ability to escape it. At first the rat tries to avoid the shock. But over time, the animal develops a "learned helplessness" and does not even try to escape; this response can be explained by looking closely at the actual nerve cells and neurotransmitters involved.

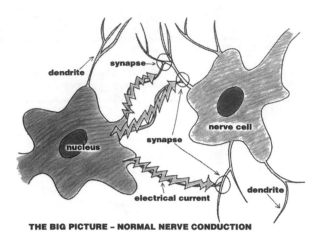

THE BIG PICTURE – NORMAL NERVE CONDUCTION

Figure 2

Feelings, thoughts, and movements occur in the body when nerves communicate with each other. In the brain, communication happens when an electrical message travels down the arm of one nerve to deliver its message to a second nerve across a synapse (see figure 2). The synapse is the meeting of two nerve endings in your body or brain (see figure 3).

In the brain, an electrical current is translated into a chemical message at the synapse. These chemicals, called neurotransmitters, are held in small vesicles in the presynaptic nerve endings. The electrical message causes a release of neurotransmitters into the space between two nerve endings. In order for the message to be transmitted, these neurotransmitters must connect with a receptor on the receiving nerve ending.

The brain prefers a relatively even flow of neurotransmitters through the intersynaptic space. Complex feedback systems regulate the flow of messages through the nerves. If the environment is too stressful, too many neurotransmitters are released in the intersynaptic space. Over time, the number of postsynaptic receptors decreases, making it more difficult for a neurotransmitter to connect with a receptor. This decrease in postsynaptic receptors is called down-regulation (see figure 4).

If there is too little stimulation, only a few neurotransmitters are released into the intersynaptic space. In order to increase the chance that each neurotransmitter finds a receptor, the brain increases the number of postsynaptic receptors. This increase in postsynaptic receptors is called up-regulation (see figure 5).

In chronic PTSD, the brain loses its ability to regulate important neurotransmitters. Imagine a child growing up in a violent home. The extremes of stress and fear initially cause a massive outpouring of neurotransmitters into the intersynaptic space. The brain will try to control the large flow of neurotransmitters by down-regulating the postsynaptic receptors—an attempt to "turn down the volume."

With continued violence, the warning messages keep flowing; but eventually, the neurotransmitters temporarily run out. The brain recognizes this depletion of neurotransmitters and will up-regulate the postsynaptic receptors. In chronic PTSD, the postsynaptic receptors get "stuck" in the up-regulated state. When the brain is again able to make adequate neurotransmitters, it does not adjust to the increase by decreasing the number of postsynaptic receptors.

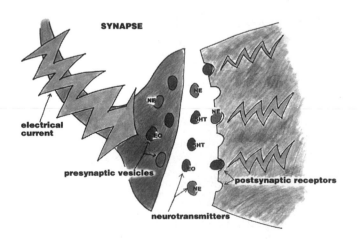

Figure 3

When a person is able to make a normal amount of neurotransmitters and then is overstimulated, large numbers of neurotransmitters are released into the intersynaptic space. Since the postsynaptic receptors are up-regulated, most of the neurotransmitters connect with a receptor. This is like amplification from turning the volume up full blast (see figure 6).

With PTSD there are alternating patterns of neurotransmitter depletion and overstimulation. These correlate with the erratic relational picture described for survivors. When flooded with chemicals, a person may react to small stimuli as if retraumatized; she may feel terrified of people around her. When depleted of neurotransmitters, she feels emotionally shutdown, with no interest or energy to reach out and connect. As even small stimuli get "amplified," people with PTSD repeatedly feel as though the violence is currently happening. They are literally chemically "locked" in the past.

In the last five years or so, researchers are beginning to measure the actual functioning of the brain through positron emission tomography (PET) scans. Although this work is still in the very early stages, there are a few curious findings:

1. There may be a decrease in hippocampal volume in some people with PTSD. The hippocampus is the area within the limbic (emotional) brain that helps one put danger signals within a context, to differentiate threats. It may be that a decrease in the size of the hippocampus indicates that this crucial area of the brain is not working effectively in PTSD—which may help explain the many observed behavior patterns of people with PTSD, including that they often are revictimized throughout their lives.
2. The amygdala in people with PTSD seems to be overactive. The amygdala is the limbic system of the brain where emotions are created. The amygdala sends danger signals—in people with PTSD it is more active than in those without PTSD. Therefore, the former's brains may send danger signals even when there is little threat of danger.
3. The frontal lobe of the brain may be underactive. One role of the frontal cortex is to help modulate the amygdala. With the frontal lobe functioning less effectively, the amygdala is able to send off "louder," more frequent messages.

This research shows that there are many areas of the brain and body that are dysregulated in the condition of PTSD. All of these imbalances conspire to keep a person with PTSD locked in a perpetual state of reliving traumas.

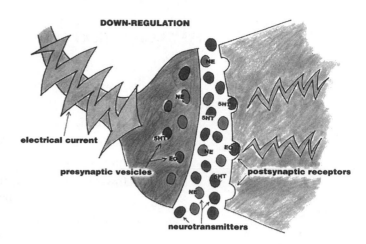

Figure 4

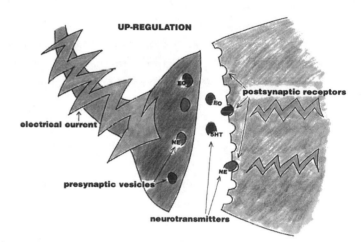

Figure 5

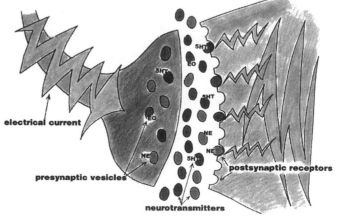

Figure 6

TREATMENT OPTIONS FOR PTSD

PTSD symptoms can be treated with a number of different modalities—cognitive behavioral therapy, trauma-focused individual and group therapy, and Eye Movement Desensitization and Reprocessing (EMDR). However, the key to healing this disorder is stabilizing the erratic brain chemistry so that individuals are then able to suspend their terror and enter into safe relationships in which healing can occur.

Psychotropic medications can be very helpful in stabilizing the dysregulated brain chemistry. However, given that there are a number of different neurotransmitter systems believed to be responsible for PTSD symptoms (norepinephrine, serotonin, endogenous opioids, dopamine, and glutamate), it can be very complicated to treat PTSD with medications. There is no anti-PTSD drug as there are antianxiety and antidepressant drugs.

The American Psychiatric Association recently published recommendations for the medication treatment of PTSD. The first line of treatment should be a selective serotonin reuptake inhibitor (SSRI) or a selective serotonin and norepinephrine reuptake inhibitor (SSNRI). These drugs have been found to have a more global effect on PTSD symptoms. They can regulate mood fluctuations, decrease irritability, decrease anxiety, and decrease some of the intrusive symptoms of PTSD. However, this class of drugs, believed to be the best, can treat only about 30 to 50 percent of the symptoms of PTSD. Frequently, clinicians are then forced to add medications to address other bothersome symptoms.

If a person has trouble sleeping even after treatment with an SSRI or an SSNRI, Desyrel, Ambien, or a sedating tricyclic antidepressant may be added. Catapres is often added to treat nightmares and flashbacks. A mood stabilizer or Catapres can be added if a person with PTSD experiences intense rage or irritability. Finally, fear and panic can be treated with a benzodiazepine such as Valium.

PTSD can be a very complicated condition to live with and to treat. However, recent and continuing research offer much hope for future understanding. It is essential that anyone seeking help for PTSD find a mental health clinician who has experience treating clients with trauma and who is familiar with the treatment options available.

—Amy Elizabeth Banks, M.D.

Body Image

How men feel about themselves is a result of many factors: their mental and physical abilities, how others view them, how effective they are. For women, it pretty much comes down to satisfaction with one's body.

Why is this? Why do we tend to be so dissatisfied with our bodies? And what is the function of this dissatisfaction, in our individual lives and in society?

WHAT WOMEN THINK OF THEIR BODIES

Look at figure 1 and pick the body shape that most reflects your own right now. Note the number. Now pick the body shape that represents how you would *like* to look. Note that number. Finally, pick the body shape that you believe men would pick as the most attractive.

If you're like most women, your ideal body shape is smaller than your actual body shape. For example, the average female college student picked the figure numbered 4 as their own body, but figure number 3 as the body they would most like to have. This was also the figure the women thought men would prefer. A 1988 Gallup poll found that the average American woman wanted to weigh eleven pounds less, stand an inch taller, and wear a dress size two to four sizes smaller than her actual weight, height, and size. In contrast, when men are asked about their actual and ideal body type, most men are happy with their weight but would like to be an inch taller and more muscular.

What do men consider the ideal woman's body? Although one out of three women want a thin body and think men do, too, men actually prefer a more average female body type. For example, the average male college student picked a figure between 3 and 4 as the most attractive.

In general, women are more concerned than men about their bodies, obsessing more about body weight, food, and eating. Women weigh themselves more and diet more. Finally, women are more likely than men to describe themselves as overweight when they are, in fact, of normal weight. A 2001 study of over 800 adults ages nineteen to thirty-nine found that 31 percent of the women who were of normal weight perceived themselves to be overweight; only 5 percent of men of normal weight had that misperception. In fact, about one out of four men of normal weight perceived themselves as underweight.

BODIES AS OBJECTS

One of the most notable aspects of women's feelings about their bodies is inherent in the very title of this chapter: body image. Women tend to view their bodies as objects, things to be evaluated and commented upon. Women seem to relate to their bodies from the outside, as the image they see in a mirror or reflected in another's eyes. Because women, from girlhood on, are constantly judged and evaluated on the basis of their appearance (beauty pageants and the lack of anything comparable for males come immediately to mind), they internalize such a perspective.

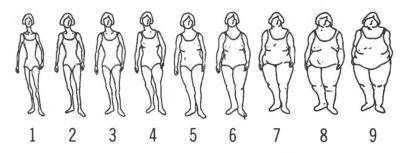

Figure 1. Female body shapes

Psychologists Barbara Frederickson and Tomi-Ann Roberts in 1997 developed "objectification theory" to understand how women learn to view their bodies as objects to be constantly monitored and evaluated. They argue that habitual self-monitoring of the body increases women's shame and anxiety while reducing awareness of internal bodily states. Identifying one's self with one's body image and the habitual body monitoring that follows make women vulnerable to a host of psychological problems, from increased depression to sexual dysfunction to eating disorders. Even on less extreme levels, body consciousness has been found to increase women's anxiety and decrease their performance on tasks requiring close attention, like math.

Looking at your body as an object is in contrast to relating to your body as a process, an experience rather than a thing. It's the difference between "feeling strong" and "looking good." When you feel strong, you're aware of what your body can do; when you look good, you're aware of your image.

ORIGINS OF THE SLENDER IDEAL

One thing we know is that women's dissatisfaction with their bodies and their desire to be thinner starts very early, with body image distortion at a peak at age eleven. This age is related to puberty and the multitude of changes that female bodies go through at this time: development of breasts and rounded hips, increased body fat, menstruation, pubic and underarm hair. Although some adjustment to their changing bodies is a commonplace experience of both boys and girls, it is telling that girls' concerns focus so heavily on their weight that 17 percent of girls ages eight and nine perceive themselves as overweight and 25 to 50 percent of ten- and eleven-year-old girls report dieting to lose weight. This percentage increases to 50 to 80 percent for females ages sixteen to twenty.

This body dissatisfaction, although common among American females across the sociological spectrum, is most pronounced in white middle- and upper-class heterosexual young women. For example, among whites, wealthier women tend to be thinner than poorer women, whereas for men, it's the wealthier ones who tend to have the biggest waistlines. In both African American and Latin cultures, the ideal body size for women tends to be larger than for white Americans. These cultures also place less emphasis on the female body relative to other behavioral and personality aspects, such as nurturing behaviors. Consequently, African American and Latina women tend to be more satisfied with their bodies than white women. In addition, lesbians tend to be both heavier and more satisfied with their weight than heterosexual women. Despite these cultural variations in body dissatisfaction, such dissatisfaction and its consequences occur in women of all races, ethnicities, classes, and sexualities.

The current slender ideal for women is a reflection of our times and culture. Historically and cross-culturally, the ideal female body has more often been more fleshy than slender, a sign of wealth and/or health. In most of human history, those who are excessively thin have more often been very ill or unable to find or afford enough food. The slender ideal for women came into vogue in the United States in the 1920s, the "flapper" era. This faded after World War II such that the cultural beauties of the 1950s (e.g., Jayne Mansfield, Marilyn Monroe) were more fleshy and voluptuous.

Starting in the late 1960s, however, the ideal female body became increasingly thinner, as represented by the model Twiggy in the 1970s. This increasingly slender ideal can be seen in the changes in two cultural representations of ideal womanhood: Miss America winners and women chosen as Playboy centerfolds. From the 1960s to the 1980s, the weight and body mass of these icons steadily decreased. This despite the fact the average body size of American women increased steadily over the same period. Since the late 1980s, the slender ideal has been augmented by increased breast size and muscle definition. Because the combination of slenderness and large breasts is an unlikely one naturally (since breast size is related to body fat), the current ideal is increasingly difficult to attain without surgery. The result: increased numbers of women who cannot look like the cultural ideal, increased body dissatisfaction, and increased numbers of breast augmentation surgeries.

As this brief historical timeline suggests, the media plays a major role in setting standards of beauty. Most women in television, movies, and magazines are ultrathin (as well as white, large-breasted, and young). Models who weighed 8 percent less than the average woman in the 1960s now weigh 23 percent less. Advertising models in particular present an unrealistic image, since their portrayal increasingly reflects computer manipulation. Thus, even the models themselves may not look like their images.

> Advertising models in particular present an unrealistic image, since their portrayal increasingly reflects computer manipulation. Thus, even the models themselves may not look like their images.

Yet these images are powerful. Research has found that looking at ads of thin models makes women feel depressed and negative about their own bodies. This occurred in 70 percent of women viewers after only three minutes of exposure! Television ads also have this effect, at least those that portray women as sex objects. The low visibility of African American and Latina models and actresses may actually be one reason girls from these cultures are less dissatisfied with their bodies than white girls.

Kim Chernin, feminist writer, and Sandra Bartky, professor of philosophy and gender and women's studies at the University of Illinois, Urbana-Champaign, and others suggest that this slender ideal is actually a form of political oppression of women. Whereas women's independence and freedom of movement used to be restricted by external constraints (from foot binding to corsets to veils), modern women are restricted by internal constraints, mainly an obsession with being thin. This obsession also restricts women's attention and energy through constant dieting, exercise, and general body dissatisfaction. Thus, it is no longer necessary to physically limit women in order to control them and limit their power; just fostering an obsession with their bodies makes

> Advertising's main goal is to get us to buy products; to do so, ads must make us feel inadequate and to perceive the product as the way to attain adequacy.

women limit themselves. This obsession also divides women from uniting with other women to work for social change since women are more encouraged to view other women as competition (for male approval and attention) than as comrades-in-arms. Thus, we have ads aimed at women with slogans like, "Don't hate me because I'm beautiful."

The slender ideal became popular in the United States at two points in time corresponding to an expansion of women's social roles. The first, in the 1920s, followed the attainment of women's suffrage and the entry of women in increased numbers into higher education and the labor force. The second, in the late 1960s, followed the second wave of the women's movement and the increased pressure for political and legal equality. As women's social and professional roles have expanded, their bodies have been portrayed as shrinking.

EFFECTS OF BODY DISSATISFACTION

Women's body dissatisfaction affects self-esteem. Women who are happy with the way they look tend to feel good about themselves. It works the other way as well: women who are unhappy with the way they look tend to feel bad about themselves. Such negative feelings make women more prone to depression and anxiety than men. In fact, women are two to three times more likely than men to suffer from depression, and almost twice as likely to suffer from anxiety disorders.

In a recent study of adolescent girls, body dissatisfaction, along with pressure to be thin and buying into this thin ideal, increased girls' risk of developing depressive symptoms one to two years later.

This overfocus on the body combined with unrealistic portrayals of women in the media makes women very prone to body image distortion. The vast majority of women overestimate their body size, thinking they are at least 25 percent larger than reality. Two out of five women overestimate their body size by a larger margin, perceiving at least one body part to be at least 50 percent larger than it actually is. The more distorted the body image, the worse women feel about themselves.

Another effect of body dissatisfaction and objectification is shame. Women, constantly presented with idealized young and slim female bodies in the media, are likely to feel like failures for not living up to this cultural ideal. Researchers have found that when women become more body conscious, shame related to their body increases. This in turn leads to more restrained and/or disordered eating.

> ✦
>
> Women's body dissatisfaction affects self-esteem. Women who are happy with the way they look tend to feel good about themselves; women who are unhappy with the way they look tend to feel bad about themselves.

Negative cultural attitudes toward overweight women add to the pressure and shame many women feel about their size. This is most pronounced among white Americans. Much more than men, overweight white women are perceived as lazier, more undisciplined, less attractive, and less intelligent than their more slender counterparts. Perhaps this is why overweight women in the workplace earn less than thinner women; in contrast, there is no pay differential for men as a function of their weight. This negative stigma of being overweight for white women contributes to their body dissatisfaction.

Black women and men do not show the same denigration of large women, especially large black women. For African American women, beauty is more about style, personality, and attitude than it is about a certain weight. Thus, the slender ideal is primarily a product of and for the dominant white culture. However, women of all cultures can aspire to this highly prized look, and indeed, minority girls and women who are most acculturated are also the most vulnerable to eating disorders.

Disordered eating is just one effect of body dissatisfaction. In fact, women spend billions of dollars and untold time and energy trying to change their bodies: dieting, exercising, buying beauty products, and undergoing elective cosmetic surgeries, such as breast implants and liposuction. The fact that the cultural female body ideal is impossible to achieve and/or maintain for the vast majority of women means that women's attempts are endless and their sense of failure and body dissatisfaction perpetual.

An example of the perpetual nature of body dissatisfaction for women can be seen in the cultural mandate that women's bodies should be hairless. Although this norm did not get firmly established in the United States until after World War II, it is now such an imperative that the vast majority of women remove their leg and underarm hair several times a week, some daily. Many go further and remove all body hair up to, and often including, the pubic hair (the "Brazilian wax" treatment). Women who do not remove their leg and underarm hair are looked upon negatively, even if there are medical reasons for not shaving. Women themselves have learned to view their own body hair as disgusting and dirty, despite the fact that it is natural and a female secondary sex characteristic. The overall message that most women have internalized is that women's bodies are not okay as they are.

This body dissatisfaction sometimes leads to drastic "remedies." Plastic surgery has become a multi-billion-dollar industry, used primarily by women. No longer confined to members of the entertainment industry, whose employability may rest on their looks, it has expanded to all those wishing to conform to the cultural ideal, at least those who can afford it. It started with ethnic minority women who used plastic surgery to look more "American," that is, white Anglo-Saxon Protestant. For example, Jewish women often had rhinoplasty (a "nose job") to reduce the size of their ethnic noses, and Asian women often had eye surgeries to add a fold to their eyelids. More recently, conforming to the cultural ideal has meant breast augmentation surgery for the big-breasted look, liposuction to attain the no-fat look, and face-lifts and Botox for the youthful look.

Not only faces can be made younger looking. Surgery is now available to women who have given birth that will restore their "youthful" labia. Then there are the stomach-stapling methods of weight loss for overweight women who lose hope of weight loss through other means. Research suggests that it is those women who have most internalized the cultural "beauty ideal" who are most willing to have cosmetic surgery to enhance their appearance.

Sometimes these attempts to conform to the slender ideal leads to serious problems. Constant dieting and excessive exercise can lead to injuries and poor nutrition as well as the development of such clinical disorders as depression, eating disorders, and body dysmorphic disorder. Even eating itself can be seen as unfeminine, so women may try to eat lightly, especially in public.

A vicious cycle of dieting and low self-esteem may ensue. Feeling bad about oneself may lead to dieting to lose weight and to improve one's feelings of self-worth. However, few di-

> A study of girls over the four-year high school period found that those who were most concerned with their weight as first-year students were at highest risk for developing disordered eating by their senior year.

ets work or work for long (most people who lose weight regain it), so dieters have frequent feelings of failure that may lead to even more extreme dieting. Severely restraining one's eating sets in motion an equally strong biological drive to eat, setting up a restraint-disinhibition cycle with habitual feelings of shame and failure.

No wonder many young females (estimates are one out of five) develop patterns of disordered eating. A 1996 study of girls over the four-year high school period found that those who were most concerned with their weight as first-year students were at highest risk for developing disordered eating by their senior year. Ten percent of this weight-concerned group developed symptoms by the end of high school compared to none of the girls who were not concerned with weight.

> We need to learn to appreciate our bodies as a process, not as objects; an experience, not just an image.

In addition to eating disorders, body dissatisfaction can be so extreme that body dysmorphic disorder develops. People with such a disorder worry about their appearance so much that it interferes with their everyday functioning. Such worry, which has an obsessive quality, also causes significant emotional distress. Feeling too fat is only one worry; people also may worry about the size of their nose, the appearance of their skin—any body feature can be obsessed over. These self-degrading thoughts are invariably distorted; for example, an anorexic woman who is all skin and bones may still be convinced she is fat. Approximately one out of fifty people suffers from this disorder, which seems to be on the rise. Most sufferers are teenaged and young adult women with low self-esteem who feel like failures for their perceived physical flaws. Although less researched than eating disorders, it is likely that body dysmorphic disorder also is related to pressure on women to monitor and modify their appearance to fit cultural norms.

Women's insecurities about their bodies do benefit many aspects of our culture, if not women themselves. American industries make more than $30 billion a year on diet and weight-loss products alone. Then there's the fitness industry (exercise clubs, tapes, equipment), the cosmetics and "beauty" industry (makeup, hair care, body care, antiaging products), and the medical profession (Botox, liposuction, and other cosmetic surgeries). Fueling all of this is the advertising industry, whose job it is to encourage and manipulate people's insecurities so that they buy the advertised products.

LOVING OUR BODIES

Reducing eating disorders and improving women's feelings about their bodies will require a major overhaul in cultural attitudes. We need to recognize that the obsession with slenderness is as restrictive as Victorian corsets and bustles: it hobbles the mind and spirit as well as the body. We need to understand the cultural messages in order to free ourselves from their negative effects and to learn to accept the body we have. We also need to learn that we are more than our bodies.

One way to break out of the cycle of body dissatisfaction is to understand that each person has a natural "set point" of weight, just as we have a natural "set point" of height. This set point is based on biological and genetic factors. We readily accept that although most people are of average height, some people are taller than average and some are shorter than average. This variation is normal and the distribution of height in the general population takes the form of a bell curve. Weight works the same way, with most people having an average set-point weight, with some having higher and some having lower set points. Although overeating or starvation may temporarily affect our actual weight, normal eating and activity levels always bring us back to our set point. This is the reason most diets fail.

We need to understand that the cultural ideal for women is a body possessed naturally by less than 5 percent of the adult female population. A woman who is healthy and of normal weight has approximately 25 percent body fat, yet the cultural ideal is less than 15 percent body fat. No wonder most women feel too fat! Thus, it is important to realize that the current aesthetic ideal is unrealistic and unhealthy for the vast majority of women.

We also need to develop a critical consciousness with respect to the media. Advertising's main goal is to get us to buy products; to do so, ads must make us feel inadequate and to perceive the product as the way to attain adequacy. Thus, ads create and prey on our insecurities. And advertising is everywhere: magazines and newspaper ads, commercial television, movies, billboards, websites, and so on. Many people make a lot of money off women's body dissatisfaction: publishers of women's magazines, cosmetic surgeons, and manufacturers of diet, exercise, and beauty products.

Finding supportive communities can be helpful in challenging the prevailing unrealistic body ideals for women. For example, African American women who are proud of being black are happier with their appearance and themselves than their sisters with a weaker racial identification. It is likely that being proud of your race is associated with evaluating yourself using more appropriate race-based standards. Local feminist groups exist that challenge the distorted portrayal of women in the media. There also are self-help groups in many communities, such as Overeaters Anonymous or body awareness groups. Those suffering from eating disorders, body dysmorphic disorder, or serious depression should seek professional help. Cognitive behavior therapy and antidepressants have been very helpful for many sufferers of these disorders. See the recommended websites in the suggested reading section at the end of the book for more information and referral sources.

Our bodies are amazing creations, capable of many activities and tasks. However, we are more than just our bodies: we have aptitudes, talents, personality traits, interpersonal styles, character strengths, soul. We need to learn to appreciate our bodies as a process, not as objects; an experience, not just an image. Our worth as human beings cannot be reduced to the numbers on a scale or on a tape measure.

—*Susan A. Basow, Ph.D.*

RELATED ENTRIES

Anxiety Disorders

Depressive Disorders

Eating Disorders and Disconnections

Eating Disorders and Disconnections

Telling the Problem
from the Solution

For most of us, learning to live comfortably and move confidently in our bodies is not an easy task. Is my body me, an aspect of me—or is it an alien other, as some experience it? Can I love it, live in harmony with it—or is it the enemy I must conquer? Can I listen to it, can I respond to my feelings of desire, or fear, or hunger—or must I ignore, numb, stuff, or swallow down these feelings that seem too much, or too dangerous, to bear?

Most women in our culture have some degree of concern about food, eating, and body image. We are bombarded with images of young, thin women who have become the standards by which ordinary women measure themselves—and find themselves lacking. We hear the drumbeat of pitches from the diet industry. We bond with friends over the dramas of battles won and lost with food. We feel virtuous and strong when we succeed in losing a few pounds, and frustrated and guilty when they return (as they do 95 percent of the time). For most of us, the result of regained weight is a bruised ego and some difficult moments in the cold light of the dressing room. Life goes on, and these concerns move into the background, subsumed by greater priorities.

For some women, however, concerns about weight, eating, and body image stay very much in the foreground. While these individuals may appear engaged and active, if you ask them they are likely to tell you that they spend almost all of their time thinking about food, eating, or their body. They are terrified of food and of gaining weight, and they are afraid of being out of control. They base their self-esteem on their size. They may binge, they may restrict food, they may purge, they may over-exercise, they may even do all these things. They feel disconnected from their hunger, their feelings, and their relationships. They find it hard to live in their skin, which has not always been a safe or comfortable place for them. These women have moved away from a healthy relationship with food and their bodies, if they ever had it to begin with, and have developed eating disorders.

Anna, seventeen, devoted considerable time to competitive ice skating. After an injury ended her career, she felt she lost a major part of her identity. To make matters worse, with the change in her activity level and her body's maturation, her weight went up fifteen pounds. She felt depressed, out of control, no longer "special" in any way. She cut out fats and other foods she once enjoyed, and started swimming daily. When she lost the fifteen pounds, people were complimentary. But she was still unhappy with her body, especially her hips and thighs. She resolved to focus her energy on losing more weight, the way she had focused on skating. By the time she lost another fifteen pounds, her periods had stopped and, although she had always been a good student, she was finding it hard to focus on her schoolwork even though she spent more time on it. Her family grew concerned, noticing that she seemed wan and irritable and no longer showed interested in friends or activities other than exercise. Anna herself felt that the only thing that gave her any relief or sense of accomplishment was seeing the numbers on the scale drop.

When Sarah was home by herself during middle school, she began to binge secretly, taking comfort in eating when she felt lonely. She had trouble letting others know when she was hurt by or angry with them, fearing she would lose friends if she stood up for herself. In high school, she felt more a part of the crowd when she was drinking; sometimes she restricted her food to make up for the extra calories. When a friend introduced her to purging, she initially felt she could "have it all." In six months, she was vomiting almost daily, sometimes even when she had not binged but just felt anxious or angry. She was reluctant to eat around others and spent more time alone. At times she was able to stop the bingeing and purging for a few weeks, until something stressful happened and she began again. Sarah's weight fluctuated rapidly; she could gain and then lose twenty pounds in two or three months. Sarah, now twenty, has always felt that she has managed to "pass" as reasonably smart, attractive, and interesting only by dint of her hard work—"I am not a natural at anything." She worried that she was a fraud, and that others would find this out and no longer like her. She came to treatment at the urging of her college roommates, who had been concerned about her even though she denied having any eating problems; she was both annoyed and relieved that they had figured out what she was doing.

Maria, thirty-two, had come with her mother and stepfather from Colombia as a child. When she developed full breasts at twelve, she felt embarrassed, awkward, like she had done something wrong. Boys made fun of her, stared at her breasts, and even tried to touch them. She found that when she binged she did not think about these things. She could count on food for comfort and distraction. When she went up three dress sizes, she felt guilty and ashamed, but she could not control her bingeing. As she became an adult the weight gain continued, and men no longer seemed to notice her body in a sexual way. Sometimes she feels terrible about this, but other times she feels like she has some insulation from their eyes, like she is in camouflage.

About 90 to 95 percent of those who suffer from anorexia and bulimia are women. According to the National Institute of Health, an estimated .5 to 3.7 percent of females suffer from anorexia and an estimated 1.1 to 4.2 percent suffer from bulimia at some point in their lives.

WHAT IS AN EATING DISORDER?

Anna, Sarah, and Maria all have eating disorders, although in many ways their lives and dilemmas are quite different. Anorexia nervosa, bulimia nervosa, and binge-eating disorder are psychiatric conditions that cause serious disturbances in the bodies, thoughts, feel-

SIGNS AND SYMPTOMS OF ANOREXIA NERVOSA

- Emaciated appearance
- Dry skin, brittle hair and nails, hair loss
- Orthostatic changes and hypotension
- Low body temperature, pulse below 60
- Yellow discoloration of skin, especially palms
- Loose-fitting, multilayered clothing
- Fatigue, muscle weakness
- Hyperactivity, anxious energy
- Excuses for skipping meals

- Playing with food, cutting it into small pieces, unusual food combinations
- Constipation
- Depression, irritability, withdrawal, personality changes
- Intolerance to cold
- Lack of concern about low body weight or other changes
- Osteoporosis

ings, and relationships of those who suffer from them. While many women have experienced one or more of the symptoms of an eating disorder, a much smaller number have a diagnosable eating disorder. About 90 to 95 percent of those who suffer from anorexia and bulimia are women. According to the National Institute of Health, an estimated .5 to 3.7 percent of females suffer from anorexia and an estimated 1.1 to 4.2 percent suffer from bulimia at some point in their lives. Binge-eating disorder is even more common, with an estimated 2 to 5 percent of the general population meeting the proposed diagnostic criteria.

Anorexia Nervosa Anna has developed anorexia nervosa, restricting type. This disorder most frequently develops in adolescence but can begin earlier or later. According to the *DSM-IV*, the essential features of anorexia nervosa are that the individual

- maintains a body weight of less than 85 percent of minimally normal body weight for her age and height
- is intensely afraid of gaining weight or becoming fat, a fear that is usually not alleviated by weight loss
- exhibits a significant disturbance in the perception of the shape or size of her body; self-esteem is highly dependent on body shape or weight, and the seriousness of the low body weight is denied
- has missed at least three consecutive menstrual cycles

The individual with anorexia nervosa is considered to be of the *restricting type* if she has not engaged in binge eating or purging, and of the *binge-eating/purging type* if she has regularly engaged in bingeing or purging behaviors.

As with Anna, the most striking and obvious symptom of anorexia is dangerously low weight. Family and friends are often unaware of this as a problem for some time. They may have offered encouragement and praise for weight loss. Only when the anorexia is entrenched is it recognized as a problem. Sometimes anorexia is mistaken for a purely medical condition; sometimes it is masked by multiple layers of clothing. Often the individual denies that there is a probem and indicates a sense of accomplishment and satisfaction about the weight loss.

Bulimia Nervosa Sarah is suffering from bulimia nervosa, which typically develops a little later than anorexia—and sometimes develops out of anorexia. Bulimia nervosa has existed as a formal psychiatric diagnosis only since 1979; many researchers think that this particular cluster of behaviors was rare before 1970 or so. The essential features of bulimia nervosa are

- recurrent episodes of binge eating, which are characterized by eating an amount of food that is significantly larger than most people would eat in similar time and circumstances, and a sense of lack of control over eating during the episode
- recurrent inappropriate compensatory behavior in order to prevent weight gain, such as self-induced vomiting, misuse of medications, fasting, or excessive exercise
- binge eating and compensatory behaviors that occur, on average, at least twice a week for three months
- self-evaluation that is unduly influenced by body shape and weight
- the disturbance not occurring exclusively during episodes of anorexia nervosa

In addition, the individual is classified as the *purging type* if she has regularly purged (vomited or misused medications such as laxatives or diuretics), or the *nonpurging type* if during the current episode she has engaged in behaviors such as fasting or excessive exercise but has not purged.

Like Sarah, the woman with bulimia will often go to great lengths to deny or conceal bulimic behaviors; this is true even of a woman who has always seen herself as basically honest. She may initially believe she has hit on an ingenious solution to "have her cake and eat it too," and therefore ignore the risks.

Eating Disorder Not Otherwise Specified As many as half of those diagnosed with eating disorders have serious problems with eating that do not precisely meet the above descriptions. For instance, a woman may meet all the criteria for anorexia but still have periods. Or another may vomit after eating small amounts of food, yet still be of normal weight. Most common in this group is *binge-eating disorder*, which has received much attention as a potential diagnosis in its own right. Binge-eating disorder (sometimes called compulsive overeating) is characterized by recurrent episodes (more than two times weekly for six

SIGNS AND SYMPTOMS OF BULIMIA NERVOSA

- Recurrent dehydration (sometimes leading to ER visits for "flu")
- Frequent significant weight fluctuations
- Abdominal pain, bloating
- Constipation
- Secretive about eating, avoids eating with others
- Swollen glands, especially parotid

- Lesions on the back of hands
- Fatigue, decreased energy
- Depression, irritability
- Dental enamel erosion, caries, periodontal disease
- Muscle weakness, peripheral edema
- Frequent trips to the bathroom, especially after meals

SIGNS AND SYMPTOMS OF BINGE-EATING DISORDER

☞ Often, though not always, overweight

☞ Preoccupation with being overweight, dieting

☞ Depression

☞ Abdominal pain, bloating

☞ Shame about body and eating

☞ Alternating between dieting (or trying to) and overeating

☞ Otherwise generally healthy appearance

months) of binge eating, as described above, but without the regular use of inappropriate compensatory behaviors that are a part of bulimia. For binge eaters like Maria, the binge episodes are associated with eating rapidly, eating until feeling uncomfortably full, eating large amounts of food when not physically hungry, eating alone out of embarrassment, and feeling disgusted, depressed, or very guilty after overeating. Thirty percent of the obese population and 2 to 5 percent of the general population meet the proposed diagnostic criteria.

Like many binge eaters, Maria uses food to cope, to comfort, to numb. For her, food is no longer about satisfying hunger or enjoyment; her eating is determined more by emotions and availability than by internal body cues. Binge eating is the most common pattern of disordered eating.

WHAT LEADS TO EATING DISORDERS?

An eating disorder is a biopsychosocial problem, one that affects and is affected by a woman's body, mind, and relationships. Why do so many women suffer from an eating disorder? Why is it so frequent in this era, in this culture?

Biological/Physical Factors Many women report that their eating disorder began with dieting. Often, the dieting becomes extreme. What are the effects of extreme dieting? In 1950, Ancel Keys conducted a study of food deprivation with male volunteers who had no apparent prior food issues. They were limited to approximately half their normal calorie intake for six months and lost approximately 25 percent of their original weight. After the weight loss, they experienced many problems, including increased isolation; difficulty making decisions; decreased libido, concentration, and motivation; increased depression; and irritability. They lost interest in activities and other people and focused increasingly on food. The symptoms that they experienced were strikingly similar to many of those experienced by women with eating disorders, suggesting that severe food restriction alone can play a critical role in a host of cognitive, emotional, and interpersonal problems common with eating disorders.

> An eating disorder is a biopsychosocial problem, one that affects and is affected by a woman's body, mind, and relationships.

When a woman has developed an eating disorder, her unusual eating patterns complicate her experience in an ongoing way. The anorectic woman restricts intake severely, which her body reads as starvation; this leads to lowered metabolic rate, as the body tries to survive and maximize use of calories. The chaotic eating that is characteristic of bulimia and binge eating results in impairment in the ability to recognize hunger and fullness. Many bulimic women eat little during the day and then, feeling deprived and physically hungry, binge all evening; sometimes they stop bingeing only by purging or by going to sleep. And the "promise" of future restraint—"I've already blown it tonight so I'll keep going, but tomorrow I will be extra good"—often leads to continued overeating for both bulimics and binge eaters. This "deprivation cycle"—learned guilt about normal eating leads to restraint, which leads to feelings of deprivation, which leads to overeating, which leads, in turn, to more guilt—is characteristic of women who binge.

> Severe food restriction alone can play a critical role in a host of cognitive, emotional, and interpersonal problems common with eating disorders.

Women whose family history includes substance abuse or eating disorders appear to be at greater risk of developing an eating disorder. While some of this may be learned behavior, a genetic component also appears to be at work. Further research is being done on the genetic factors in eating disorders, which may have many implications for future diagnosis and treatment.

Psychological/Developmental Factors Women with eating disorders generally feel unhappy with themselves, out of control, and ineffective. Close to half report depression or anxiety before the onset of the eating disorder, and about a third report obsessive-compulsive symptoms. A large subgroup of women have a history of substance abuse or trauma as well. Perfectionism, difficulty with change, and all-or-nothing thinking are other common characteristics. These women are frequently keenly attuned to others' feelings and expectations, yet profoundly out of touch with their own real feelings or desires—feelings and desires that are about much more than food.

How do these patterns develop? The relational model of development discussed by Jean Baker Miller and Irene Stiver in *The Healing Connection* gives us one way of understanding how relationship issues that start in childhood may contribute to the development of eating disorders.

When people in our lives are basically genuine, responsive, and empathic, we learn to feel connected to them and to our own feelings and desires; we feel energy and interest in engaging with other people and other pursuits. When our thoughts, feelings, and perceptions are responded to as irrelevant or wrong (and possibly dangerous), we experience a profound disconnection. Major disruptions in development occur when positive connections are rare and disconnections are more severe and more chronic. Unable to change the relationship but yearning to save the connection, a young girl in this situation may then focus on changing (or blaming) what she can: herself. In order to be accepted in an unaccepting relationship, she may exclude whole aspects of herself from relationships—and thus from the opportunity to learn and to grow. This

> Women with eating disorders are frequently keenly attuned to others' feelings and expectations, yet profoundly out of touch with their own real feelings or desires.

leads to Miller and Stiver's central paradox: People will do almost anything to keep a relationship, including keeping more and more of themselves out of the relationship.

An eating disorder represents a literal attempt to make oneself "shrink to fit" the expectations of others. Women may go through physical and emotional contortions in an effort to appear as they believe they should appear, to do and say as they should. We develop, based on personal experience, images of how relationships work. Women with eating disorders tend to blame themselves for difficulties, to conclude that "I am the problem." It is an easy step to seeing one's body (and its desires) as a major part of the problem. This sense of inherent badness or wrongness connects to a strong sense of shame about one's very being, which leads to feelings of unworthiness and further isolation. Isolated and unsatisfied, feeling unworthy of human care or contact, these women may find it safer and more predictable to turn to food—or restriction—as a "solution." They may think:

- I would have died without my eating disorder.
- I protect myself by my heaviness, so people will not see who I am.
- I'm worthless, I don't deserve to eat.
- My eating disorder is the only thing that keeps me safe.

Sociocultural Factors Contemporary American culture seems to be fertile ground for the development of eating disorders. Almost any magazine displays the dominant body type: thin, tall, "toned," and preferably white. While variations exist between cultural and ethnic groups, it generally appears that the more a woman is tied into our dominant culture and its values, the more at risk she is for an eating disorder. The "superwoman" who thinks she needs to do it all is a woman in danger of developing an eating disorder. Let's consider some of the major cultural strands that are particularly influential.

Historic Western Culture. One of the earliest stories many of us learned is that of Eve: She hungered for the apple, gave into temptation ... and paradise was lost to humankind. From many beliefs and stories in our culture, we have learned to think of our psyche and our soma as separate and in conflict. As women we have been taught to think of the body as both vulnerable and bad, less a source of pleasure or general power than a source of danger and sexual power. Having imbibed these lessons, some women seek approval or love through their body, while others try to be invisible and desireless.

Societal and Media Culture. Being thin is for many not simply about perceived beauty; thinness is equated with success, control, and love. Women once had as their primary reference points other women they knew. Women of today are surprised to see how "heavy" idealized women from other eras are, whether they are looking at an impressionist painting by Renoir or a movie star from the 1950s like Marilyn Monroe. Now women compare themselves with media images of extremely thin women who are apparently happy and successful. Over the last few decades, the discrepancy between women's real and "ideal" weights has steadily grown. The idealized body type has gotten steadily taller and thinner while the average American woman has gotten larger—a prescription for distress.

> An eating disorder represents a literal attempt to make oneself "shrink to fit" the expectations of others.

Yet another way in which media may contribute to the growth of eating disorders is the frequent high-profile coverage of celebrities who have eating disorders, generally anorexia or bulimia. While the ostensible purpose of these stories is to express shock or sympathy, they can sometimes create a glamorous aura about disorders that are, in real life, heartbreakingly unglamorous.

Ethnocultural Influences. For many years the stereotype has been that eating disorders occur primarily in young, white, high-achieving, financially comfortable women. This is no longer the case. As young women from other cultures assimilate into our thin-obsessed culture, they become fearful of being fat and show more symptoms of eating disorders, especially bulimia and binge eating. D. J. Harris and Sue A. Kuba suggest a relationship between conflicted identity and eating disorders in a 1997 study with women of color.

> Some women seek approval or love through their body, while others try to be invisible and desireless.

Some have considered lesbian women to be relatively protected from eating disorders, since as a group they seem to be less invested in social expectations about appearance (conversely, gay men are generally seen as being more at risk than men in general because of greater emphasis on appearance). While there is some truth to this, at least one study indicates that gender trumps sexual orientation as a risk factor. Lesbian women are at somewhat less risk than most women, but they have still absorbed many of our society's expectations and pressures in regard to food and appearance.

Family and Peers as Cultural Influence. In addition to being influenced by the broader culture, many women feel pressure from their family or peers. In a family where Mom is worried about her weight and appearance, and members tease about weight, daughters will be vulnerable. If a woman belongs to a group where appearance or low weight is valued, such as dancers or athletes, her risk of an eating disorder is again increased. Some college-age women face dorm suites in which several roommates have eating disorders, making it feel almost normal to binge and purge.

HOW ARE EATING DISORDERS TREATED?

If you have an eating disorder, your condition seriously affects your body, mind, spirit, and relationships; you need to get both a medical and a psychological evaluation. These evaluations are the first steps in developing a coordinated plan for treatment, which often involves working with an interdisciplinary team. In addition to individual therapy, family and group therapy is often helpful. Your therapist or physician may also suggest that you meet with a dietitian, who can look closely at your eating patterns with you and help you develop a better relationship with food.

Medical/Biological Treatment Your physician needs to know if you have an eating disorder. He or she can then evaluate the effects of the eating disorder and establish whether any other medical conditions need to be treated. A complete physical examination, which may include blood work, an EKG, and other tests, will provide such information. If your eating disorder is active but you are not in immediate medical danger, your physician may ask you to come in weekly or even more often, although visits usually will not be this frequent.

Monitoring your electrolyte levels, weight, and vital signs is particularly important, since problems in these areas indicate that your body is in immediate trouble. The great majority of eating disorder problems are treated on an outpatient basis. If, however, you are in medical danger or if your eating disorder is accompanied by severe psychiatric difficulties, hospitalization may be recommended.

Many women who are being treated for eating disorders benefit from medication. A psychiatrist generally prescribes it, although your physician may as well. Antidepressants, which are commonly used, appear to be helpful with symptoms of bingeing and purging. Since many women with eating disorders also have symptoms of depression, anxiety disorders, and obsessive-compulsive disorders, antidepressants also may be helpful in treating these symptoms. The use of medication is somewhat less common in treating anorexia nervosa; many believe the patient should first gain weight and let the psychological symptoms due to starvation itself begin to improve.

Psychotherapy Most people begin treatment by meeting with a therapist who specializes in eating disorders. Because the quality of the therapy relationship is an important part of healing, you need to work with a therapist who is responsive and empathic to your current concerns and perspectives. A good therapy relationship can help you address both the symptoms of your eating disorder and the reasons the disorder developed. It can help you create better connections with your body, with your feelings, and with other people.

> ✦
>
> A good therapy relationship can help you address both the symptoms of your eating disorder and the reasons the disorder developed.

Because the consequences of eating disorders can be dangerous, even life-threatening, most therapists agree that symptoms—bingeing, purging, restricting, having a distorted body image, and related difficulties—should be addressed directly in therapy. (The notable exception is those practicing interpersonal therapy, which has demonstrated some lasting results by focusing on interpersonal issues only.) Cognitive-behavioral approaches—learning to identify and change the thoughts and behaviors that are a part of your eating disorder, thus learning to develop healthier eating patterns and to change distorted beliefs about food, body, and yourself that underlie the eating disorder—have been particularly effective. Therapists of different orientations frequently use the following techniques.

Journal Writing. You might be asked to keep a food journal. Entries could include when, where, and what you eat, whether you consider it a binge, if you purge, and the circumstances, thoughts, and feelings connected with your eating. The purpose is to see the patterns in your eating, not to count calories. Journal writing can help both you and your therapist be more aware of what is actually happening, and it can help you begin to make links between your eating, your thoughts and feelings, and the events in your life.

Psychoeducation. Your therapist may provide you with information about such topics as the physiological effects of food restriction, purging, and bingeing. You may also discuss cultural and other factors involved in eating disorders.

Self-Care Activities. Many women with eating disorders feel guilty when they take time to do things for themselves, making them feel deprived, which then leads them to turn to the eating disorder as a way of comforting or distracting themselves. One of the ways to break this deprivation cycle that fuels eating disorders is to find non-food-related ways of comforting and giving to yourself. These activities can also be used as ways of postponing or avoiding bingeing and purging.

Developing Regular Eating Patterns. Women with eating disorders frequently skip meals and often describe their eating patterns as chaotic. Most therapists recommend that you begin to have three meals and two or more snacks daily. While such a change in your eating habits may be difficult at first, it is an important step in learning to be responsive to your body's needs and signals, including feelings of hunger and satiety; many women find this an important step in reducing urges to binge as well. If you have been avoiding certain foods, your therapist may suggest ways for you to gradually begin eating them again.

Setting Realistic Goals for Yourself. Your therapist may ask you to create weekly goals for yourself in terms of bingeing, purging, and other areas. If you are a perfectionist, you may be tempted to set your goals too high. For instance, it may be more realistic to begin with a goal of bingeing one fewer time than eliminating bingeing for the week.

Improving Body Image. Developing a critical awareness of the cultural pressures to be thin will help you learn to think differently about your body. Your sense of who you are, and what makes you worthwhile, should come from qualities other than appearance. You will learn to appreciate your body for what it can do rather than for how it looks, to approach exercise for enjoyment and health rather than for weight loss. Challenge your negative thoughts about your body, and spend time with people who help you take a loving, respectful approach to your body. Question the importance that our culture places on women's size and appearance, and challenge the enormous prejudice that heavy women face every day.

Identifying and Changing Negative Thoughts and Feelings. Women with eating disorders tend to have basic beliefs ("I must be perfect," "Everyone must love me"), and reasoning errors (all-or-nothing thinking like "I've already messed up by eating a cookie, I might as well finish off the box"), and emotional reasoning ("I feel fat, so I must be fat") that get in the way of self-esteem. By identifying and challenging these thoughts, you can begin to notice how you talk to yourself and how you can relate to yourself in a more encouraging, realistic way.

Increasing Mutual Relationships, Decreasing Isolation. Isolation puts you at greater risk for depression and eating disorders, and it is often linked to images or models of relationships in which you see others as unresponsive or even dangerous and yourself as unworthy. By learning through therapy that new kinds of relationships are possible—that, for instance, relationships can be a source of support, safety, and growth—you become more able to recognize and create good, mutual relationships in your life. Group and family therapy can be helpful in this work, as can community self-help groups.

—*Jane MacDonald, Ph.D.*

RELATED ENTRIES

Depressive Disorders

Anxiety Disorders

Body Image

Cognitive Behavioral Therapy

Insight-Oriented Therapy

Growth in Connection

Women and Addictions

While addiction itself is a discrete, freestanding problem, addictive behaviors exist in a complex network of relationships. The addiction is in part a response to these relationships, creating many of the issues that can actually bring a woman to treatment. The traditional model of substance abuse treatment treats addiction as a primary disease that *causes* conflict in love and work, but, in reality, women who become addicted often do so *because* their lives are somehow impaired, and the addictive behavior is one way of coping. The following vignette illustrates some of the common themes running through the lives of substance-dependent women.

Joanie was a thirty-eight-year-old divorced mother of two when she sought counseling for help with her current boyfriend, Steve. She described feeling unloved, overwhelmed, sad, and anxious much of the time for the past decade or so, and these ongoing emotions were complicating her relationship with Steve.

"No wonder he's such a jerk to me, when I'm such a mess with my moods and all," she said during our first session. She described a childhood with a strict, verbally abusive, alcoholic father and a mother "who couldn't defend herself, never mind me or my sister." Joanie said her first husband was a lot like her father, making her feel so horrible that she finally mustered up the strength to leave him. Unfortunately, she had a "horrible breakdown" after the divorce, making her doubt her ability to care for her kids even now. Joanie sobbed as she reported this.

In her current relationship, she thought she had found a kind, gentle man. But then their fights started, sometimes violent fights, after which Joanie experienced a sense of detachment, "a kind of numbing out when it all got to be too much." Upon further discussion, Joanie explained that she felt ashamed when she drank "too much wine sometimes while out with Steve," usually when she was feeling "weird in her relationship with him," which always led to "bad sex and an argument." Before Steve, she also recalled that she'd probably had unprotected sex a few times with "all the wrong kind of guy" typically after drinking too much, which left her, in the days and weeks following, scared about HIV.

"I know better," she said, "and I'm not that kind of girl, really ..." Joanie also told me that she took a "Valium or something" to help her sleep when her anxiety threatened to keep her up at night. This sometimes made her oversleep, so she had been late to work four times this month and was now feeling like she was on "shaky ground there."

There was a lot going on for Joanie when we met. She clearly was dealing with issues that go beyond alcohol and Valium misuse. Joanie is at least equally concerned about her current relationship, her rough childhood with an abusive and alcoholic father, an unprotecting mother, domestic violence within her first marriage, the possibility of losing her job, her fears of HIV infection from her mystifying reckless behavior, and most troubling to her, doubts about her parenting ability. Let's take a closer look at some of these issues.

CAUSES OF ADDICTION

Early Traumas and Substance Abuse Although not all women who become addicted have experienced early traumas, early and chronic scars on the psyche do seem to predispose the victim to a wide variety of self-destructive or addictive behaviors. Charlotte Kasl, in *Women, Sex, and Addiction,* writes that "childhood abuse, along with poverty and oppression, underline numerous addictions, addictions that may operate alternately or simultaneously. In many instances, misuse of food, sex, alcohol, work, and money either occur together or interchangeably as an individual desperately tries to quell an inner emptiness created by some form of childhood abuse or neglect."

B. A. van der Kolk also looks at this relationship, in *Psychological Trauma,* though through a slightly different lens, speculating that childhood deprivation may predispose the victim for a large variety of addictive disorders in an attempt to relieve painful feelings.

We all possess natural painkillers, called endorphins, that are secreted from cell to cell within our bodies. Endorphins are pharmacologically similar to opiates, and they are pumped out in huge supply during extreme digression or during times of extreme pleasure. van der Kolk and others speculate that a person with an early history of trauma may strive to stimulate her own endorphin production to relieve a constant sense of suffering. Food bingeing, reckless love affairs that produce their own short-term "high," workaholism, and, of course, substance use all cause the reward centers in our brains to glow, but only briefly. Then the person in pain seeks more—more work, more love, more sex, more drugs, and so the cycle goes round. To further complicate matters, a mechanism called "neural adaptation" causes the brain, when it is regularly supplied with external opiates, to stop producing its own endorphins; the person comes to rely all the more on the outside source. The person becomes "addicted," but we can see how the addiction grew from seeds of pain.

Joanie's story shows us how her early experiences with a "strict, abusive, alcoholic father" and "unprotecting mother" started her off in a place with little safety or security. Her early substance use became her protector, as we'll see more of later. Early and prolonged injuries to the forming psyche are important to consider as a driving force in the establishment and continuation of many addictive behaviors. They also often act as a complicating factor in many traditional treatment settings for addictions where the focus is solely on the substance misuse, and the underlying issues are often relegated to another treatment setting for much later exploration.

> Women who become addicted often do so *because* their lives are somehow impaired, and the addictive behavior is one way of coping.

In these traditional treatment settings, where addiction is considered the cause as opposed to the consequence of suffering, a woman seeking help may find herself shortchanged. M. Harris and R. D. Fallot note in their article "Designing Trauma-Informed Addictions Services" that because addictive disorders are so common among women who have experienced prolonged sexual and physical abuse, it is especially important to design addictions services that meet the needs of the trauma survivor. And finally, while becoming sober is a crucial step for entering treatment, ignoring the causes of the behavior can set women up for early treatment failures and hopelessness about long-term change.

Social Class Even the most conservative researchers agree that poverty is a real risk factor for addiction. In a series of studies using rats at Simon Fraser University in Canada, Bruce Alexander and others demonstrated how environment contributes to addiction. In his research, Alexander addicted two sets of rats to morphine. He then housed one group in cramped, individual, tenement-like cages, and the other group in a stimulating and comfortable "rat park" with lots of space, exercise equipment, companions of both sexes, and even a scenic painting of a forest along the walls. He then offered both sets of rats morphine-laced water and plain water. The rats housed in the park, even though already "addicted," displayed little interest in the morphine-laced water once in the park; the caged rats continued to prefer the morphine-laced water for as long as they were confined to the small cages.

Genetics Studies have concluded that alcoholism does, in fact, run in families. N. S. Cotton and D. W. Goodwin explored this idea as early as the mid-1970s. Goodwin found that male children of alcoholics are four times more likely to become alcoholics than children raised in non-alcoholic households. However, from their research, it is unclear whether the behavior arose because of genetics or because of the environment in which they were raised, or both. In their 1994 outline of direct and indirect genetic links to addiction, Edward Kaufman and others listed parental or other family member addictions as direct. They concluded that indirect links to addiction—which include temperament, anxiety, depression, and mental illness—may also leave a child vulnerable to addiction.

> While becoming sober is a crucial step, ignoring causes of addictive behavior can set women up for early treatment failures and hopelessness about long-term change.

Later studies of twins by R. W. Pickens and others demonstrated that identical twins developed addictive behaviors more often than fraternal twins, leading once again to the belief of a genetic basis to addiction. In spite of challenges in accounting for unequal environmental conditions between identical and fraternal twins, this increasing body of research has been useful and has strengthened the possibility of a genetic component in addictions.

CONSEQUENCES OF ADDICTION

Addiction and Domestic Violence One of the dangers of addictive behaviors, especially substance misuse, is that they are often linked with domestic violence. The cycle of violence is complex. The Substance Abuse and Mental Health Services Administration Clearinghouse for Alcohol and Drug Information explains that alcoholism and battering share similar behavioral profiles: both may be passed from generation to generation, both involve denial or minimization of the problem, both involve isolation of the family, and both are intertwined as causal and mitigation factors. In addition, the shame that comes from many addictive behaviors—whether it be substance misuse, compulsive sex, or overeating—further isolates a woman and hinders her power to care for and protect herself and her children.

Through sharing her story, Joanie realized how her alcohol use repeatedly put her in a compromised state, leaving her vulnerable to abuse and victimization in her first marriage, in her fleeting relationships, and then in her current relationship with Steve.

She went on to describe how her shame about the use and the abuse made her feel isolated and alone. This cycle of abuse can exacerbate addictive behaviors and vice versa, while avoiding blame that can bring further shame and hopelessness about the possibility for change and growth.

Addiction and Impact on Work While addictions oftentimes stem from underlying life issues, they also create chaos in the user's universe. According to the National Clearinghouse for Alcohol and Drug Information in 1992, an estimated $82 billion in lost potential productivity was attributed to alcohol and drug abuse. This amount accrued in the form of work not performed—including household tasks—and was measured in terms of lost earnings and household productivity. These costs were primarily borne by the drug or alcohol abusers and by those with whom they lived.

Further, the 1997 National Household Survey on Drug Abuse found that workers who reported current illicit drug use were more likely than those who did not report illicit drug use to have skipped one or more days of work in the past month. And they found that workers who reported heavy alcohol use were about twice as likely as those who did not report such use to have worked for three or more employers in the past year and to have skipped one or more days of work in the past month. These figures came to life as Joanie told her story, having missed several days of work in the fall and having been late for work four days in the month before we met, due to her Valium use and fights with Steve.

> ✦
> Studies over the past decade have shown a direct link between major depression and female alcoholism.

Addiction and Parenting Addiction can consume oneself and one's family. In the words of Lisa Montanye, LCSW, a clinical social worker in East Boston who works primarily with drug-addicted women and their families, "addictions, and the related mental illness and chaos, can tear apart a family."

Studies over the past decade have shown a direct link between major depression and female alcoholism. Findings from Johns Hopkins in 2001 highlight that single mothers receiving welfare payments are at a heightened risk for depression, and thus addiction. Other studies, such as the one in 1999 completed at the Research Institute on Addictions in Buffalo, New York, suggests that women with alcohol and drug problems are more likely to be punitive toward their children.

Other consequences of addiction on parenting success, Montanye points out, include "lack of nurturing communication, lack of healthy role modeling, and less attention to diet and exercise." As Montanye explains, "Even the most well-intentioned moms can get thrown off track by the pushes and pulls of addiction, poverty, domestic violence, and overall stress.... Unfortunately, this leaves the children to often pay the price."

TOLERANCE AND WITHDRAWAL

Tolerance and withdrawal are important factors in addiction. Over time and with regular use, a user's tolerance increases, requiring more and more of the drug or behavior to get the desired effect.

Increased tolerance means an increased risk for overdose for two reasons. First, every drug has a main effect (the effect the user wants) and side effects (effects that the user does not want). Tolerance to all effects of a drug does not develop evenly. For example, barbiturate users develop tolerance to the desired mood-altering effect of the drug faster than they do to the side effect of depressed breathing. When the user increases the dose to get the desired effect, they risk taking enough to cause them to stop breathing, which of course would cause death. Second, if a user has not used for a while, tolerance will decrease and the dose the user had previously used when her tolerance level was elevated may now be enough to cause an overdose.

Withdrawal is related to physical dependence and tolerance. After repeated use over a period of time, the body adjusts itself to function normally with the presence of the drug; perhaps it produces less of a chemical used in the brain that the drug imitates, or it develops more receptors in the brain to handle the drug. The body might start producing enzymes to break the substance down, and hormone levels could change to make that happen.

> Alcoholic women had significantly smaller volumes of both gray and white brain matter, as well as greater volumes of sulcal and ventricular cerebral spinal fluid, than nonalcoholic women.

When drug use suddenly stops, the body fails to function normally because "normal" now includes the presence of the drug; this abnormal functioning is felt as withdrawal. The higher the degree of tolerance and dependence, the worse the withdrawal symptoms will be. Withdrawal to different drugs varies in unpleasantness, severity, and risk of death. Withdrawal from heroin is reportedly one of the most unpleasant withdrawals, but withdrawal from heavy barbiturate or alcohol use has a greater risk of death, according to studies by N. Miller and M. Gold. Withdrawals vary widely from person to person and substance or activity.

Knowing the signs and symptoms of drug withdrawal can save an addict's life, since immediate medical treatment may be required, especially with delirium tremors, which often begin 72 hours after the last alcoholic drink and can lead to death if not treated.

ADDICTION'S TOLL ON THE BODY

Research shows the effects of alcohol and other substances on women may be vastly underreported. According to researchers at Dalhousie University in Nova Scotia and the University of Calgary, Alberta, the same standards are often applied to define "use" in women and men, in spite of differences in body mass index. What is clear is that the risks are serious. D. W. Hommer, in a report in the *American Journal of Psychiatry*, found that alcoholic women had significantly smaller volumes of both gray and white brain matter, as well as greater volumes of sulcal and ventricular cerebral spinal fluid, than nonalcoholic women. The men studied had similar findings, but to a lesser degree, leading the researchers to believe that on average, women alcoholics tend to drink as much in volume as alcoholic men.

Other permanent changes to the brain have been attributed to chronic substance use. According to figures posted on Psychiatry Online in 2001, approximately 10 percent of chronic alcohol-dependent people develop dementia due to alcohol, placing approximately 1 percent of the entire population at risk. An additional 5 to 15 percent of alcohol-dependent people develop mild cognitive impairments that do not meet the criteria for dementia. Additionally, addictive behaviors produce countless risks to women's reproductive health and the health of the fetus during pregnancy, including increased risk of sexually transmitted diseases due to addiction-driven sexual behavior. A team from the University of Washington Medical Center found that a substantial number of women treated in

SIGNS AND SYMPTOMS OF DRUG WITHDRAWAL

Drug	Peak Period	Duration	Signs	Symptoms
Alcohol	1–2 days	5–7 days	Elevated blood pressure, pulse, and temperature, hyperarousal, agitation, restlessness, cutaneous flushing, tremors, diaphoresis, dilated pupils, ataxia, clouding of consciousness, disorientation	Anxiety, panic, paranoid delusions, visual, auditory, and tactile hallucinations
Benzodiazepines and Other Sedatives/Hypnotics	Short-acting: 2–4 days Long-acting: 4–7 days	Short-acting: 4–7 days Long-acting: 7–14 days	Increased psychomotor activity, agitation, muscular weakness, tremulousness, hyperpyrexia, diaphoresis, delirium, convulsions, elevated blood pressure, pulse, temperature, tremor of eyelids, tongue, and hands	Anxiety, depression, euphoria, incoherent thoughts, hostility, grandiosity, disorientation, tactile, auditory, and visual hallucinations, suicide
Stimulants (Cocaine, Amphetamines)	1–3 days	5–7 days	Social withdrawal, psychomotor retardation, hypersomnia, hyperphagia	Depression, anhedonia, suicidal thoughts and behavior, paranoid delusions
Opiates (Heroin)	1–3 days	5–7 days	Drug seeking, mydriasis, pilorection, diaphoresis, rhinorrhea, lacrimation, diarrhea, insomnia, elevated blood pressure and pulse	Intense desire for drugs, muscle cramps, arthralgia, anxiety, nausea, vomiting, malaise
PCP/Psychedelics	Days to weeks	Days to weeks	Hyperactivity, increased pain threshold, nystagmus, hyperreflexia, hypertension, tachycardia, eyelid retraction (stare), agitation, hyperarousal, dry skin, violent self-destructive behaviors	Anxiety, depression, delusions, auditory and visual hallucinations, memory loss, irritable and angry mood and affect, suicidal thoughts

obstetrics have unrecognized and untreated psychiatric and substance abuse disorders. Psychiatric and substance abuse problems during pregnancy could have detrimental effects, in terms of both poor pregnancy outcomes and increased costs of care.

LIFE'S DEMANDS INTERFERING WITH HELP

Joanie came to treatment because her relationship with Steve was falling apart, she was feeling vulnerable about her job, and she was scared of not being a capable mother. For her, substance abuse came after all of these other issues. In earlier attempts to get help, Joanie's substance abuse had been the sole focus of treatment. Treatment had eventually failed each time to meet her goals, and she had dropped out feeling she had too many things on her plate—most especially her children and their needs.

Once before her therapist had referred her for short-term inpatient treatment for substance use, but she had been unable to participate due to her immediate child-care and housing needs. Her therapist, she said, told her she was "in denial and not serious about getting help" and pushed her to have her parents care for the children during the 28 days of inpatient treatment. This suggestion did not take into consideration Joanie's own terrifying experience with her parents; she dropped out of treatment and tried to handle her problems alone again.

> Often, having access to safe and reliable child care and transportation and a work schedule that allows the person to continue earning an income will enable a woman to face an addiction and get help.

It was crucial for Joanie to have *her needs* heard at this point. Instead of designing a treatment plan that immediately included abstinence, urine screens, mandatory attendance at twelve-step meetings, or leaving children in her parents' custody while she received inpatient treatment, we explored what her *immediate* needs were. We did this even though we both suspected her substance misuse was making her circumstances worse.

Joanie defined communicating better in her relationship, maintaining her job so she could remain independent financially, and protecting her children as her primary initial goals. This approach may be helpful with anyone trying to assist an addicted loved one. Problem solving on these issues can be done together; you can break down the barriers to getting help, avoid misunderstanding, and keep good communication lines open. Often, having access to safe and reliable child care and transportation and a work schedule that allows the person to continue earning an income will enable a woman to face an addiction and get help.

In Joanie's case, we first defined her immediate needs, worked on how to meet her goals, and began to problem solve together. Having become aware of how certain behaviors were exacerbating her problems, she expressed her willingness to change the behaviors. For example, Joanie was able to see how her drinking interfered with her ability to communicate clearly with Steve about how she felt or what she needed in the relationship, resulting in continued disappointments. She then began to practice spending evenings with Steve without drinking by keeping her goals in the forefront. She began to feel more self-empowered in the relationship, more confident in her day-to-day life. As these feelings evolved, she found she needed the substance use less.

Addictive behaviors often meet the needs of more than one person in the home. Oftentimes, a client will begin to make changes only to find their partner, family members, or friends resisting or, worse yet, sabotaging their efforts. Joanie found that Steve grew increasingly verbally abusive as she began to express her needs and defend her self-worth. His behavior contributed to her relapse on two occasions, until she understood that Steve was attempting to keep the status quo. Oftentimes, as with Joanie and Steve, couples therapy or physical separation may be necessary during this process as new communication tools are developed, styles of relating change, and boundaries and respect are built.

THE JOURNEY THROUGH CHANGE

Whether we are thinking about starting a diet, making a change in our career, or kicking a heroin problem, people face real change in predictable ways, according to J. Prochaska, C. Clemente, and J. Norcross. In their article "In Search of How People Change: Applications to Addictive Behaviors," they describe five basic stages of change:

1. Pre-contemplation
2. Contemplation
3. Preparation
4. Action
5. Maintenance

During the pre-contemplative stage, you may not be thinking about change. You may feel out of control with a large amount of denial and may be minimizing the seriousness of consequences related to the damaging behavior. Addicts often end up in mandated treatment at this point, having been referred by a legal, employment, or relational source. In the pre-contemplation stage, you may express only passive wishes for change and may have very different priorities for treatment than your clinician or loved one.

Clinicians must work to join the person on common ground at this point—to find shared genuine goals that may include avoiding legal consequences, reducing anxiety, maintaining housing, or "sorting out these problems with my boyfriend," as in Joanie's case. With the goal of increasing awareness, the person struggling in this stage may need to answer, "What would have to happen for you to know this is a problem?" or "What warning signs would let others know there is a problem?"

Contemplation occurs when you begin to weigh the benefits and costs of the behavior. Ambivalance to change is normal. Typically, addressing change head-on at this stage isn't successful; in fact, if the consciousness of the person facing change isn't raised first, according to Patt Denning, relapse and treatment failure is common. This consciousness comes through answering such questions as "What are my reasons for not changing?" or "What are the barriers to change?" and "What might help eliminate those barriers?" The goal of these questions is to examine the benefits and costs of changing the behavior and to begin building the supports you need to maintain change once it happens.

In the preparation stage, a person facing change will experiment with small changes. For instance, during this stage, Joanie limited wine to one very small glass with dinner ("just for the taste"), stopped smoking marijuana altogether, and switched from Valium to Benadryl to help her sleep at night when feeling anxious.

During the action stage, attempts at change are evident enough to be noticed by others. A defined goal has often been identified. At this point in Joanie's treatment, she outlined that she wanted to stop her alcohol use entirely and learn new relaxation and meditation skills to manage her anxiety at night to reduce her use of sleep aids.

Maintenance of new behaviors over time occurs most successfully when the person has learned and integrated new coping skills and relationship patterns. With practice come confidence and skill in the new behaviors and patterns of relating.

Keep in mind that relapse is a normal part of change. This fact is often minimized, which leaves people feeling demoralized when relapse occurs. How often have you slipped while on a diet and begun to feel hopeless about losing that last ten pounds? Both patient and clinician must actively prepare for relapse throughout the treatment relationship.

> Keep in mind that relapse is a normal part of change. This fact is often minimized, which leaves people feeling demoralized when relapse occurs.

Disease theorists, who see addiction as a lifelong illness, would disagree, but Patt Denning describes termination as when the behavior no longer intrudes on daily life and an evaluation and celebration of the change occur. Remaining flexible, creative, and open during this process is critical, as change is fluid.

Understanding the process of change helps everyone involved with a woman with an addiction: the clinician, family member, loved one, or friend, and certainly the woman herself. Together they can develop interventions to initiate, support, and maintain the desired changes.

UNEARTHING AN ADDICTION OR TWO

As Joanie's story teaches us, an addiction can be buried within a mountain of other life issues. A better understanding of how people change can help the person struggling with an addictive behavior to be more successful as she works her way through treatment.

Some key questions to ask yourself or someone you feel might be in trouble with an addiction might include:

- Was there ever a time in your life when you (insert behavior) too much or in unsafe ways?
- Has anyone close to you ever said you have a problem with (insert behavior)?
- Has (insert behavior) ever caused problems for you? What sort?
- Because of the (behavior), how often have you missed work, had trouble at school, or not taken good care of the children?

When Joanie answered these questions we determined that the alcohol, marijuana, and Valium use had contributed to her problems and was inhibiting her from meeting her goals. She came to see that while she had long ago become dependent upon these substances for the comfort and pain relief they provided, they were now causing her continual problems.

According to the *DSM-IV*, abuse is considered the continued use of alcohol, drugs, or addictive behavior in spite of negative consequences. Dependency or addiction is defined as use that a) causes social and occupational trouble in a woman's life and b) causes a compulsive need to keep using despite the increasing chaos. While physical dependence, tolerance, and withdrawal are often signs of addiction, they cannot be sole determinants.

Cocaine, for instance, causes no physical dependence, but it can be addicting. Some addicts are able to rather easily withdraw from heroin, but this doesn't mean the heroin use did not cause severe problems in their lives. On the other hand, a cancer patient may develop a tolerance to morphine and need very high doses to obtain relief, but this does not mean she is destined to continue using morphine addictively once the pain ceases or her condition improves. In fact, in a study of morphine and pain, patients revealed that addiction rarely results, even when high doses are used consistently. Why is this so? Some speculate that painkillers have a different pharmacological effect when used for the relief of pain rather than the pursuit of pleasure. Others take a different view, suggesting that a cancer patient usually uses opiates for a very discrete reason; when the reason no longer exists, use ceases to be compelling. A substance abuser, however, often has not a discrete physiological problem but a snarl of internal and external stressors that resists unraveling.

Through the process of exploring the effects that her use had on her goals, Joanie found she had been requiring increasing amounts and frequency of the substances she used to relieve her pain and suffering. She realized she had grown truly dependent on these substances, even without daily use.

DOES THIS MEAN I HAVE A DISEASE?

In 1960, E. M. Jellinek presented a comprehensive disease model of alcohol addiction. Jellinek's model described a progression from initial drug exposure to drug use resulting in a high, to development of an irresistible appetite for the drug, to continued use of the drug despite negative consequences, and, finally, to progressive deterioration resulting in physical, moral, and spiritual bankruptcy. Key to Jellinek's disease model is that one is powerless to stop the progression toward addiction.

Several important professional bodies followed suit in recognizing addiction as a disease, including the World Health Organization, the American Psychiatric Association, and the American Medical Association. Jellinek's model opened up thinking about the genetic and physiological issues in addiction treatment. The relationship between the widely accepted self-help program Alcoholics Anonymous and the disease model explains the model's durability, despite claims that Jellinek's research contained many flaws and did not include any female subjects. In his book, *Love and Addiction*, S. Peele argues that the disease model has continued to exist because it has become profitable: its application has spread to gambling, overeating, shopping, and almost every other form of self-destructive behavior.

An alternate to the disease model, the adaptive model, states that substance use develops out of traumatic, highly stressed, or faulty upbringing, environmental inadequacy, or genetic unfitness. From these negative points come a sense of self-hate, depression, and poor social integration, with substance misuse compensating for the painful feelings. Addiction to illicit and licit drugs, gambling, food, sex and love, criminality, or fanaticism may develop. A key to the adaptive model is that a choice is theoretically made to cope with one's internal and external circumstances through the addictive behavior. If addictive behavior can be one choice, then other behaviors can be chosen if circumstances and understanding change.

No single model is absolutely the right model. What matters here is what fits for the woman who is experiencing distress. Joanie at first found that the disease theory resonated most with her experiences but in the end viewed her substance abuse problem more through the adaptive lens.

HOW DO I GET HELP?

A range of treatment options exist if you are seeking help for addiction: self-help groups, outpatient treatment, partial day treatment, and inpatient and residential treatment.

Some key questions to ask yourself or someone you feel might be in trouble with an addiction might include:

✦ *Was there ever a time in your life when you (insert behavior) too much or in unsafe ways?*

✦ *Has anyone close to you ever said you have a problem with (insert behavior)?*

✦ *Has (insert behavior) ever caused problems for you? What sort?*

✦ *Because of the (behavior), how often have you missed work, had trouble at school, or not taken good care of the children?*

Which treatment setting would work best for you depends upon the severity and potential lethality of the addictive behavior, day-to-day difficulties like child care and housing demands, and where you are in the change process.

Self-help groups include Alcoholics Anonymous (AA), Sex Addicts Anonymous (SAA), Narcotics Anonymous (NA), Overeaters Anonymous (OA), Women For Sobriety (WFS), Self Management and Recovery Training (SMART), and Rational Recovery (RR). These groups vary in their target behavior, approach, and orientation but are usually free and available in most areas. The twelve-step groups, such as AA, NA, OA, and SAA, are based on an abstinence model in which you admit to powerlessness over the targeted behavior and change begins from there by working your way through the twelve steps toward heightened spirituality with the support of the group community.

Twelve-step self-help groups have helped thousands of people remain safe and sober, and they can provide an effective and helpful complement to other treatment for the recovering person. The twelve-step format does have problems, however. Some people are turned off by this approach of admitting to powerlessness and accepting of a "higher power," often referred to as "God" in the meetings. Further, many feminists, including Charlotte Kasl, believe the steps should be rewritten for women to build on self-empowerment and rejecting blame, while maintaining recognition that the symptom (drinking, sexual acting out, drug use) can lessen one's power and overall success. Women For Sobriety grew out of these concerns; behavioral changes are promoted through positive reinforcement, cognitive strategies, and body work, which is facilitated through dynamic group participation.

Others have rejected twelve-step groups for labeling the participants as addicts and for the nonrational approach to addiction's problems. Programs such as Rational Recovery and SMART emphasize development of a rational, cognitive-behavioral approach to change. SMART acknowledges that the dysfunctional behavior/substance use often began as a means to cope with life's problems, but that it has now become counterproductive and impractical. SMART groups utilize rational emotive behavioral therapy techniques, based on the work of Albert Ellis, to help reverse self-destructive behaviors.

Many women first get help for addiction through outpatient treatment. They enter treatment to deal with relationship problems or to reduce stress, only to discover in the course of treatment that their substance abuse/addictive behaviors are continuing their problems; they then begin to focus on those behaviors. Individual counseling or group work may be done in outpatient settings via a private practitioner or community-based mental health/substance abuse clinic. A mutual peer aid group, a trusted friend, or a well-trained

Self-help groups include:

- Alcoholics Anonymous (AA)
- Sex Addicts Anonymous (SAA)
- Narcotics Anonymous (NA)
- Overeaters Anonymous (OA)
- Women For Sobriety (WFS)
- Self Management and Recovery Training (SMART)
- Rational Recovery (RR)

therapist may provide help. Finding the right fit for your needs is important, so don't be afraid to interview a few providers.

Partial day, inpatient, and residential treatment exist for those needing more structure and support, to ensure safety and facilitate very difficult change. Specialty programs such as those targeting people with a dual diagnosis (mental health and substance abuse issues) are increasingly available and are often well suited for addressing both the addiction and the coexisting symptoms of trauma, depression, and/or anxiety.

Detoxification with medical supervision may be required for those facing change in use of physiologically addictive substances or when withdrawal could trigger life-threatening symptoms. One of the most serious detoxifications is that for alcohol, where withdrawal can be life-threatening if not monitored.

Group work is considered a vital component of most people's path to recovery. The group process helps break through denial but also provides a vital sense of community and support that may be lacking after years of using and isolation due to dysfunctional patterns ofrelating, domestic violence, and/or family care-giving demands.

Many options exist for sculpting a sound treatment and support system for a person facing change of their longstanding behaviors or addictions. For Joanie, an outpatient detox followed by intensive outpatient services and then regular outpatient work met her needs for stabilizing and eventually ending her use, while maintaining her ability to work and care for her children. Whatever the plan, the person facing change must be involved in its development and implementation in order to increase commitment and ownership of the process.

—*Kathryn Davis, B.A., LICSW*

RELATED ENTRIES

Depressive Disorders

Anxiety Disorders

Women and Trauma

Poverty and Women's Mental Health

Schizophrenia

The Brain under Siege

Schizophrenia means literally "split brain." Often misconstrued as "split personality," this heterogeneous, enigmatic illness is more properly characterized as a division of the self, a splitting of thought from perception, of internal from external realities. Once afflicted, most often in late adolescence, schizophrenics are driven by intrinsic, invisible demons that confound their senses, befuddle logic, and render social interactions impossible to negotiate.

Perhaps because the illness so often intrudes at the beginning of adult life, just as its victims are embarking on careers and families of their own, it is particularly painful, poignant, and destructive. A relatively small percentage of people with schizophrenia make a full recovery. The majority improves, but live a life of concession to the illness with impaired social relations, lower levels of career and academic achievement, and persistent or intermittent battles with mental trickery. In the last ten years, a new generation of antipsychotic medications has made schizophrenia more livable, but, as with so many psychiatric illnesses, a cure still eludes us.

EPIDEMIOLOGY

Schizophrenia is among the most democratic of diseases, occurring with about equal frequency in England and Ethiopia, Hong Kong and Haiti. All told, the illness afflicts just less than one percent of the world population. There is some evidence that rates are higher in urban than in rural populations; analogously, outcomes appear to be better in developing than in developed countries. (Some have postulated that the better prognosis reflects a stronger network of social support.)

Schizophrenia comes with enormous costs: in the United States, the financial burden of schizophrenia is greater than that incurred by all cancers, combined. The prevalence of the illness is greatest among the lowest socioeconomic classes, and it is estimated that one-third to one-half of homeless persons are afflicted.

Women and men develop schizophrenia at about the same rate. However, the onset of the illness and its subsequent course may differ between the sexes. For men, there is a sharp peak in incidence between the ages of seventeen and twenty-seven. For women, risk similarly increases at age seventeen, but thereafter plateaus until about age thirty-seven.

Women are also at greater risk for developing schizophrenia in midlife or old age. In some cases, the affected person has been noted to have certain pre-existing personality characteristics, such as a tendency to be isolative and introverted; however, in other instances the onset of illness is abrupt and unheralded.

SIGNS AND SYMPTOMS

Mr. C. is a forty-one-year-old man with chronic paranoid schizophrenia. He enters the office wearing a blue cotton sweatshirt beneath his corduroy sport coat; he explains that he avoids synthetic fabrics because they cause cancer. He states that it took him longer than usual to get here today, because six Russian agents forced him off the city bus and searched his backpack, looking for a hidden microphone. When asked how he is feeling, he responds, "There's too much resistance."

The hallmark of schizophrenia is a gross disturbance in sensory perception, such as visual or auditory hallucinations. Visual hallucinations may include animals or people, animate or inanimate objects, images that are mundane or monstrous. Auditory hallucinations typically comprise voices that comment on or instruct the patient's behavior, music, messages from God or some other power. Also common are delusions: People may believe they have the ability to fly, to read others' thoughts, to cause or reverse natural disasters or global events (such as 9/11). They may believe they are being persecuted, spied upon, that their homes are being broken into. One woman I knew wore an aluminum helmet, to protect against alien mind control.

Along with hallucinations and delusions, there are often disturbances of thought and speech. Paralleling the mind's disarray, schizophrenic language becomes fragmented, illogical, and eventually undecipherable. Words flit erratically here and there; the train of association is terminally derailed. Asked to complete the sentence, "A man fell on the street," a schizophrenic man replied, "because of World War II." In some cases, language becomes so disjointed that only the speaker discerns any semblance of meaning.

In addition to these manifest disturbances, which are also called the "positive symptoms" of schizophrenia, the illness is characterized by more subtle or covert behavioral changes. The so-called negative symptoms of schizophrenia include apathy; social withdrawal; lack of motivation or initiative; stereotyped, repetitive behavior; decreased speech; or mutism. Other possible symptoms include frozen posturing (catatonia), disorganization, or frenzied activity. Absorbed in their usually hostile inner worlds, schizophrenics are typically unaware of the social implications of their behavior.

SYMPTOMS OF SCHIZOPHRENIA

Visual or auditory
  hallucinations
Delusions
Disjointed use of language
Apathy
Social withdrawal
Lack of motivation or initiative
Repetitive behavior
Decreased speech
Frenzied activity

ETIOLOGY

The cause of schizophrenia is not known. Clearly there is a genetic component: Children of a schizophrenic parent have a risk that is five to ten times greater than that of the general population, and children with two schizophrenic parents have a 35 percent chance of developing the illness. However, 90 percent of people with schizophrenia have no family history of the disease. This suggests that whatever inherited risks may be present, there must be environmental or developmental factors that influence the expression of illness. A number of possible factors may be implicated, including influenza infection, birth and preg-

**RELATED
ENTRIES**

*Antipsychotic
Medications*

nancy complications, or in utero exposure to a viral agent. One mechanism that these diverse pathways may share is an increased level of stress hormones. In one study, women who had been exposed to a tornado during pregnancy had an increased risk of having a child with schizophrenia. In another trial, children whose mothers did not want to be pregnant also had an increased risk of developing schizophrenia. Pregnant women whose partners die before the birth are more likely to have children with schizophrenia, as well as with other psychiatric illnesses.

Researchers have long noted the coincidence of schizophrenia with adolescence and have postulated a link between reproductive hormones and a deleterious effect on brain structure and function. Just which structures or processes are influenced remains unclear. As with many medical conditions, our understanding of the immediate causes of schizophrenia largely stem from observations of drug effects on the brain. Drugs that increase levels of the neurotransmitter dopamine, such as cocaine and amphetamines, can cause a paranoid psychosis that resembles schizophrenia; meanwhile, drugs that block dopamine can alleviate the symptoms of the illness. The first class of medicines used to treat schizophrenia comprised such dopamine-blocking agents as Haldol, Mellaril, and Trilafon. Current theories suggest that serotonin, the same neurotransmitter involved in depression, may also be implicated in schizophrenia, but in excess rather than deficient amounts. The newer antipsychotics, including Clozaril, Seroquel, and Risperdalare, are modeled on this theory of serotonin overactivity.

COURSE AND PROGNOSIS

The course of schizophrenia varies, but the prognosis is too often guarded, if not ominous. A number of factors seem to be associated with improved outcome, for example, a rapid onset at a later age, fewer negative symptoms, and the presence of a good social adjustment before becoming ill. It seems that if an individual is able to learn a framework for relating to others before she develops schizophrenia, the odds of maintaining an integrated life improve.

> There is little evidence that chronic schizophrenia will respond to behavioral interventions, or attempts to reason one's way out of paranoid psychosis.

Medications, too, have had a considerable impact: With drug treatment, only 10 to 15 percent of patients relapse per year, versus 65 to 70 percent without treatment. John Nash (the topic of the book and movie *A Beautiful Mind*) notwithstanding, there is little evidence that chronic schizophrenia will respond to behavioral interventions, or attempts to reason one's way out of paranoid psychosis. Even with medications, about one-third of schizophrenics remain chronically ill. Spontaneous recoveries do occur, but in most case remission, rather than cure, is the foremost treatment goal.

—*Susan Mahler, M.D.*

Marriage and Motherhood

Married American and European women in the twenty-first century at long last hold the right to choose their own partners, to control reproduction, to own property, to work outside the home, to divorce. The law does not tolerate physical abuse and unwanted sexual acts. And yet, despite these victories—surely enviable in a place like Istanbul, where a woman is not allowed to leave the house unescorted, or Nigeria, where the authorities threaten women with punishment of death by stoning for adultery—studies show that marriage is still better for a man's mental health than for a woman's. What is it about the matrimonial union, the beginning of which we customarily celebrate with champagne and lace, that makes it hazardous for women?

Dalma Heyn, author of *Marriage Shock: The Transformation of Women into Wives*, thinks that women submerge a central part of themselves when they marry. Is this the reason that newlywed women think often about death, as one study found? When a woman exchanges her own surname for her husband's, relocates for his job, and cuts back on her career when the children arrive, it's not difficult to see why she has trouble holding on to her sense of self. A part of her *has* died.

Women submerge a central part of themselves not only in life decisions but also in the day-to-day compromises and adjustments that living closely with another person necessarily entails. She likes the house neat and orderly while he is oblivious to his surroundings; she listens to country western tunes while he demands news of the world; he leaves the toilet seat up, she requires it down. Women, who tend to be highly relational and therefore sensitized to the needs of others, are more likely than men to compromise and accommodate. In an intimate partnership, one that requires deep and delicate negotiation, women may be more comfortable submitting to someone else's needs than standing up for their own, especially if that other person has a willful or dynamic personality. In other words, when it comes time to live with a man, she is more likely to pick up his clutter, to demur that her radio show is not so important, to learn to contain and restrain, to time after time bend down to adjust the toilet seat. And after so many years of bending and bending, she no longer maintains her own true shape. She becomes pressed down—in other words, depressed.

David Popenoe and Barbara Dafoe Whitehead, codirectors of the 1999 report from the Rutgers University National Marriage project, found that young women today, especially teens, are fairly disenchanted with marriage. They are marrying later—at median age of twenty-five as opposed to a median age of twenty in 1960. They are pessimistic, not so much about committing themselves to a lifelong partner but about finding a man suitable enough.

Popenoe and Whitehead found that young women especially want a man who will have a high capacity for emotional intimacy in marriage, as well as a vested involvement in child-rearing and household work. And women's growing economic independence means they are not as willing as they once were to put up with an unsatisfactory husband out of sheer economic dependence. Popenoe and Whitehead's conclusions explain not only why young women today are increasingly reluctant to marry, but also why nearly 50 percent of contemporary marriages dissolve.

> In an intimate partnership, one that requires deep and delicate negotiation, women may be more comfortable submitting to someone else's needs than standing up for their own.

Most dangerous to a woman's health, of course, is domestic violence. Surveys of American couples show that 20 to 50 percent have suffered violence in their marriage. Between 2 and 4 million incidents of domestic violence are reported every year. One quarter of all murders take place within the family. Once wife beating occurs, it is likely to happen repeatedly, and family life is lived in a cycle of tension, explosion, and forgiveness that a woman, especially if she is economically or emotionally dependent, will find difficult to leave.

And yet, we continue to hear wedding bells. Even pessimistic marriage researchers predict that up to 85 percent of women will marry at least once by age forty-five. Early, late, once, twice, three times, in churches and synagogues and function halls and city halls, we continue to join our lives to a man's. We continue to vow ourselves to another. We continue to hope.

How can a woman make marriage a healthier place for her mental health?

Bookstores and libraries supply shelf after shelf of marital advice. Some examples: Best-selling author Judith S. Wallerstein, in *The Good Marriage: How and Why Love Lasts*, describes four kinds of marriages—Romantic, Rescue, Companionate, and Traditional—and nine tasks that must be mastered in a good marriage. John M. Gottman, Ph.D., a psychologist and author, has devised seven principles to make marriages work harmoniously and be long lasting. Cheryl Jarvis, in *The Marriage Sabbatical: The Journey That Brings You Home*, proposes that a woman can maintain health in both her self and her marriage by spending time away from her husband developing her own talents and interests. Richard Schwartz, M.D., and Jacqueline Olds, M.D., write in their book *Marriage and Motion: The Natural Ebb and Flow of Lasting Relationships* that any two people in an intimate relationship will naturally navigate periods of closeness and distance. A good marriage is dependent upon accepting that ebb and flow and, moreover, learning to grow and deepen with the tides.

> Most dangerous to a woman's health is domestic violence. Surveys of American couples show that 20 to 50 percent have suffered violence in their marriage.

Good advice, all. Helpful, no doubt, to many. But maybe the problem with marriage cannot be broken down into steps and principles. Maybe the problem lies with our expectations. In today's fairy tale, doesn't living happily ever after mean having it all—appliances, orgasms, and a lifelong soul mate?

What we expect from marriage is socially and historically constructed. For example, diamonds have not always been a girl's best friend. In 1939, De Beers Consolidated, the South African diamond company, was high on supply and short on demand. It mounted an aggressive advertising campaign to convince consumers that a diamond ring could express love. In fact, one could argue that romantic love has always been bought and sold. For much of human history, marriage was not necessarily about love but was instead a legal contract to maintain the social order, transfer property, and provide a stable environment for raising children. Romantic love first sprang into being in the Middle Ages, when it began to be popularized by troubadour love songs. For the troubadours, romantic love was an idealized passion, one that existed outside both marriage and carnal knowledge. A knight might worship his master's lady. Dante immortalized his love for Beatrice despite having seen her only three times in his entire life. By the sixteenth century, romantic lovers consummated their passions, but always outside marriage. Shakespeare, that great love poet, is primarily an adultery poet. By the nineteenth century, romantic love, still adulterous, was cautioned against. Passion brought suffering. Lovers could die for their transgressions. Ethel Spector Person, in "Romantic Love: At the Intersection of the Psyche and the Cultural Unconscious," parallels the rise of romantic love with the rise of the autonomous, free-willed individual in society.

> Perhaps we would experience greater marital happiness, by which I mean reduced feelings of disappointment and inadequacy, were we to set the bar lower.

Romantic love, which psychologists say we model on the mother–infant dyad, and which depends on a deep yearning for the idealized beloved, claims that you are unique and irreplaceable in the other's eyes, even as it privileges the primacy of your emotions. To require the intensity of this love before and during marriage is a relatively new development in Western society. To maintain this intensity through a lifetime fraught with challenge and change is difficult indeed. Perhaps it is the demand itself—our romanticization of the married relationship—that should be questioned. Perhaps we would experience greater marital happiness, by which I mean reduced feelings of disappointment and inadequacy, were we to set the bar lower. Men are complicated beings. Women are complicated beings. Children are complicated beings. To live together in harmony and intimacy is sometimes possible. Other times, marriage is a segment of the ordinary human unhappiness that Freud posited as a natural, even enviable state of mind. Marriage, a profound laboratory for human emotion, brings us up against an other, and ourselves, and from this we learn. When we marry, we sign up for the whole human catastrophe—by which I mean birth, sickness, death, fortunes made and fortunes lost. And how it all turns out is often a matter of luck.

> If you have a child, especially a preschooler, it is better for a woman's mental health to be married than not.

One aspect of marriage that has not changed with history is its effectiveness for bringing up children. The only population with an even higher incidence of depression than married women is single mothers with young children. If you have a child, especially a preschooler, it is better for a woman's mental health to be married than not. Motherhood, however, runs an even higher risk of undermining a woman's mental health than does marriage. Motherhood can knock a woman off her feet as surely as it can transform her life.

For starters, a woman can suffer postpartum psychiatric illness. Postpartum blues—a few weeks of weeping, irritability, and moodiness—affects up to 80 percent of new mothers. A tiny percentage—1 in 1,000—will contract postpartum psychosis, the new mother's brain turning hallucinatory, delusional, with thoughts of her own suicide and her baby's death paramount. Each year, over 400,000 women in the United States alone, an estimated

13 percent of new mothers, suffer from postpartum depression. PPD can overtake a woman anywhere in her baby's first year. Susan Kushner Resnick, whose memoir *Sleepless Days* chronicles her experience with PPD four months after the birth of her second child, describes the illness thus:

> It causes insomnia, mood swings, anxiety, fear of losing control, weird thoughts of hurting the baby that you never intend to carry out but that scare the hell out of you nonetheless, thoughts of suicide, and a general feeling of being overwhelmed, disconnected from everyone you love, and desperately wanting to be mothered. All those tender nurturing feelings you expected or felt before the depression began—are absent most of the time. You can't seem to locate your old self, although you're aware enough to know she's missing and remember who she was.

Postpartum depression can be difficult for a mother to admit, and difficult even for medical professionals to diagnose, so interwoven are its symptoms with most new mothers' experiences of jittery exhaustion. Although the disease itself is not new, its naming and treatment have been around only since 1994. Like many other similarly stricken women, Resnick recovered with the help of antidepressants, sleeping medication, and a therapist experienced with PPD.

For those who do not experience a clinical mental illness in the first year of motherhood, there is always garden-variety sleep deprivation, identity crisis, marital discord, stress, fatigue, and loneliness. Most women find that the first year of motherhood is monumental and transformative to their psyche. Iris Krasnow, in *Surrendering to Motherhood: Losing Your Mind, Finding Your Soul*, likens the daily work of mothering to the Zen challenge to Be Here Now and testifies to the soul growth available to a woman who "surrenders" to motherhood.

During my son's first year, a year that included broken sleep, thousands of diapers, four baby colds, two cases of maternal mastitis, nine months of breast-feeding, countless interrupted meals, and twenty-five hours per week of paid relief from child care, I found myself appreciating and reconnecting to my own mother for the first time in twenty years. Instead of the fault finding and blaming I'd engaged in ever since adolescence—an exercise laden with self-pity for the person I'd become—I suddenly found myself grateful, on a visceral level, that my mother had heaped such unconditional love on my infant self, for surely this was the same love I could give to my own baby. In the context of my becoming a mother, I could again enjoy my own mother's company. I knew she was proud and happy to see me as a mother and I knew that she, too, loved my son. I felt gratified seeing my mother become a caring and involved grandmother.

An acquaintance, however, found her entry into motherhood quite painful. During her child's first year, realizing that her own mother was as profoundly unequipped to mother a grandchild as she had once been unable to care for a child, this self-supporting graphic designer broke irrevocably with her mother. Many women I know experienced equally profound changes in their identity as they seriously rethought their commitments to work and family. Some discovered they were not the stay-at-home cookie-baking moms they'd imagined themselves to be, while others realized they were no longer the ambitious, briefcase-carrying professionals they were before the baby arrived.

A full 50 percent of mothers with preschool children experience symptoms of intense emotional distress on a regular basis.

The problem with motherhood and mental health, says Susan Mushart, sociologist, mother of three, and author of *The Mask of Motherhood: How Becoming a Mother Changes Everything and Why We Pretend It Doesn't,* is that we millennial women—94 percent of whom will choose to become mothers—cling to an overly romanticized notion of motherhood, the same as we do to marriage. We expect to run the board meeting and be home in time to read *Goodnight Moon* to our children. We expect our husbands, those same men beside whom we studied in graduate school, whose bodies we once found on par with Adonis, and on whose mean spaghetti sauce we rely, to be an equal partner during the parenting years.

The reality of motherhood, says Mushart, is very, very different from what we envision. A full 50 percent of mothers with preschool children experience symptoms of intense emotional distress

> Instead of the fault finding and blaming I'd engaged in ever since adolescence, I suddenly found myself grateful, on a visceral level, that my mother had heaped such unconditional love on my infant self.

on a regular basis. These mothers report shock, panic, chronic fatigue, feeling unprepared, feeling overwhelmed, and in general, difficulty coping. What's worse, Mushart argues, is that instead of speaking the truth about the difficult challenges and very real price we pay for having children, we too often wear a mask to pretend that everything about this daunting task is effortless and under our control. Unmasking motherhood, says Mushart and others, is the final task of feminism.

Any analysis of the stresses and surprises of motherhood and their effect on women's mental health would be remiss without mention of Arlie Hoschild's widely acclaimed and groundbreaking work in *The Second Shift* and *The Time Bind.* Hoschild's research points out that while women have been gaining parity in the workplace (almost two-thirds of U.S. women with preschoolers work for pay), they have done so in addition to their substantial unpaid labor in the domestic sphere. When they come home from their job, a full second shift awaits—cooking, cleaning, getting the children to bed, organizing, laundry—repetitive tasks psychologists relate to anxiety and depression. Mushart calls this "the juggled life" and a "chronic-fatigue lifestyle." In households where couples try to divide the chores more equitably, the men often end up doing work like repairs or yard work—chores that, because they can be postponed, are less stress inducing. Even so, a woman who works outside the home, either full or part-time, has a higher rate of self-esteem than a full-time, stay-at-home mom who does not work for pay. The working mom appears to have greater emotional reserves for caring

> Although the stay-at-home mom *seems* to have a more leisurely lifestyle, the social isolation and lack of status can often make her increasingly irritable, depressed, and even emotionally unstable.

for her children and reports fewer symptoms of depression. Although the stay-at-home mom *seems* to have a more leisurely lifestyle, the social isolation and lack of status can often make her increasingly irritable, depressed, and even emotionally unstable.

A major factor endangering a full-time mother's mental health is the schizoid and perilous way we as a society construct motherhood. Mythologically speaking, we venerate motherhood. We sanctify the child's need to attach to an attentive, loving, constant, and well-informed primary caregiver mother; we call for a return to family values; we bemoan too many hours of day care; we pledge that breast is best. Rightly or wrongly, these belief systems are alive and well in parenting magazines, in the media, in pediatricians' offices, and, most important, in women's heart of hearts. The very great problem, says Ann Crittenden in her consequential book *The Price of Motherhood: Why the Most Important Job in the World Is Still the Least Valued,* is that public policy and public opinion undermine our ability to carry out these beliefs. Changing the status of mothers in the twenty-first century, says Crittenden, is "the great unfinished business of the women's movement."

Crittenden, a Pulitzer Prize nominee in journalism, who left her job as a reporter at the *News York Times* to raise her son, has assembled an impressive arsenal of facts to back her thesis. She estimates that over her lifetime, a college-educated woman who has a child will pay a "mommy tax" of more than a million dollars in foregone income. Stay-at-home mothers—who essentially provide childrearing, cooking, cleaning, shopping, chauffeuring, dispute mediation, financial planning, appointment making—perform services conservatively valued at $100,000 per year. But our society makes no adjustments to these economic realities. Zilch. Staying at home with the kids is routinely referred to as "doing nothing." Nannies earn Social Security credits; stay-at-home moms do not. American mothers have smaller pensions than either men or single women. In short, women today are penalized for taking seriously the very job, motherhood, that society takes such pains to worship. And the penalty for living within this contradiction is often psychological as well as financial.

> Nannies earn Social Security credits; stay-at-home moms do not.

What is needed, says Crittenden and other thinkers, is for caretaking—not only of children, but of the elderly and the disabled as well, whom women also care for disproportionately—to be conceptualized as *work*. Women who perform the necessary job of caretaker must demand that they be treated as productive citizens, with all the ensuing social and economic rights. Crittenden calls for major changes in social policy, such as giving every parent the right to a year's paid leave after the birth of a child, equalizing social security for spouses, providing universal preschool for three- and four-year-olds, and providing free health care coverage for all children and their primary caregivers. Changes like these would benefit not only mothers and children, but also our well-being as a nation.

European nations are already way ahead of the United States in truly valuing motherhood. France offers preschooling to all three- to five-year-olds at little or no charge. In Britain, new mothers receive home visits from a nurse. Scandinavian countries offer generous paid parental leave opportunities for mothers and fathers, as well as affordable day care.

> Women who perform the necessary job of caretaker must demand that they be treated as productive citizens, with all the ensuing social and economic rights.

What would motherhood look like were we to offer even some of these changes?

During my son's first year, I became friends with a Norwegian mother. Ingunn's son was born three weeks after mine, and we met often in the park as together our children learned to crawl, then walk. Married to an American, she spoke often of being homesick for Norway and displayed with pride the long underwear and raingear her relatives sent so her son could be comfortable outdoors in any weather. Highly educated, trained as an economist, my friend chose to care full-time for her son that first year. I detected subtle differences, inflections really, like the accented English she spoke so fluently, between Ingunn and the other new mothers I knew.

She viewed this year as a discrete and temporary period of time, one in which she would above all be present for her child. Although she was as interested as any American mother in discussing, for example, at what age to introduce solid foods, there was less of the competitive, compulsive behavior that other professional moms often exhibit in mastering motherhood as a new project. Although she, too, complained about lost sleep, there was less self-pity and more a sense that these were difficulties that went with the job. She took no pains to present herself as the perfect, pulled-together mother; more often than not, her clothes were wrinkled and her hair uncombed. But she took care of herself in ways more essential than grooming. She allowed herself to experience wholeheartedly and unambivalently the joys, fears, tedium, rewards, and challenges of becoming a mother. Unlike American mothers I knew, she did not agonize over the emotional ramifications of not working at a paying job. She did not feel demoted by society. She did not fear losing her intelligence. Although she and her family lived closely that year on her husband's salary as a medical resident, she simply assumed that it was important to sit in the park and watch her child pour sand into a pail. Had she been caring for him in Norway, she would be entitled to nine months maternity leave at her original salary. Her husband, too, would be entitled to four weeks off, also with pay. Just the awareness of these facts seemed to make Ingunn a less conflicted mother.

Soon the year would be over. She'd been accepted for a position at the Central Bank of Norway. Her son would be in day care across the street from her office building, where she could visit on her lunch break. Reluctantly, we said goodbye. I had learned a lot just by being around Ingunn and her son. I was losing a friend unafraid to think *and* mother, no small juggling act. Two years later, I received a Christmas card from Ingunn. Unsurprisingly, she had remained in Norway. Her new baby smiled from the photo. She was spending another year at home.

Marriage and motherhood are brave, exciting, soul-deepening, challenging enterprises. The human race literally depends on our willingness to give ourselves to their engagements. The problem is when our imaginary constructs, both individual and collective, become impossible goals, ones that hurt rather than help us in our lives; when women cannot script plots other than those they have absorbed from media and society.

Yet too often the story turns out so differently from what we imagined. The man turns cold and distant, a wage-earning machine relegated to the margins of family life, available to neither the wife nor the child he loves. The woman turns sad and resentful, overtaxed by loads of laundry and inflexible work hours, with little left to give the children and husband she loves, and even less to give herself.

If women talk openly about themselves and to one another, we can connect in larger networks, write articles, rants, books and speeches, make demands, draft legislation. Again and again we must ask the fathers to change diapers and make school lunches, and not criticize them for doing it differently than we do. Women are ferociously strong. How else could so many of us hold three jobs simultaneously: paid work, marriage, motherhood?

—*Karen Propp, Ph.D.*

RELATED
ENTRIES

*Intimate
Relationships*

*Postpartum
Depression*

Postpartum Depression

You feel unplugged. Nothing's connected anymore. Not you with your baby or you with your husband or you with the dream you had of motherhood. You're flagging, and it's not just because of those nighttime feedings. You don't want to get out of bed, but you must, because nobody else can take care of the baby like you can. You don't want to stay awake another instant, but your body seems to have lost the ability to sleep. When that happens, you feel the opposite of unplugged. You're supercharged and there's a buzzing inside, a buzzing in your blood, as if the cells are being electrocuted. You can't stop the buzzing; not with deep breaths or long walks or anything that used to soothe you. Not that you want to do anything pleasurable. You can't read anymore. If you have sex, it's just to prove you're alive. And forget about television. The actors are too happy, so you hate them. Or they're so loving—those women on *Sesame Street*, especially—that you just want them to step out of the screen and take care of you. But they can't. So you cry while your baby sucks in milk, his terry-cloth PJs soaking up the tears.

You can't stop crying. Everything seems so, so sad. Your youth is over, your baby hates you, you're an utter failure at this mothering gig. No one would miss you if you died, because you don't matter to anyone anyway. Or it's all unbearably frightening. What if the baby stops breathing? What if you drop him down the stairs by accident? What if you drop him down the stairs on purpose? What if the shaking and sweating and spastic stomach never stop? What if you have to spend your life white-knuckling the kitchen table as you wait for yet another anxiety attack to pass? And worst of all, what if somebody finds out that you're cracking up? Then, surely, some heartless official will take the baby away.

This is all irrational. You realize this once in a while, because, oddly, there are moments, even days, when you feel totally normal. Days when you convince yourself, *oh, I just felt that way because I needed more sleep,* or *I was having a bad attitude, but now I'll be fine.* Even on the bad days, you occasionally realize that all these thoughts and feelings are not normal. Because inside, beneath the crazy woman, lies the old you. She can't get out, but she can occasionally send a signal. Sometimes she reminds you that you're not completely nuts—yet. If you're lucky, she'll goad you into getting some help.

It isn't easy telling someone what's going on. In fact, it's quite shameful. This wasn't supposed to happen. You were supposed to be happy. Happy, happy, happy. Everyone else is happy. The baby smiles. The father beams. Your sister, when she had a baby, freaking glowed. But you need to surrender to the authorities. Sometimes help is an illusion. The doctor tells you to take a vacation. Your mother tells you it's tough on everyone, but buck up, Baby, because at least you don't have five brats running around. Other times, help comes right away. Your OB, or the baby's pediatrician, or the lady who rented you your breast pump gives you the number of a shrink. This woman, they say, has experience treating postpartum depression.

Postpartum depression? That's not what I've got. I've only had a little trouble sleeping. I've just been under stress. It's not easy having a baby. I …

This woman, they say, call her.

You do. You tell her what's going on and she says she'll see you the next morning. Gee, you think, she must not have many patients if she can see me that soon. But what you don't know is that she heard your desperation, and she knows what happens to the women who don't get help. She knows you need her immediately. You sit in her office the next morning and do nothing but cry. The baby lies in his car seat by your feet and you catch him flirting with the therapist. He coos and cuddles and fetchingly gnaws his fist. Does the shrink wonder how much this behavior irritates you? It's worse than his crying jags. Those, at least, you can relate to. But when he's happy like this you feel as if he's mocking you. The baby is supposed to wail and the mother is supposed to coo with joy, not the other way around. But you wouldn't dare share your resentment with the doctor because you know it's despicable to be bitter with your baby. Just contemplating it multiplies your already oppressive burden of guilt.

> ✦
>
> You can't stop crying. Everything seems so, so sad. Your youth is over, your baby hates you, you're an utter failure at this mothering gig. No one would miss you if you died, because you don't matter to anyone anyway.

At the end of the hour, you contemplate a sit-down strike. I will not move, you imagine saying, until I am better. The shrink—or social worker or psychiatric nurse (these helpers come with a variety of degrees)—understands you. She makes you feel safe, safer than you've felt since the baby was born. If you could just stay here, you believe, everything would be fine.

You leave her office with a prescription. If you're ready to start the healing, she'll prescribe something to help you sleep right away and some kind of antidepressant that will take a few weeks to kick in.

> ✦
>
> This wasn't supposed to happen. You were supposed to be happy. Happy, happy, happy.

They've done studies, and now they know that even nursing mothers can take some medications. If you're not ready to slay your dragon, if you still insist that you can handle this yourself or that only crazy people take antidepressants or that those pills are a crutch, maybe you'll leave with just a recommendation for a book. Getting a book isn't so hard. Most of them are even written in bite-sized pieces, so people wracked with anxiety can read a tiny bit at a time. Here is what you find out:

You aren't alone. Fifteen to 20 percent of all new mothers suffer from postpartum depression (PPD). That's at least 400,000 American women a year. It usually strikes within the first three to six months after birth, but PPD can wait in the wings until a year after delivery. Eighty percent of new mothers get "the blues." Those lucky stiffs have a period of crying every day—usually at the same time—for about two weeks after delivery. It's unpleasant, like an intense bout of premenstrual syndrome, but limited. The moodiness, weepiness, nervousness, sleeplessness, and general yuckiness come and go quickly. One out of a thousand mothers gets postpartum psychosis (PPP). They lose touch with reality, sometimes hurt their babies, sometimes end up on the news. There's a checklist to see whether you're one of them: Do you want to kill yourself or your baby? Do you hear voices or see things no one else sees? Are you confused, incoherent, manic, paranoid, or irrational? If so, you read in big letters, get to an emergency room.

You don't think you have any of the symptoms of PPP. But you have thoughts of suicide. You haven't thought of *doing* it, but you've worried about losing control. *What if all this gets worse and I lose control and I become suicidal or homicidal? What if this is how those mothers on Oprah felt before they went over the edge?* If I've had that thought, you reason, then maybe I should go to the ER. Then you start obsessing. *Am I suicidal? I don't want to die. I just want to feel good again. But then why did that ugly word even pop into my head? There it is again.*

Obsession. That's one of the symptoms on the PPD list. If you have some of these, seek help as soon as you can: sadness, guilt, anxiety, poor concentration, shakiness, upset stomach, extreme agitation, insomnia, trouble breathing, heart palpitations, hopelessness, worthlessness, despair, feeling too worried about the baby or not worried at all, resentment, shame, fear of losing control, excessive exhaustion, panic attacks, feeling as if you're going crazy, thoughts of suicide, and bizarre thoughts. The bizarre thoughts are the worst. All of a sudden, an unbearable image pops into your mind: your baby's head smashed against the glass coffee table. It's just one nightmare of a slide in a relatively benign presentation, one that you didn't put there intentionally, but one that causes extreme shame and terror. *What kind of mother would think that?* Now you know you're going crazy.

> It was supposed to be beautiful, with sunlight gilding the nursery. But the fantasy hasn't materialized for you.

But you're not. You're sick, certainly, but not crazy. Crazy people aren't usually so aware that something is wrong with them. You know something's up, it's just hard to accept that motherhood has actually made you ill. It wasn't supposed to be like this. It was supposed to be beautiful, with sunlight gilding the nursery and wisdom oozing from your pores. But the fantasy hasn't materialized for you. You want to know why.

There are a lot of theories on what causes postpartum depression. There's the hormonal theory that blames biology. Some research has shown that the sudden drop in estrogen and progesterone that occurs as soon as the placenta is removed might bring on PPD. Estrogen, in laboratory studies, has been shown to be a mood enhancer. When drizzled onto the exposed neurons of rats, it literally puts a zip in the cells, causing them to liven up and jig. This may be why so many women actually claim to feel good during pregnancy. You're on an estrogen high, and then you deliver and your own personal placenta gets pulled out from under you. The baby falls, and she's caught in the doctor's cool, gloved hands. You fall, and nobody catches you, which seems more than a little unfair.

If estrogen is so good at perking up cells and energizing animals, then common sense would say it's the perfect postpartum drug. Give the weepy woman a dose of that estrus hormone, for goodness sakes; inject it into her, and she should feel better, yes? Researchers have tried that intervention, giving women with PPD shots and tablets and creams containing the estrogen elixir, with mixed results. Some women claim to feel tranquil and sane after the hormone treatment. Others claim to just feel nauseous. The results, all in all, are not impressive, or not impressive enough to warrant the risk of using estrogen as an antidepressant when there are so many other nonhormonal choices available.

Lack of estrogen isn't the only hormonal theory as to what causes PPD. Other research points to the increase in prolactin, the hormone that stimulates milk production. Most recently, researchers have found that women with certain thyroid antibodies during pregnancy were almost three times as likely to develop PPD.

> Researchers have found that women with certain thyroid antibodies during pregnancy were almost three times as likely to develop PPD.

But PPD doesn't often occur simply for biological reasons. Usually, there's a psychological component, too. If you're having trouble reconciling the old, independent you with the new maternal you, or if having a baby makes you flashback to your own traumatic childhood, PPD could be your booby prize. An upsetting birth experience, one bad enough to cause Post-Traumatic Stress Disorder (PTSD), could tempt a case of PPD. The list of possible causes is long: a family or personal history of depression or obsessive compulsive disorder, severe sleep deprivation, a difficult pregnancy, history of infertility or miscarriage, money problems, marital problems, isolation, a recent death in the family, a recent move, and a hostile relationship with your mother. In essence, PPD is a mystery. So far, the experts haven't been able to pin the cause down to one thing. PPD seems to need a combination of factors, sort of a pu-pu platter of maladies, to emerge.

The cure isn't so mysterious, though. Your doctor tells you that some people can lick PPD with therapy, but most need therapy and antidepressants. If you don't get either, the depression should resolve itself in a year, but it's bound to catch up with you. You think of your mother and all her friends, with their migraines and martinis and mother's little helpers. Maybe they all had PPD, too, but were never treated. So, they spent their lives battling

SYMPTOMS OF PPD

- Sadness
- Guilt
- Anxiety
- Poor concentration
- Shakiness
- Upset stomach
- Extreme agitation
- Insomnia

- Trouble breathing
- Heart palpitations
- Hopelessness
- Worthlessness
- Despair
- Feeling too worried about the baby
- Feeling no worry about the baby
- Resentment

- Shame
- Fear of losing control
- Excessive exhaustion
- Panic attacks
- Feeling as if you're going crazy
- Thoughts of suicide
- Bizarre thoughts

POSSIBLE PSYCHOLOGICAL TRIGGERS OF PPD

- Family or personal history of depression or obsessive compulsive disorder
- Severe sleep deprivation
- A difficult pregnancy
- History of infertility or miscarriage
- Money problems
- Marital problems
- Isolation
- A recent death in the family
- A recent move
- A hostile relationship with your mother

madness. Still, you're hesitant, until your doctor uses the diabetes analogy. If you had diabetes, she says, you'd take medication to treat it. And you wouldn't blame yourself. So, why are you doing it now?

When you start taking antidepressants, not much happens at first. You may doubt the medication and will probably obsessively ask your shrink questions about it. But the medicine for anxiety and sleep started working right away, so in those areas you're starting to feel slightly human. Eventually, steadily, when the antidepressants kick in, you will start to feel better. Your brain, which felt like it had been chopped in two, now begins to close, as if with a zipper. Your old self makes more frequent appearances.

On the neuron level, what's happening is largely mysterious. The smiles are there, but how the medicine helps to produce those smiles is still anyone's best guess. Some research suggests that such drugs as Prozac help the brain to literally repair itself; depression, this research states, is neurotoxic and antidepressants stimulate the growth of new nerve cells. That's far from proven, though. Other research posits that antidepressants are just uppers with a seal of social approval on them; anyone who takes them will feel better. However, studies have disproved this. Most people who take Zoloft feel nothing—no high, no buzz. Those who feel something usually feel better, because their baseline emotional state was bad to begin with.

Your baseline has been bad, and then you take the drugs, and one day you smile. Another day you sing along with the car radio. You like the baby again. You stop counting the bad days. You stop blaming yourself because you can see that it was a real sickness—not a character flaw—that brought you down. And you start talking about what you've been through.

> Studies show that talk therapy in combination with antidepressant treatment has the most long-lasting effect.

You might wonder whether drugs are really all it takes. Is there a way to get through PPD without resorting to pills? Here we go again. Yes, there is. There's a way of getting through war wounds without resorting to bandages, but you'll heal slowly, and with infections. Drugs are not an easy answer. They are, just simply, one answer among many. You can wait it out. You can stay sad. You can decide depression is authentic and drugs just camouflage that reality. All of these are appropriate responses, but none of them will actually help you get back on your feet, to be a mother and a woman again. Ultimately, for PPD, drugs are the most pragmatic and humane response, although, as new nonpharmacological treatments develop, that may change. Someday, we may be able to treat depression with electromagnetic fields or with implanted electrodes. There are new options emerging from beaker-filled laboratories. There's reason for you to hope, and for your younger sisters and daughters to hope, too.

In addition to swallowing pills, you should also talk to someone. Someone with a soft chair in an office with pastel walls who takes notes once in a while. Studies show that talk therapy in combination with antidepressant treatment has the most long-lasting effect. And, indeed, talk therapy is always relevant. Even if your PPD is purely biological, it has undoubtedly upset your life and caused you to question yourself in new ways. That's fodder for a shrink. For most of us, however, our PPD points to longstanding and unaddressed problems within ourselves and our families; PPD is the curse that reveals, and by revealing offers us a chance to flourish. Like it or not, PPD will dissolve the sugar coating that got you through life so far. What you will find underneath may be bitter, but it may also be rich and it will almost certainly bring you to a different place. You will find in your new terrain some valuable things. Some invigorating things. Some struggles and secrets now worth telling.

You might decide one secret now worth telling is the fact of the PPD itself. People will say they had no idea anything was wrong with you. Many PPD sufferers, it turns out, are masters of deception. Other people will confide that they, too, had PPD. You will start to wonder if there are any new mothers who *haven't* had it.

You might question whether to have more children. Now that you're an expert, you know you're likely to suffer from PPD again. But there are ways to head it off. You can stay on your antidepressant throughout pregnancy or go on it during the last trimester or the moment the umbilical cord is snipped. You can hire a baby nurse or demand a relative's help so you can heal properly. You can be nicer to yourself next time. Or you could move to a different continent.

You wouldn't have had this problem if you lived in another part of the world. A "primitive" part, with huts and animal skins, where all the women in a village take care of the new mothers after birth for about forty days while she nurses her baby and lets her torn parts knit together. Or an industrialized part, like China, where many women still "do the month," which means following traditional postnatal customs (avoiding wind and eating lots of chicken among them) while your mother and mother-in-law fawn over you. But you don't live in a slice of the world where the new mother's vulnerability is taken into account. You live in the United States, where women compete to see who's the best mother and who's back at the desk or treadmill soonest. The wimps stay in bed. Real women kill themselves trying to appear perfect.

You bought into that once, too. But now you know better. You now know that your mental health comes first, because that's what makes you a superior mother. You know that *rest* is not a dirty word, that childbirth is a hell of an undertaking, that there's no shame is getting sick, and that people will help if you ask them to.

—*Susan Kushner Resnick*

RELATED ENTRIES

Antidepressants

Becoming a Mother

Depressive Disorders

> You now know that your mental health comes first, because that's what makes you a superior mother.

Menopause and Psychiatric Illness

The time between perimenopause and menopause, known as the climacteric, marks the transition from a reproductive to a nonreproductive stage of a woman's life. Menopause is defined as the cessation of menstrual periods and is considered to be complete when a woman has not menstruated for an entire year. Perimenopause includes the process of declining ovarian function that precedes menopause and continues for several years following the cessation of a woman's menstrual cycle. Women vary considerably in the age of onset, duration, and physical and emotional experiences associated with this transition. On average, however, menopause occurs between the ages of forty-five and fifty-five, and the entire process typically ranges from five to ten years.

Menopause culminates from a complex interplay of neuroendocrine functions involving both the ovaries and the brain. The onset of this phase in life is thought to be triggered by decreasing amounts of ovarian hormones, mainly estradiol and progesterone. The pituitary responds to this change in hormonal milieu by releasing greater amounts of follicle-stimulating hormone (FSH) in an attempt to release an egg. These fluctuations in hormones cause menstrual irregularity as the ovarian follicles steadily decline in number until, ultimately, the amount of ovarian hormones is insufficient to sustain the menstrual cycle. Age-related changes in hypothalamic function have also been implicated in the timing of menopause.

Although the precise mechanisms that cause all of this change in function remain unclear, it is believed that the physical and emotional symptoms experienced by many perimenopausal women are due to these changes in hormonal levels and hypothalamic functioning. Common symptoms include hot flashes; changes in vaginal tissue that can lead to dryness, itching, and painful intercourse; sleep disturbances; irritability; forgetfulness; and, possibly, symptoms of anxiety and depression. As stated previously, these experiences vary greatly from woman to woman in terms of frequency, intensity, and duration.

MENOPAUSE AND MENTAL HEALTH

Until recently, there has been little systematic scientific inquiry into the relationship between hormonal events and women's mental health, and even less attention to this relationship during menopause. Fortunately, this appears to be changing, in part due to an increase in women's average life span. Before the first decade of the twenty-first century ends, the number of postmenopausal women will approach an estimated sixty million in the United States alone.

Adolescent and adult women are twice as likely to experience major depression as men in the same age range. This gender differential appears to be most pronounced during the reproductive years. Sociocultural factors, social learning theory—which examines the impact of role modeling on shaping behavior—and feminist perspectives that consider the subjugation of women throughout history have all been used to explain why women have such a high rate of depression. In addition, hormonal factors are increasingly implicated as playing a mediating role in the expression of mood disorders in women. Each of these variables may explain a piece of a complex puzzle, yet none provide a complete picture.

Contrary to popularly held beliefs, menopause is not associated with an increase in psychopathology among women in general. However, perimenopause does appear to be a time of increased vulnerability, particularly for women with a history of a mood disorder. Women who experienced the onset of or an exacerbation of psychiatric symptoms with other reproductive or hormonal events, such as menarche (the initial menstrual period), the premenstrual phase, pregnancy, the postpartum stage, or the initiation of oral contraceptives or other synthetic hormones, are also vulnerable.

Research on other psychiatric disorders and the hormonal changes associated with perimenopause and menopause is sparse and inconclusive. Some evidence indicates a slight increase in psychotic episodes for women with schizophrenia during periods of low levels of estrogen. This is believed to result from the loss of the protective effects that estrogen provides the brain, making it unsurprising that the fluctuating and ultimate declines in ovarian hormones associated with this transition would pose a potential risk in women who are predisposed to psychiatric difficulty during hormonal events.

THE RELATIONSHIP BETWEEN HORMONES, MOOD, AND COGNITION

The relationship between hormones, neurotransmitters, and the structure and function of the brain is fascinating and complex. Neuroscientists, psychopharmacologists (psychiatrists who specialize in medication), and endocrinologists are only beginning to understand the intricate and multidimensional connections between these variables. Estrogen, progesterone, and testosterone receptors are found in many regions of the brain and affect various neurotransmitter systems. Estrogen, for instance, influences the concentration and availability of several brain chemicals, including monoamines, serotonin, norepinephrine, and dopamine, as well as endorphin levels (natural opiates in the brain that play a role in decreasing pain), all of which affect mood, energy, and cognition.

In recent years, there has been a surge of research examining the relationship between estrogen and cognitive functioning. Early observational studies suggested that estrogen might exert a neuroprotective role and possibly slow the progression of Alzheimer's disease. However, results from well-designed randomized clinical trials examining the relationship between hormones and cognition have been inconsistent, and recent evidence from the Women's Health Initiative study points in the opposite direction. In particular, the findings indicate that an estrogen/progestin combination did not improve cognitive function in postmenopausal women but rather increased the risk of both dementia and stroke in this population. Over the past several decades, the thinking and recommendations made by physicians regarding HRT has fluctuated dramatically. While the research suggests important trends, decisions about initiating, continuing,

> Menopause is not associated with an increase in psychopathology among women. However, perimenopause does appear to be a time of increased vulnerability, particularly for women with a history of a mood disorder.

or tapering HRT should take into account your unique symptoms and medical history. Although the Women's Health Initiative is the best-designed and largest study to date, its findings will not be the final word on this very important topic.

HORMONE REPLACEMENT THERAPY

Hormone Replacement Therapy (HRT) is simply replacing diminishing natural hormones with synthetic hormones prescribed by a woman's doctor. The decision of whether to take HRT is a personal one and should be made with the help of a trusted medical provider. In light of the early termination of the Women's Health Initiative, a large-scale, federally funded, well-designed, randomized clinical trial study, the topic of hormone replacement therapy has received a great deal of attention. The findings of this study indicated that the risks of cardiovascular disease and breast cancer outweighed HRT's benefits of protection against colon cancer and osteoporosis. In particular, the higher likelihood of cardiovascular disease was in direct contrast with earlier epidemiologic studies and years of recommended clinical treatment. When considering that at the time of the release of the study's results close to 40 percent of menopausal women in the United States were prescribed HRT, this finding was alarming to both medical providers and women alike.

> Once menopause is complete, women who have struggled with psychiatric difficulties throughout most of their reproductive life often experience a decrease in symptoms.

As a direct consequence, many women were told to stop their HRT—and many began to experience a resurgence of bothersome menopausal symptoms. Upon closer scrutiny, however, the increased incidence in cardiovascular disease was specifically linked to overweight women who began HRT in their sixties and seventies, a finding that may or may not be relevant to healthy women in their forties and fifties who are actively experiencing menopausal symptoms.

A consideration of the woman's whole being must be taken into account when deciding whether to initiate or continue HRT. Risks and benefits should be discussed openly with a thorough understanding and consideration of each woman's unique medical and psychiatric history. From a mental health perspective, particular attention should be given to prior symptoms around earlier hormonal and reproductive events, as well as current clinical presentation. If a woman chooses to explore HRT, she has a multitude of options; preparations vary in terms of hormonal combinations, dosages, and route of administration.

> The importance of restorative sleep, adequate nutrition, and moderate exercise cannot be overestimated; they directly affect the brain and the body to decrease symptoms of depression and anxiety, improve energy and mental clarity, and enhance overall well-being.

It is generally agreed that HRT is helpful in treating mild depression as well as many of the physical symptoms that often accompany the climacteric. However, with more moderate or severe depression, HRT is typically not sufficient, and antidepressants are warranted. For some women, HRT has been useful in augmenting or increasing the effectiveness of an antidepressant medication or other psychotropic drug. Most HRTs are composed of both estrogen and progesterone, although progesterone may induce dysphoric mood states such as agitation or depression. Some medical providers may consider prescribing unopposed estrogen (estrogen without progesterone) for a period of time and slowly adding progesterone to see how it is tolerated. However, this option requires close monitoring, including periodic biopsies, as endometrial hyperplasia (thickening of the endometrium) may result and has been associated with endometrial cancer. Limited anecdotal evidence also shows that estrogen may destabilize some women with bipolar disorder by increasing mood cycles. Although testosterone is not frequently prescribed to perimenopausal or menopausal women, it has restored libido and orgasm and enhanced general well-being in some women.

Women who suffer from mood disorders or other psychiatric conditions and experience an exacerbation of symptoms during the transition from perimenopause to menopause should ask their medical providers (primary care physician, gynecologist, and psychiatrist) to work closely with each other in order to monitor, fine-tune, and find the optimal treatment regimen. The good news is that once menopause is complete, women who have struggled with psychiatric difficulties throughout most of their reproductive life often experience a decrease in symptoms. This reduced reactivity of the brain, which may be experienced as a calming, is often welcome.

THE IMPORTANCE OF SELF-CARE

The field of behavioral medicine focuses on the mind-body relationship and emphasizes behavioral strategies for coping with medical and mental health concerns. In the groundbreaking book *Women's Moods: What Every Woman Must Know about Hormones, the Brain, and Emotional Health*, Deborah Sichel, M.D., and Jeanne Watson Driscoll, M.S., R.N., C.S., recommend their NURSE Program, which emphasizes the importance of Nourishment, Understanding, Rest and relaxation, Spirituality, and Exercise. With regards to nutrition during menopause, they recommend a low-fat diet, consuming foods high in phytoestrogens (such as soy products), and supplementing with calcium, antioxidants, and omega-3 fatty acids.

The importance of restorative sleep, adequate nutrition, and moderate exercise cannot be overestimated; they directly affect the brain and the body to decrease symptoms of depression and anxiety, improve energy and mental clarity, and enhance overall well-being. Some women may benefit from learning strategies to decrease physiological arousal through meditation, relaxation exercises, hypnosis, or biofeedback. Finding a health routine that is flexible and realistic and fits one's style, schedule, and unique rhythms is paramount to increasing and maintaining wellness.

The end of the reproductive years often marks a time in a woman's life when we become less concerned with others' perceptions or expectations of who we should be or how we should act. This time can initiate a process of reevaluation, of taking stock of our lives, shifting our priorities, focusing on those relationships that are meaningful, and creating more room to nourish our souls. We may embark upon creative endeavors or revisit earlier passions that we put aside to focus on the multiple roles women often juggle. This postmenopausal phase of life is considered by many as a time of greater wisdom, clarity, intuition, and ability to truly embrace who we are as women.

—*Allyson Cherkasky, Ph.D.*

RELATED ENTRIES

The Fires of Menopause

Aging and Its Effects on Mood, Memory, the Brain, and Hormones

Depressive Disorders

Anxiety Disorders

Pregnancy as a Life Passage

Aging and Its Effects on Mood, Memory, the Brain, and Hormones

As life expectancy increases, quality of life issues related to aging and the prevention or slowing of degenerative diseases become of increasing importance and interest to us all. One of the greatest challenges in neuroscience research today is to find ways to help maintain intellectual and emotional functions throughout our advancing years.

As women age, they enter perimenopause, an important physiological stage of life that involves a steady decline in the levels of the reproductive hormones, including estrogens, progesterone, and testosterone. Perimenopause is a natural process involving gradual menstrual and hormonal changes that eventually result in the end of menstrual cycle (i.e., the menopausal phase). This process may continue for at least the first year after menopause. All women who live long enough will eventually begin the menopausal phase of life, which generally occurs between the ages of forty-five and fifty-five, with fifty-one years being the average age of onset.

As the life span of women in the United States continues to increase, the number of years spent in the postmenopausal state also increases. This means that understanding the physiological effects of this new stage of life and their influence on the mind and moods is a matter of growing importance for women.

Emotional disorders sometimes occur for the first time during or after the perimenopausal years. They can also become significantly worse, especially during menopause itself. During this time, women may experience depression, anxiety, agitation, restlessness, mood swings, irritability, fears, insomnia, memory dysfunction, and weight loss. Although the majority of women pass through the menopausal stage of life without a problem, a significant minority develops disabling emotional symptoms. Hormonal factors may have a lot to do with this. On the one hand, the pattern of hormonal changes that occur during the perimenopausal and menopausal phases is relatively common to all women. On the other hand, these changes may be highly variable in their duration and magnitude when you compare one individual woman to another. For example, the average duration of the perimenopausal phase is 3.5 years, yet nearly 10 percent of women will have no symptomatic perimenopause transition at all and will have regular menstrual cycles until their cycles abruptly end.

So why do some women have a more difficult time during this phase of life than others? One possibility is that there may be a special feature of the brain that predisposes some women to develop hormonally related depression or anxiety. This feature can manifest as an unusual sensitivity of the brain to hormones or hormonal changes. Certain markers indicate a predisposal to hormonal sensitivity. These markers include (1) being left-handed or having an immediate family history of left-handedness, (2) having a neurological (i.e., brain) disorder, (3) the presence of skeletal asymmetry between the two halves of the body, and (4) having a mood disorder or even a family history of a mood disorder. Another indirect marker is the presence of an electrical disturbance in the brain, which can be detected by a brain wave test (EEG), particularly if this occurs in the brain's emotional centers. Essentially, then, mood disorders related to the perimenopausal years and beyond can result from age-related hormonal changes, having a brain that has an increased sensitivity to hormones, or both.

The specific part of the brain that may be particularly sensitive or dysfunctional in this setting is known as the temporolimbic system, the region associated with the emotions. Unique circuits connect this area of the brain with the hormone centers in the brain, the hypothalamus, and pituitary gland, and additional circuits that connect the hypothalamopituitary system with the ovaries. The result is that ovarian production of the estrogens and progesterone can be indirectly affected by temporolimbic dysfunction. This amazing network of neurohormonal communication links can have profound effects on a woman's well-being if the system doesn't work properly.

Other age-related changes further complicate the picture. As one ages, there is a gradual loss of nerve cells and the connections between these cells in specific regions of the brain. Interestingly, studies have shown that while some connections are lost, others of these branch-like connections actually grow with age and may help to make up for the age-related loss of nerve cells. This unique compensating feature of the brain is known as neuroplasticity. Various chemicals and neurotransmitters in the brain, such as serotonin and dopamine, also decline to some extent with age. These and other neurotransmitters make it possible for us to perform a variety of functions and are key players in helping to regulate emotions, mood, behavior, and memory.

The reproductive hormones can have powerful effects on various types of neurotransmitters. In general, the estrogens have neuroexcitatory, antidepressant effects, whereas one of the bioactive components of progesterone has powerful neuroinhibitory, antianxiety effects.

The emotional changes that can occur during the perimenopausal state are quite diverse and may include different forms of depression as well as anxiety disorders such as panic attacks, phobias, and obsessive-compulsive disorders. It is important to distinguish the various manifestations related to these conditions since different emotional changes may be associated with specific types of hormonal disturbances. For example, during the natural perimenopause, a decline in progesterone levels typically occurs before estrogen levels start to decline. This can occur even as women continue to have regular menstrual cycles and may be evident for many months before the estrogen levels begin to decline as well. When progesterone declines before the estrogens do or even if the estrogens are just starting to decline, a condition occurs in which there may be a relatively high ratio of estrogens to progesterone, potentially causing depression with agitation and irritability components or anxiety disorders.

At the other end of the spectrum, either during late menopause or after a hysterectomy with removal of both ovaries, there is a loss of production of both types of hormones. This

Certain markers indicate a predisposal to hormonal sensitivity, including

1. being left-handed or having an immediate family history of left-handedness,

2. having a neurological (i.e., brain) disorder,

3. the presence of skeletal asymmetry between the two halves of the body, and

4. having a mood disorder or even a family history of a mood disorder.

can result in vegetative depressive symptoms, such as having a poor appetite, decreased energy level, and feeling tired and unusually emotional. If these distinctions are not carefully considered, the potential benefits of hormonal therapy in helping to treat mood disorders may be overlooked. Unfortunately, this happens all too often. I have seen many cases in which women have been told by other physicians that their emotional disturbances are "in their head" and have no physiological basis when, in fact, the symptoms they are experiencing are related to what is going on in the brain and actually do have a neurohormonal basis.

HORMONAL THERAPIES

Generally, the whole intended purpose of taking long-term hormone replacement therapy is to preserve health and prevent disease. During the summer of 2002, the results of a study pertaining to the safety of hormone replacement therapy were reported by the Women's Health Initiative (WHI) program. The study was the first randomized primary prevention trial that looked at how a particular combination of synthetic estrogen and progestin replacement affected the health of women. The part of the study that compares estrogen alone with placebo in women with hysterectomies is still in progress. However, the part of the study that compares estrogen/progestin with placebo was terminated early for several reasons. The data and safety monitoring board (DSMB) recommended discontinuing this part of the trial because women receiving the combination of estrogen and progestin had an increased risk of invasive breast cancer, and an overall measure suggested that the treatment was causing more harm than good. The decision to stop the trial was made after an average follow-up of 5.2 years (planned duration, 8.5 years). Clearly, more research studies are needed to determine whether other types of estrogen and progesterone replacement, particularly those that are bioidentical to women's natural hormones, may have beneficial effects in preserving health, preventing disease, and improving well-being.

While any course of treatment should be carefully discussed with your physician, here is a brief look at the use of hormones to treat disturbances of mind and emotion.

Estrogen replacement can enhance mood and lead to a subjective improvement in well-being; small studies in menopausal women have shown a correlation between positive mood states and circulating estrogen levels. The antidepressant effects of estrogen may also contribute to the frequently associated improvements in cognitive function. Studies have shown that cognitive function, such as memory, tends to worsen with negative mood or depressive symptoms. There has also been some evidence that depressed mood may be a risk factor for developing a memory disorder, including Alzheimer's disease.

Alzheimer's disease is a degenerative brain disorder that results in progressively worsening memory loss, impairments in language, and changes in personality. There may be benefits to memory and intellectual functions with the use of estrogen therapy, especially for verbal material. There are also gender differences in the occurrence of Alzheimer's disease (AD). AD affects 1.5 to 3 times more women than men, and this notable gender difference is present even after the difference in longevity between women and men is taken into account. Some, but not all, recent studies suggest that postmenopausal estrogen replacement therapy may provide protection against the development of Alzheimer's disease. Estrogen has also been used to treat women with established dementia. In general, the results show that long-term estrogen therapy is associated with a progressive but modest improvement in cognition during the course of one year of treatment and that the progression of Alzheimer's disease can be delayed for up to two years.

Progesterone therapy can be helpful in the treatment of anxiety disorders and the agitated form of depression. Even though the synthetic progestins may be more commonly prescribed by physicians, they affect the brain and behavior differently than natural progesterone. Specifically, natural progesterone is converted in the brain to a chemical known as allopregnanolone, while the synthetic progestins are not. This chemical has antianxiety and antiagitation effects that are more potent than some of the most powerful sedative medications and comparable to some of the most potent benzodiazepines (e.g., Valium). The important message here is that women, particularly during the perimenopausal phase, may benefit from natural progesterone therapy if they have symptoms related to an anxiety disorder or the agitated form of depression.

Testosterone therapy may act in conjunction with the estrogens to improve depressive symptoms or even cognitive function. This occurs as a result of the partial conversion of testosterone into estrogen, which results in increased estrogen levels. A recent study showed that women had an improvement in well-being and fewer hot flashes when testosterone was included with estrogen replacement therapy. Testosterone has energizing effects and is the most important hormonal factor in promoting sexual desire. However, excessive testosterone influence can promote aggressive, impulsive, and hypersexual behavior.

—*Mark N. Friedman, D.O.*

PART THREE

Getting Help

PSYCHOTROPIC MEDICATIONS

Antidepressants

Selective Serotonin Re-Uptake Inhibitors (SSRIs)

BRAND NAME	GENERIC NAME
Celexa	Citalopram
Lexapro	Escitalopram Oxalate
Prozac	Fluoxetine
Luvox	Fluvoxamine
Serzone	Nefazodone
Paxil	Paroxetine
Zoloft	Sertraline
Desyrel	Trazodone

Combination Norepinephrine, Serotonin Re-Uptake Inhibitors

BRAND NAME	GENERIC NAME
Remeron	Mirtazapine
Effexor	Venlafaxine

Tricyclic Antidepressants

BRAND NAME	GENERIC NAME
Elavil	Amitriptyline
Anafranil	Clomipramine
Norpramin	Desipramine
Sinequan	Doxepin
Tofranil	Imipramine
Pamelor	Nortriptyline

Monoamine Oxidase Inhibitors

BRAND NAME	GENERIC NAME
Nardil	Phenelzine
Parnate	Tranylcypromine

Other Antidepressants

BRAND NAME	GENERIC NAME
Wellbutrin	Bupropion
Zyban	Bupropion

Mood Stabilizers

BRAND NAME	GENERIC NAME
Tegretol	Carbamazepine
Neurontin	Gabapentin
Lamictal	Lamotrigine
Lithium	Lithium
Trileptal	Oxcarbazepine
Depakote	Valproic Acid

Anxiolytics/Hypnotics (Sleep Medications)

Benzodiazepine Anxiolytics

BRAND NAME	GENERIC NAME
Xanax	Alprazolam
Tranxene	Chlorazepate
Librium	Chlordiazepoxide
Mitran	Chlordiazepoxide
Klonopin	Clonazepam
Valium	Diazepam
Ativan	Lorazepam
Serax	Oxazepam
Centrax	Prazepam

Nonbenzodiazepine Anxiolytics

BRAND NAME	GENERIC NAME
Buspar	Buspirone
Atarax	Hydroxyzine
Vistaril	Hydroxyzine

Benzodiazepine Hypnotics

BRAND NAME	GENERIC NAME
ProSom	Estazolam
Dalmane	Flurazepam
Doral	Quazepam
Restoril	Temazepam
Halcion	Triazolam

Nonbenzodiazepine Hypnotics

BRAND NAME	GENERIC NAME
Sonata	Zaleplon
Ambien	Zolpidem

Beta-Adrenergic Drugs

BRAND NAME	GENERIC NAME
Tenormin	Atenolol
Inderal	Propranolol

Antipsychotics: Atypical

BRAND NAME	GENERIC NAME
Abilify	Aripiprazole
Clozaril	Clozapine
Zyprexa	Olanzapine
Seroquel	Quetiapine
Risperdal	Risperidone
Geodon	Ziprasidone

Antipsychotics: Typical

BRAND NAME	GENERIC NAME
LOW-POTENCY	
Thorazine	Chlorpromazine
Serentil	Mesoridazine
Mellaril	Thioridazine
MID-POTENCY	
Trilafon	Perphenazine
Loxitane	Loxapine
Moban	Molindone
HIGH-POTENCY	
Prolixin	Fluphenazine
Haldol	Haloperidol
Navane	Thiothixene
Stelazine	Trifluoperazine

Stimulants

BRAND NAME	GENERIC NAME
Adderall	Dextroamphetamine
Dexedrine	Dextroamphetamine
Desoxyn	Methamphetamine
Concerta	Methylphenidate
Ritalin	Methylphenidate
Provigil	Modafinil
Cylert	Pemoline

Others

BRAND NAME	GENERIC NAME
Straterra	Atomoxetine
BuSpar	Buspirone
Catapres	Clonidine
Revia	Naltrexone
Topamax	Topiramate
Ambien	Zolpidem

Antidepressants

Though medications for depression have been around for a half century, the last two decades have seen a proliferation of new treatment options. The first drugs available were the tricyclic antidepressants (TCAs), a class of medicines with significant side effects and with a high risk of lethality when taken in overdose. Next to emerge were the monoamine-oxidase inhibitors (MAOIs). These medications eliminated many of the side effects of the tricyclics, but proved problematic because of the need to adhere to strict dietary restrictions.

With the advent of the newer selective serotonin-reuptake inhibitors (SSRIs) in the 1980s, antidepressant medications became more easily tolerated as well as safer to use. For these reasons, the SSRIs are now considered the first line of treatment for depression. Another growing category of medicines called "atypical antidepressants," which do not fit neatly into any of the preexisting classes, are increasingly used as alternatives to the SSRIs when these are unsuccessful or poorly tolerated.

TRICYCLIC ANTIDEPRESSANTS (TCAs)

The tricyclics were the earliest class of antidepressants, and they remain equally effective as the SSRIs in treating depression. These medications act primarily by increasing the availability of the neurotransmitter norepinephrine at the receptor sites. The most commonly used TCAs are Tofranil, Anafranil, Norpramin, and Pamelor.

The side effects of the tricyclics include *anticholinergic* effects, such as dry mouth, constipation, and urinary retention, and *antihistaminic* effects, such as sedation and weight gain. Tofranil and Elavil are more apt to cause these side effects than are Norpramin and Pamelor. The tricyclics also have effects on cardiac function, which contribute to their dangerousness in overdose.

Toxicity from TCAs can result from relatively low doses of medication; as little as a week's supply can prove lethal. For this reason, physicians often monitor blood levels of patients taking these medications. Symptoms of overdose include fever, blurred vision, confusion, seizures, and coma. In addition, there may be abnormalities of cardiac conduction, causing arrhythmia and death. Overdose with any quantity of tricyclic antidepressants is considered a medical emergency.

Despite these risks, the tricyclics remain highly useful in the treatment of depression, as well as other disorders. In fact, they may be more efficacious in treating certain types of depression, including "melancholic," or agitated, depression; they also may be more effective in treating depression in men than SSRIs. Anafranil, a TCA with strongly serotonergic properties, is highly effective for the treatment of OCD. All of the tricyclics are effective in treating anxiety disorders, as well as depression and dysthymia.

SELECTIVE SEROTONIN-REUPTAKE INHIBITORS (SSRIs)

When the SSRIs first colorfully and exuberantly appeared in the early 1980s, critics mused that we all would soon be consuming these medications. They appeared to be without side effects and they seemed to make people "better than well." Although the SSRIs remain the most commonly prescribed psychotropic medications, it is now clear that they are neither cure-alls nor side effect-free. (Thus proving the popular joke among psychiatrists that one should prescribe a drug when it first comes out, while it still works.) The SSRIs appear to work by blocking the reuptake of the neurotransmitter serotonin, thereby prolonging its effects. However, long-term changes also appear, including alterations in protein synthesis and gene expression. As noted elsewhere, these changes may prevent loss of neurons or even induce the synthesis of new nerve cells.

The SSRIs include Prozac, Paxil, Zoloft, Celexa, and Luvox. These drugs differ somewhat in their relative activity on serotonin and norepinephrine receptors. They also differ somewhat in the time during which the drug remains active in the body (called the "half-life"). For instance, the half-life of Prozac is four to six days, while the half-lives of Luvox and Paxil are less than a day. Drugs with shorter half-lives have a greater risk of causing withdrawal symptoms when stopping medication.

> Side effects are very individual, and some that appear at the beginning of treatment fade over time.

All of the SSRIs are equally efficacious; they all also have the potential to cause the same side effects, although some adverse effects are more commonly associated with some drugs than with others. On the whole, the most common side effects include nausea, decreased appetite, excessive sweating, headache, insomnia, jitteriness, sedation, dizziness, and sexual dysfunction. It is quickly apparent that many of these side effects are contradictory; it is difficult to be both jittery and sedated. The important point is that side effects are very individual and that some that appear at the beginning of treatment fade over time. In addition to these side effects, some people report an affective "blunting," or difficulty in accessing emotion.

Like the tricylics, the SSRIs are used for a variety of disorders, including anxiety and eating disorders, as well as depression. Unlike the TCAs, however, these drugs are relatively safe when taken in overdose, making them the preferred choice for suicidal persons.

MONOAMINE-OXIDASE INHIBITORS (MAOIs)

The MAOIs are a lesser-known class of drugs that exert their effect on the enzyme monoamine oxidase, a protein responsible for the breakdown of certain neurotransmitters, including serotonin, dopamine, and norepinephrine. By interfering with the actions of this enzyme, the MAOIs increase the concentration of these neurotransmitters, an effect thought to be responsible for the alleviation of depression. The MAOIs are more effective than the TCAs in treating "atypical" depression, characterized by increased sleep and appetite, fatigue, and "mood reactivity," or a responsiveness of mood to external conditions. The most common side effects of these drugs are lightheadedness (due to low blood pressure), insomnia or agitation, weight loss, dry mouth, and constipation.

The chief difficulty with the MAOIs is that their actions are not specific to the nervous system. The enzyme monoamine oxidase is also found in the intestine, where it is responsible for the breakdown of certain amino acids, including tyramine. When this breakdown process is inhibited, the amino acids build up to toxic levels at the nerve terminals. The result is termed a "hypertensive crisis" and is characterized by fever, dangerously elevated blood pressure, and cardiac arrhythmia. When untreated, these episodes are frequently life threatening.

In order to avoid the occurrence of a hypertensive crisis, people on MAOIs must follow a specialized diet that is low in tyramine as well as several other amino acids metabolized by monoamine oxidase. The principal restriction is against all forms of cheese except cream and cottage cheese; for this reason, the hypertensive crisis is also called the "cheese effect." Other prohibited foods include fermented or dried meats (e.g., pepperoni), yeast extract, fava or broad bean pods (not the beans themselves, just the pods), sauerkraut, soy sauce, and other soy products. In addition, foods to be consumed in moderation include alcoholic beverages, dried fruits, caffeine, and chocolate. Certain medications, including some cough medicines, decongestants, and Demerol, also have potentially dangerous interactions with the MAOIs.

> ✦
> The MAOIs are more effective than the TCAs in treating "atypical" depression, characterized by increased sleep and appetite, fatigue, and "mood reactivity," or a responsiveness of mood to external conditions.

The most commonly used MAOIs are Parnate and tranylcypromine Nardil. In addition, there has been a recent resurgence of interest in Eldepryl, a medication also used for treatment of Parkinson's disease. This medicine is interesting because at low doses it acts selectively on the monoamine oxidase in the brain, avoiding the unwanted intestinal effects, and thereby obviating the need for strict dietary restrictions. However, research on the effectiveness of this medicine for depression is limited; furthermore, there is some evidence that antidepressant effects are obtained only at higher, nonselective doses.

ATYPICAL ANTIDEPRESSANTS

The atypical antidepressants are a diverse class with a broad range of actions on several neurotransmitter systems. The dissimilarity of this group yet their comparable effectiveness suggests more complexity to depression than was previously supposed. These atypical medications include Effexor, a medicine that is SSRI-like in its actions on both serotonin and norepinephrine. The side effects of Effexor parallel those of the SSRIs and include nausea, sedation, dizziness, and sexual dysfunction.

> ✦
> It is important to note that all of these agents may require up to eight weeks for a full effect.

Nefazodone (Serzone) and trazodone (Desyrel) are similar agents, which act primarily on serotonin reuptake. Desyrel is the more sedating of the two and is most often used as a sleep medication rather than as an antidepressant. The side effects of Serzone are similar to those of the SSRIs, except that it is less likely to cause sexual dysfunction.

Remeron has effects on both the serotonin and norepinephrine systems. This medication also has antihistamine effects, including sedation, weight gain, dry mouth, and constipation. The sedating effects are thought to be worse at lower doses. Sexual side effects are rare with Remoron.

Wellbutrin is unique in that it averts the serotonin system completely. Instead, it works by increasing levels of dopamine and norepinephrine. Wellbutrin, which has also been used in smoking cessation, also has a somewhat unique side-effect profile; the most common adverse effects are agitation, tremor, weight loss, and insomnia.

APPROACH TO TREATMENT

The choice of an antidepressant is determined by many factors, including patient preference, the symptoms exhibited, and concurrent medical conditions. For example, an older man with agitated depression might do better on a tricyclic; a woman with mood reactivity and low energy might respond preferentially to SSRIs; another with sexual problems might be more appropriately treated with Wellbutrin or Serzone. It is important to note that all of these agents may require up to eight weeks for a full effect. Further, people who don't improve on one medicine have a 60 percent chance of improvement when switched to another class of drugs. The dose at which an individual responds is quite variable and does not necessarily correlate with the degree of depression.

The use of antidepressants in pregnancy and lactation has been the subject of much debate and recent research, though without definitive findings. The largest body of research concerns the tricyclics, which demonstrate no significant increase in congenital malformations. There is some evidence, however, that infants born to mothers on these drugs are prone to develop a withdrawal syndrome, involving difficulty breathing, cyanosis (bluish skin due to oxygen deficiency), and feeding difficulties. Prozac has also been studied fairly extensively in this regard; here again, the bulk of evidence documents no increase in fetal anomalies or spontaneous pregnancy loss. Follow-up studies of preschool children exposed in utero to Prozac have found no differences in temperament, mood, activity, intelligence, or language development. However, here again there are conflicting reports: individual studies have suggested more perinatal complications in women taking Prozac. All psychotropic medications are secreted into breast milk, albeit in trace amounts.

The use of MAOIs, in contrast, is clearly contraindicated in pregnancy. Not only can these medications worsen pregnancy-related hypertension, they also may interfere with drugs used during labor and delivery.

The decision to use antidepressants by pregnant or nursing women should be an informed one, jointly made by women and their physicians. The detrimental effects of depression on the developing fetus may be much more severe than the effects of using psychotropic medications.

—Susan Mahler, M.D.

Antianxiety Medications

Just as anxiety disorders represent a diverse constellation of syndromes, so too, the drugs used to treat anxiety are disparate and distinct in their actions. As a group, these drugs, known as the anxiolytics, have evolved empirically, as the beneficial effects of various medicines were recognized somewhat fortuitously. The drugs used for anxiety now include anxiolytics/hypnotics (benzodiazepines), antidepressants (serotonin reuptake inhibitors [SSRIs], monoamine-oxidase inhibitors [MAOIs], tricyclic antidepressants [TCAs], atypicals), and newer agents. An older class of medications, the barbiturates, has fallen out of use for anxiety because they are highly addictive and potentially lethal when combined with alcohol.

BENZODIAZEPINES

The benzodiazepines are the most commonly prescribed medications for anxiety. Some of these drugs, such as Valium, Xanax, and Librium, have popular recognition, while others (Ativan, Restoril, Serax) are lesser known. All of these medications act similarly; they differ in the speed of onset and duration of action. These differences partially account for their different utility in treating illnesses like Panic Disorder and Generalized Anxiety Disorder. As a group, however, they act quickly and effectively to control symptoms of anxiety.

This class of drugs affects the same neurotransmitter system as alcohol; therefore, they produce the same range of effects, both desirable and adverse. The side effects of benzodiazepines include sedation, poor coordination, memory impairment, and withdrawal symptoms (e.g., tremor). Like alcohol, these drugs also have the potential to be abused. For this reason, people with a history of drug or alcohol addiction should avoid these medications.

The benzodiazepines are useful for many, though not all, of the anxiety disorders. High-potency benzodiazepines, such as Klonopin and Xanax, are equally as effective as antidepressants in treating Panic Disorder. They are the preferred treatment for Generalized Anxiety Disorder (GAD) and may be helpful as well in Social Phobia and Post-Traumatic Stress Disorder. However, their efficacy in Obsessive-Compulsive Disorder (OCD) is uncertain.

The benzodiazepine Valium has been shown to cross the placenta and may be associated with fetal abnormalities such as cleft lip and palate. Women are advised against using these drugs during the first trimester; during the second and third trimesters, they should be used with caution.

ANTIDEPRESSANTS

In the early 1960s, just as the tricyclics and MAO inhibitors were earning their stripes as antidepressants, they were also discovered to be equally effective for symptoms of anxiety. When the next generation of antidepressants, the SSRIs, emerged, the stage was already set for their application in anxiety disorders. Currently, the first line of treatment for Panic Disorder is an SSRI, such as Prozac, Paxil, Zoloft, or Celexa. The atypical antidepressants Effexor, Serzone, and Remeron have also been shown to be effective. The antidepressants are now standard treatment in Generalized Anxiety Disorder and Social Phobia and are more effective than benzodiazepines for treating OCD. However, they may require several weeks for a full effect, during which time patients may need treatment with a faster-acting drug.

The tricyclic imipramine was the first drug proven to work against Panic Disorder; the tricyclics, despite their side effects, remain viable alternatives to the SSRIs in most anxiety syndromes. The MAOIs are equally useful; they have also been shown to be the most effective drugs in treating Social Phobia.

ALTERNATIVE MEDICATIONS

A host of other drugs is currently used for anxiety; these medicines are heterogeneous in their actions and side effects. They also are quite individualized; what works for one person may not make a dent in another's symptoms. These diverse medications include the following:

Antihistamines Benadryl and Vistaril are included in this class. Common ingredients in cold medicines, these drugs are nonaddictive and, unlike most other medications, are proven to be safe if ingested during pregnancy. They tend to produce sedation and anticholinergic side effects, such as dry mouth and constipation.

Beta-blockers This class of medicines acts to decrease heart rate and lower blood pressure, which accounts for their use as antihypertensives. These effects also account for their use in anxiety disorders, particularly panic attacks and post-traumatic stress disorder. They are also frequently used to treat performance anxiety. These medicines may cause dizziness or lightheadedness.

Buspar Buspar is nonaddictive and less likely to cause drowsiness than the benzodiazepines. Although it is slower to act (days to weeks), it may be as effective as the older drugs in the treatment of Generalized Anxiety, Social Phobia, and OCD.

—Susan Mahler, M.D.

Mood Stabilizers

Mood stabilizers is a somewhat general term, referring to a diverse group of medications used to treat some, but not all, mood disorders. The current bible of diagnosis for mental health practitioners, the *DSM-IV* (*Diagnostic and Statistical Manual, Fourth Edition*), presents criteria for single episodes of depression and various types of manic states. This manual provides for the diagnosis of the mood disorders themselves through the lens of patterns of such episodes. While mood stabilizers are not typically used for single episodes of depression, they are called upon for single episodes of mania in their acute states and for the ever-widening range of the bipolar disorders. Mood stabilizers are also being investigated for their usefulness in other disorders for which mood volatility and impulsive behavior are also problematic.

Lithium was the first substance to be used as a mood stabilizer and has remained the standard to which other mood stabilizers are compared. It is a naturally occurring substance, right there on the periodic table posted on the wall of any chemistry classroom: symbol Li, element number 3. As an element, lithium is as simple as table salt and, in fact, has been used in some "lite" salts by people who have needed to restrict their sodium intake.

Lithium made its medical debut in the early 1800s: it was tried in the treatment of gout, diabetes, and epilepsy. It was not particularly effective in treating any of these disorders and, subsequently, was used more often merely as a solvent for other more effective substances.

In 1949, an Australian doctor, John Cade, a man without heavy research experience but eager to help the suffering of his patients, speculated that there might be some toxic substance building up in the bodies of patients with mania. He took the urine from some of these manic patients, where he presumed this substance might be present, and injected it into guinea pigs to see if it induced manic-like behavior. The guinea pigs died. Thinking that the components of the urine needed to be more soluble (more liquid, not crystallized), Cade added lithium to the mix. The characteristically high-strung guinea pigs became lethargic. When they were turned over on their backs, a position that generally evoked frantic scrambling to right themselves, they remained placid. A remarkable difference. He tested it on himself for safety and then injected it into his patients. Ten of his actively manic patients all improved dramatically, and some of his agitated schizophrenic patients were calmed.

Dr. Cade published his results in an Australian medical weekly, where they lay relatively fallow until a Danish researcher, Mogens Shou, found the report in 1952 and did his own studies with very promising results. At the time the United States was focusing on the development of antidepressants and did not pick up on this research. Furthermore, the pharmaceutical industry, which provides heavy financial backing for research, showed comparatively little interest in lithium—as a naturally occurring mineral, it held far less promise for profitability than other synthetic compounds. Finally, a few decades of a growing body of evidence for lithium's efficacy in Europe led to its use in the United States.

Today, lithium has been investigated in the treatment of all phases and types of episodes found in the wide range of bipolar illnesses with consistent and, at times, dramatic effectiveness. As newer agents are researched and developed, their efficacy is generally rated in comparison to that of lithium. Some of these newer agents include some drugs originally developed as anticonvulsants. A few of the newer antipsychotic agents have shown mood-stabilizing properties as well.

But lithium has remained the gold standard for mood stabilizers. It is effective in acute manic states, either alone or when given in combination with other sedating medications or with antipsychotic medications. It is also used when the acute episode is the other "pole" of bipolar, depressive. Lithium remains effective as the acute episode settles down and in the so-called maintenance phase, where it serves to help prevent or mitigate recurrences of other episodes, be they manic, mixed, or depressive.

Kay Redfield Jamison—professor of psychiatry at Johns Hopkins, author of many books about manic-depressive illness, and arguably one of the world's foremost researchers in this field—speaks compellingly about lithium's effectiveness. Jamison is herself bipolar, which she has written about in a memoir, *An Unquiet Mind*. She says:

I cannot imagine leading a normal life without both taking lithium and having had the benefits of psychotherapy. Lithium prevents my seductive but disastrous highs, diminishes my depression, clears out the wool and webbing from my disordered thinking, slows me down, gentles me out, keeps me from ruining my career and relationships, keeps me out of a hospital, alive and makes psychotherapy possible.

Lithium has what is called a "narrow therapeutic window"; too little is ineffective, too much is toxic. Frequent blood tests are necessary to monitor its level in the blood. Even within the therapeutic range there are side effects, which tend to be dose related; sleepiness, cognitive impairment, a slight hand tremor, and some coordination impairment have been experienced by some people. Gastrointestinal side effects can include stomach irritation, nausea, and diarrhea. The kidneys, stimulated by a new salt to excrete, may increase thirst and urination. Weight gain is also fairly common and can be significant. This is not just a cosmetic issue since weight gain in general is associated with elevated blood pressure, increased cholesterol levels, and all the problems that those conditions can cause. Many of these side effects can be reduced by using the lowest possible effective dose. Again, this is a delicate balancing act, for there is no absolutely clear standard for what that level might be.

Significant increase in the severity of side effects is an early sign of lithium toxicity. When lithium is present in toxic levels, all of these side effects can progress from nuisances to dangerous situations, including cardiac instability. Such toxicity can progress to seizures

> Lithium was the first substance to be used as a mood stabilizer and has remained the standard to which other mood stabilizers are compared.

and coma, with a significant risk of permanent neurological damage. Close attention to the development of side effects from lithium use as well as actual blood levels is critical.

Other medications are also used in the treatment of mood disorders. Depakote—alone or in the form of Divalproex, a combination of a sodium salt of valproate and valproic acid—is another first-line medication for acute states. It appears to be even superior to lithium when the acute state is a mixed one, or when the person has suffered many prior mood episodes (when four or more episodes occur within one year's time, it is known as "rapid cycling"). Some studies suggest that it may be more effective in women than in men. Depakote may often be preferred because it has a wider therapeutic range than lithium, making the potential for toxicity less. Many of its side effects are also dose related, including gastrointestinal (GI) distress, tremor, and sedation. It, too, can cause weight gain as well as mild hematologic and liver abnormalities, which are generally benign. However, it does pose a risk for rare idiosyncratic reactions that can be fatal. Liver failure, sudden loss of white blood cell production, and hemorrhagic pancreatitis have all been reported in association with this medication. Though the incidence of such reactions is rare, their occurrence has quelled some people's enthusiasm for Depakote and its offshoots.

Tegretol, another anticonvulsant, has been used as a first-line mood stabilizer for acute manic states in the past, but now has more of a secondary role. Its efficacy is not consistently on a par with lithium and Depakote, and it appears to have a somewhat higher risk of serious idiosyncratic adverse effects. Dose-related side effects include fatigue, blurred or double vision, unsteadiness, and nausea. Weight gain is also a problem with this medication. There are some benign, mild decreases in white blood cell and platelet production, as well as mild interference with liver enzymes. However, the risk of disastrous hematologic conditions and liver failure is not insignificant. It can also cause a rare, potentially fatal skin condition (Stevens-Johnson Syndrome) as well as pancreatitis.

Other anticonvulsants are also under investigation for their mood-stabilizing properties, including Trileptol (related to Tegretol), Lamictal, Neurontin, and Topimax. Lamictal shows efficacy as a first-line mood stabilizer on a par with lithium when the acute episode of the bipolar disorder being treated is a depressed one.

Some atypical antipsychotics have been shown to have mood-stabilizing properties. Zyprexa has shown effectiveness as a first-line mood stabilizer for acute manic and mixed states. Its side effects can include sleepiness, constipation, and dry mouth and can cause a person dizziness when getting up quickly. Zyprexa can also increase one's appetite and cause weight gain. Other atypical antipsychotics are being studied for their potential efficacy, including Risperdal, Seroquel, and Geodon.

G. B. Bloom, a Washington, D.C.–area writer, recently shared her experience with bipolar illness and these medications in the *Washington Post*. Her experience is, unfortunately, not unusual. First she found it difficult to accept the diagnosis of bipolar illness, for her surges of energy and bouts of depression had seemed normal to her. Once she accepted her diagnosis, she was reluctant to take medications. "No way was I going to poison my body or mess around with my brain chemistry," she told her first psy-

A comparison of mortality ratios in people suffering from bipolar disorder reveals that suicide is the most frequent cause of death: more frequent than cancer, heart attacks, stroke, or accidents.

chiatrist. Each medication she ultimately agreed to try caused side effects, some tolerable, others not. When she had periods of well-being, she figured she didn't need them anymore. Eventually she learned that she couldn't toss out her medications and expect to maintain mental and emotional equilibrium. She became, she wrote, determined to manage the disorder rather than letting it manage her—adding, with some ruefulness, "easier said than done."

Bipolar disorder can be devastating. Statistics cannot adequately convey the suffering or its effects on relationships and work life. However, statistics do speak clearly to the issue of suicide. A comparison of mortality ratios in people suffering from bipolar disorder reveals that suicide is the most frequent cause of death: more frequent than cancer, heart attacks, stroke, or accidents. More significant, perhaps, is that statistics strongly suggest that taking medications can reduce the rate of suicide by as much as 80 percent.

Taking mood stabilizers means living with irritating side effects as well as close monitoring for toxicity. It is a major commitment. But mood stabilizers, as writer Bloom found, can mean the difference between managing bipolar disorder or letting it control, or even end, one's life.

—*Martha Brown Martin, M.D.*

Antipsychotic Medications

Who would ever have predicted that the experimentation with ways of anaesthetizing surgical patients at a military hospital in Tunisia in the 1930s would give rise to the world of medications for people suffering from psychosis? There, surgeons saw that chlorpromazine (brand name: Thorazine), a drug related to antihistamines, exerted a striking calming effect on their agitated patients. This observation was reported in the medical literature and led psychiatrists in Paris in the 1950s to try it on their agitated psychotic patients. It had a remarkably good effect. This was the beginning of antipsychotic medication, which would become a mainstay in helping people suffering psychotic disorders to live far more connected and productive lives.

What are these antipsychotic medications specifically treating? Traditionally, the target symptoms have been those that virtually define *psychosis:* hallucinations (sensory experiences that others around the person don't share, most often voices or sounds) and delusions (beliefs held that are not shared by others of a similar culture, like the sense of being pursued or of feeling immensely important). These are often referred to as "positive" symptoms—symptoms that are present in a person's life when they shouldn't be. Often, a degree of agitation goes along with these experiences.

But in psychotic illnesses such as schizophrenia, there are other sets of symptoms that are equally important to attend to, if not more so. This group is called the "negative" symptoms and represents a deficit in normal functioning. Many schizophrenic people suffer from apathy, a lack of motivation; they can be emotionally flat, withdrawn from other people, with little to say. Often there is some degree of cognitive impairment—deficits in the ability to pay attention, in memory functions, and in judgment. Not surprisingly, negative symptoms account for a significant amount of impairment in psychosis, which means that controlling the more dramatic positive symptoms is not enough.

Consider the experience of Josephine. In her junior year of high school, she began to isolate herself from her family, something her parents assumed was typical for an adolescent. When the principal of her school called home to talk about a decline in Josephine's participation and performance, her folks gently confronted her; she simply avoided them and others more. Chalking it up as a "phase" she was going through, they left her alone. Then the principal called again, this time to report peculiar comments Josephine was making to her teachers and classmates. Her mother looked through her room. She found lots of papers filled with writing that was almost incoherent but seemed to indicate that Josephine was feeling controlled by alien forces. There were many pairs of sunglasses that had numbers written on them; a small notebook had entries rating each pair as to its efficacy in blocking the gamma rays the aliens were using to influence her. Her parents took her to the hospital that afternoon. Josephine was terrified and highly agitated in the emergency room; this all felt like part of the aliens' plot, now involving her parents. She was hearing voices damning her. An initial set of lab tests showed her to have a low level of alcohol in her system. She said she had been tapping into her parents' wine cellar to try to calm herself so that she could better resist the aliens' control. Though entirely convinced of the veracity of her perceptions, she was willing to accept treatment in the hope that it would make the voices, the most tormenting part of her experience, go away. Treatment consisted of hospitalization and medication.

Antipsychotic medications are grouped into two broad categories: the conventional ones, also known as the *typical* antipsychotics, and the *atypical* antipsychotics, or the second-generation antipsychotics. The first class is the older ones, most closely related to the original chlorpromazine: these tend to be related chemical compounds, to work on the same sets of neurotransmitter receptors, and to have similar profiles of efficacy and side effects. What distinguishes them from one another is their potency, the amount of medication that must be used to achieve beneficial effect. The typical antipsychotic agents listed on page 276 are grouped in order of relative potency, with both the brand names and generic names included.

The newer antipsychotic agents, the atypical antipsychotics (see page 276), have been developed more recently. Clozaril was the first of this second generation of antipsychotics. As a class, these drugs are more diverse in terms of their chemical structures. While they affect dopamine receptors as do the older drugs, some also affect the serotonergic receptors, and to various degrees of each.

In the brain, there are many neuronal pathways and networks that involve dopamine, a neurotransmitter in the brain. Researchers have identified some that may be related to the positive symptoms, others that may be responsible for the negative symptoms, and still others that are connected to the side effects that can emerge. Medications that are aiming for the pathways felt to be responsible for the target symptoms, of course, also bathe other nontargeted dopamine-mediated neuronal networks, leading to side effects. It has been the mission of psychopharmacologic researchers to fine-tune the medications to target the pathways causing the problems with minimal effect on others.

Among the conventional agents, the principal set of side effects is in the realm of physi-

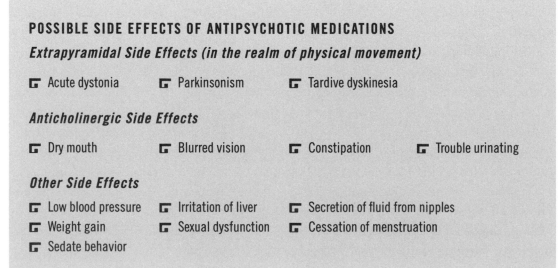

POSSIBLE SIDE EFFECTS OF ANTIPSYCHOTIC MEDICATIONS

Extrapyramidal Side Effects (in the realm of physical movement)

- Acute dystonia
- Parkinsonism
- Tardive dyskinesia

Anticholinergic Side Effects

- Dry mouth
- Blurred vision
- Constipation
- Trouble urinating

Other Side Effects

- Low blood pressure
- Irritation of liver
- Secretion of fluid from nipples
- Weight gain
- Sexual dysfunction
- Cessation of menstruation
- Sedate behavior

cal movement: These are called the *extrapyramidal* side effects. Many practitioners prescribe the highly effective antidotes for these side effects right along with the first dose of the antipsychotic, particularly when they are giving a medication that is more likely to cause these kinds of side effects (the high-potency conventional antipsychotic agents) in people who are more likely to get the side effects (young agitated men seem to be at the highest risk). Psychosis is terrifying enough, and so many practitioners want to prevent these movement side effects from occurring at the very outset of treatment.

The most dramatic and uncomfortable of these extrapyramidal side effects is an acute *dystonia*—a sudden painful muscle spasm, often involving the neck, the back, the eyes, and the tongue. There is also a condition called *akathisia* that these medications can induce, which can be almost unbearable: it is an intense feeling of restlessness, particularly in the legs. Some people taking conventional antipsychotics can develop a pattern of movement that looks so much like Parkinson's disease that it is dubbed *parkinsonism:* a slowness in walking, a stiffness in one's limbs, a tremor in the hands and arms. As the psychotic symptoms start to recede, the medications given to prevent these side effects can be gradually withdrawn. They can be completely discontinued if they are not needed, or started up again should any of these side effects emerge.

> The newer generation of antipsychotic medications, the atypical antipsychotics, holds great promise for those people suffering from psychosis.

A late-developing side effect, tragic in its occurrence as there is not as much success in treating it, is *tardive dyskinesia*—late-onset abnormal movements generally in the face and tongue. There are a number of remedies but no absolute cures for this, and it can develop after years of treatment with conventional antipsychotics. Most doctors try to avoid exposing people to these medications over the long haul for just this reason.

There are other side effects that can occur with any of these conventional medications but which tend to occur with greater frequency in people who are taking the lower-potency antipsychotics. Some people become sedate. Some get a dry mouth, blurred vision, constipated, and sometimes have trouble urinating—these are called *anticholinergic* side effects and can be great nuisances. Some people experience low blood pressure, noticed particularly when they stand up too quickly—no mere nuisance, for it can cause dangerous falls, particularly in the elderly. With many of the agents, there is a tendency for weight gain—on average, fifteen pounds, but some folks gain more than that. This is more than a cosmetic issue: increased weight increases the risk of the development of diabetes and elevated cholesterol, which can lead to life-threatening heart disease.

Male or female, pregnant or not, the dopamine blockade aimed at reducing both positive and negative psychotic symptoms can also stimulate the production of prolactin, the hormone responsible for milk production in mammals. It reveals itself by the secretion of fluid from the nipples—both in men and in women. Furthermore, the elevation of prolactin can also cause problems through the intricate and elaborate cascade system of hormonal balance in our bodies, yielding sexual dysfunction or a cessation in periods in premenopausal women. Over time, this can lead to osteoporosis due to the suppression of estrogen.

Any of these antipsychotic medications can cause irritation of the liver, the organ responsible for their metabolism and excretion. And because many other medications are also metabolized by the liver, drug interactions can occur. These can be both anticipated and monitored. Additionally, there are a number of idiosyncratic rare side effects associated with many of these medications.

The newer generation of antipsychotic medications, the atypical antipsychotics, holds great promise for those people suffering from psychosis. Each has been determined as offering at least equivalent efficacy for treating the positive symptoms of psychosis as the older medications. Importantly, some of these medications have been shown to alleviate the negative symptoms of psychosis (the emotional flatness, the apathy, the cognitive impairments) that the conventional antipsychotics do not tend to help. Some of the newer medications appear to have mood-stabilizing properties as well.

Because these medications are not as closely related to one another as the members of the conventional category, it is harder to make generalized statements about their side-effect profiles. However, as a group, they are significantly less likely to cause extrapyramidal symptoms, and some of them appear to have no effect on prolactin production. Each one, however, does present its own profile of potential side effects.

Although you might wonder why anyone would take any of these antipsychotic agents with the possibility of so many side effects, you would not have to look far beyond the intense suffering that psychosis causes to see that it would be worth it. Josephine's experience is not unusual. Within a few days of starting on antipsychotic medication, the voices Josephine was hearing were completely gone. It took a little longer for her delusions about aliens to recede. She was gradually able to reconnect with classmates and returned to her high level of academic performance. However, she grew to hate the side effects that came along with the benefits, especially the weight she had gained. She secretly stopped taking the medication and her delusions began to return. She and her psychiatrist decided to try a different agent with less of a tendency to cause weight gain. Within a few months, she had another psychotic episode. She was switched to yet another agent, which appeared to help her psychosis clear more rapidly and which seemed to have fewer of the side effects she didn't like.

Josephine and her psychiatrist strive to find the most effective agent with the fewest side effects. This is a challenge facing the many folks who suffer from psychosis and the practitioners trying to help them. Research efforts are dedicated to developing even better new medications to alleviate psychotic symptoms with fewer side effects as well as finding the mechanisms underlying psychosis that will help in targeting these mechanisms with the most appropriate treatment.

—Martha Brown Martin, M.D.

Polypharmacy

Wendy had everything going for her: a solid career as an accountant, many supportive friends, and a wedding planned for the following year. But her past haunted her. Wendy had not slept through the night in many months. She was smothered by fear as she tried to fall asleep at night and tortured by a recurrent nightmare when she finally did get to sleep. In the dream, she was a young child and a large black dog was chasing her. She usually woke up just as he was about to catch her. Morning was a relief, but she always awoke more tired than when she had gone to bed. The sleeplessness was beginning to affect her work; she could not concentrate for long periods of time and she was distracted and irritable with her colleagues. At times she was afraid for no apparent reason. Many days, images of her older brother sexually assaulting her would pop into her head at the most inopportune times.

Wendy was thirty-one years old before she finally tried to get some help. Seeking help was the only alternative to suicide, though there were many days when suicide seemed like the only solution. Wendy's primary care physician referred her to a close colleague for an evaluation. Her physician was the only one in her life who knew about the abuse and about some of her fears, who knew that she was not the "together person" she appeared to be to the rest of her world. The psychiatrist specialized in treating trauma survivors.

The first consultation lasted about an hour. Wendy could hear, as if at a distance, her own voice reporting the details of her life. She remembered saying she did not want to take a medication, so she was stunned to walk out of the office with not one but three prescriptions. After she left, questions flooded her mind. The most important one was whether being prescribed three different medications meant she was "really sick." She was also not sure she could safely take them all together.

Wendy had become a "victim" of polypharmacy. *Polypharmacy* is simply a medical term for taking more than one medication at a time. Though most physicians and psychiatrists would prefer prescribing only one medication at a time, in reality polypharmacy is something that is practiced quite regularly.

There are many reasons causing therapists to prescribe more than one medication for the same condition. The main reason is the therapeutic limits of drugs available to treat psychiatric problems. There is no drug for any psychiatric problem that is 100 percent effective in 100 percent of the people who use it. More than one medication is given when in the following situations:

1. The illness in questions is only partially treated with one medication.
2. Another medication is added to counteract the side effects of the original medication. For example, although some of the selective serotonin reuptake inhibitors

(Paxil, Serzone, Zoloft, Celexa, Prozac) can significantly improve symptoms of depression or anxiety, some people experience a side effect of sedation while on these drugs. It is often easier to add something to counteract the sedation, perhaps a more stimulating drug like Wellbutrin or Provigil, rather then change medications all together and risk losing the positive response along with the undesirable side effect.

3. Some conditions like Post-Traumatic Stress Disorder are known to involve many different neurotransmitter systems—serotonin, norepinephrine, dopamine, glutamate. There is no one medication that treats all of these areas of the brain at the same time. Therefore, it is up to the clinician to try to listen to the symptoms and come up with the smallest number of medications that will lead to the biggest reduction in overall symptoms.

Polypharmacy has a long and interesting history in psychiatry. For the most part, the practice has been criticized, particularly in the period from the 1960s to the 1980s. During this period, psychotherapy or "talk therapy" was much more popular in the field of psychiatry; medications were a second line of treatment. It was difficult to consider putting someone on one medication, let alone three. But the nineties saw a big boom in the growth and development of drugs, particularly for individuals with mild to moderate depression and anxiety. The selective serotonin reuptake inhibitors (SSRIs) introduced in the late 1980s treat both of these conditions. These drugs were also relatively safe and easy to use. With an increased knowledge of brain chemistry came an increased comfort level with many of these medications. There also developed a growing understanding that even therapy worked more effectively when the individual was not severely bothered by symptoms of depression and anxiety.

> *Polypharmacy* is a medical term for taking more than one medication at a time.

When Wendy returned home later that evening and thought about the appointment, she was confused by the drugs prescribed: Prozac, Desyrel, and Ativan. She was not sure how she should take any of them. She went online to find out more about medication use, particularly about these three medications. There was little information about taking multiple medications, though what she did find was scary: "Do not combine medication for fear of causing severe, perhaps even lethal, side effects." Not reassuring. She went to a chat room for other trauma survivors to find out about their experiences. This was a group she visited often, and she felt she could trust them. She was startled to find that almost all of them were on some combination of medications. Most, like her, did not like this, but had to admit that the additions did seem to make a positive difference in their overall ability to function. With this information in hand, she went back to the psychiatrist to find out more about the combination of drugs she was to take.

> From the 1960s to the 1980s "talk therapy" was much more popular in the field of psychiatry; medications were a second line of treatment.

Dr. Kimball walked her through the pros and cons. The benefits were clear. Because she had been diagnosed with Post-Traumatic Stress Disorder and Major Depression, it was unlikely that any one medication alone would work. She had been given Prozac, an antidepressant for both the depression and the PTSD symptoms. However, Prozac took four to eight weeks to take full effect and Wendy seemed to need some relief now. She desperately needed to sleep. She was given the Desyrel, in a relatively small quantity (50 mg qhs), to help her sleep. This would work right away, which was quite reassuring to Wendy. Finally, she was to take the Ativan only when needed—which in her case would be when feelings of terror interfered with her ability to manage her work. She was told that she did not need to take this antianxiety medication unless she felt really overwhelmed, but that when she did take it, she would feel remarkably calmer, though perhaps a little sleepy, within fifteen minutes. Wendy was skeptical about the promise of immediate relief.

> ✦
> The downside of taking multiple medications is the possibility of drug interactions.

The downside of taking multiple medications is the possibility of drug interactions. Whenever you combine two or more drugs, your body is forced to work overtime to break down the medication to clear it out of your system. Most of this work is done by the liver. Medications can get "backed up" waiting to be metabolized, resulting in elevated drug levels of any and all of the drugs you are taking. There is an extensive enzyme system within your liver that breaks down many common psychiatric medications (particularly the SSRIs), the cytochrome P450 enzyme system. Within this enzyme system are subgroups of enzymes, isoenzymes, which work on different, very specific drugs. This does not mean that you can't combine medications that are broken down by the same enzyme, but that when you do, you need to assume that the drug levels in your body will be higher than expected. This may be to your benefit, as you may have a response on a lower dose, or it may work against you, giving you more severe side effects at a lower dose.

The other problem with combining medications is that if there is a response, you may not know which medication is causing it. You may then be in the vulnerable position of trying to take away medications one at a time to find the culprit. And in doing so, you might stop taking the medication that is doing the most good.

Based on her analysis of the evidence she had gathered, Wendy decided she would go ahead with the medications. She slept like a baby the first night on the Desyrel and found herself to be less irritable at work the next day. She took the Prozac for the first time that morning and found that with more sleep she only needed the Ativan for the worst conflicts at work or for evenings when she was totally stressed out and alone. At her one-month fol-

---

If you have seen a psychiatrist who is recommending more than one drug, you should ask the following questions:

☞ What exactly is each drug being prescribed for?

☞ When should I expect to see an improvement with each drug?

☞ What would be the risk of waiting and adding the second drug at another time?

☞ What are the potential drug interactions between all the medications I am taking—including any I am taking for medical conditions?

☞ In what ways should the drugs overlap in terms of side effects?

☞ How long should I expect to be on each drug?

low-up appointment, Wendy reported improvement in most areas of her life; she was particularly impressed with the amount of sleep she was getting, although on the weekends, she could sleep up to fifteen hours at a time. She admitted this was excessive, but she felt she was simply catching up for lost time.

Eventually, Dr. Kimball suggested that they begin to take some of the medications away to see if they could find a way for her to feel emotionally better without being so sedated. At this suggestion, Wendy had the opposite of her initial reaction: She did not want her "happy pills" taken away. She did agree, however, that the sedation was becoming more of a problem. Dr. Kimball described the dilemma to her: She was on three different medications, all of which had the potential to cause sedation, even though Prozac is better known for causing agitation. It was not going to be easy to take one away to see if they could improve the sleepiness. Dr. Kimball had an alternate plan: She could add yet another more stimulating medication to counteract the sedation. Wendy worked with numbers; she could see where this was heading. She decided to come off the Desyrel for a week to see if the sedation improved.

In conditions that are difficult to treat, including PTSD, severe depression, and anxiety, polypharmacy can creep up on both the client and the clinician. Many well-meaning psychiatrists will add medication after medication in the hopes of stumbling on something that will reverse the malignant course of illness. The clinician may be able to see a small amount of improvement, but not enough for the client to feel she is functioning adequately. It may seem too risky to pull away a drug that is helping even a bit, so another is added, and then another, and another. Clients, particularly those with severe PTSD, can end up on a medication from each available class of drugs and still not feel great. As a client you have the right and obligation to put a stop to this kind of practice.

If you have seen a psychiatrist who is recommending more than one drug, you should ask the following questions:

1. What exactly is each drug being prescribed for?
2. When should I expect to see an improvement with each drug?
3. What would be the risk of waiting and adding the second drug at another time?
4. What are the potential drug interactions between all the medications I am taking—including any I am taking for medical conditions?
5. In what ways should the drugs overlap in terms of side effects?
6. How long should I expect to be on each drug?

The bottom line is that polypharmacy is currently routine in psychiatry. In many instances it can be done safely and effectively and, in fact, may represent the most effective treatment for your condition. You must be working with a psychiatrist who is respectful of your questioning and respectful and responsive to any report from you of effects and side effects from the medication prescribed. It is ultimately up to you as the consumer to ask questions and to monitor what is going into and out of your body.

—Amy Elizabeth Banks, M.D.

Medications in Pregnancy

The myth of the "happy pregnancy" is omnipresent in our society. Women are supposed to be delighted about their pregnancies, calm and tranquil, and ever hopeful about entering into a new and blissful stage of their lives. For some lucky women, thankfully, this is the case. But for others, pregnancy is accompanied by feelings of apprehension, depression, and anxiety.

Sometimes this is due to a biological vulnerability to a mood disorder that continues during pregnancy or is even exacerbated by some of the hormonal changes that occur during pregnancy. Sometimes it is because a baby means a dramatic and stressful change in one's life. Conflict in the relationship of the parents-to-be is a common source of psychological distress as are financial pressures, child care concerns, and career changes. The pregnancy may be unplanned or there may be concerns about the health of the fetus. The unrelenting time clock of the developing pregnancy can intensify psychological difficulties.

Because of the myth of happy pregnancy, women are often resistant to seeking help while pregnant. Women may be ashamed of having depressed feelings at a time when they think they should be happy, or they may feel hopeless that anything will be able to help them. They are often paralyzed at the thought of contacting a mental health professional and explaining, "I'm twelve weeks pregnant, and I'm miserable." Women who have been in treatment previously and have already established a trusting relationship with a mental health professional are often the ones who feel safe enough to ask for help quickly when they are pregnant. Women who have had a previous postpartum depression and who were helped by psychiatric treatment often plan proactively for changes in mood and anxiety that may come with a subsequent pregnancy.

The other reason that a woman may be resistant to getting help during pregnancy is fear about the effects of any potential medications on her developing child. Women are often exquisitely careful about protecting their developing babies and doing everything possible to ensure the baby's health, even if it means sacrificing their own needs. Very real cases in recent history of fetal malformations related to drugs such as thalidomide and DES (diethylstilbesterol) have added powerful images and real-life examples to these basic instinctual fears and concerns.

Difficult as it may be to ask for help during pregnancy, it is enormously important during this time of dramatic transition in a woman's life. She will never be the same biologically, psychologically, or socially. And since caring for a baby requires so much emotional and physical energy under any circumstances, one needs to be at one's best.

A woman's state of mind during pregnancy is intimately connected with the psychological milieu of the child's birth and development. Depression during the pregnancy is strongly associated with postpartum depression and there is a preponderance of evidence that postpartum depression has a great impact on the child's cognitive and emotional development.

It is also crucial during a woman's pregnancy that the stability of her life not be sacrificed, such as her relationship with her partner, her job, and her family. Psychiatric illness can threaten these aspects of a woman's life and affect her future ability to care for her children.

Thus, the conflict: Women are hesitant to seek psychiatric care during pregnancy, and especially to take medications, yet it is an incredibly crucial time for a woman to be as psychologically well as possible—to care for herself, to keep important relationships stable, and to prepare to care for a child. It is always prudent to minimize the use of medications during pregnancy by using and optimizing other types of therapy, and it has been repeatedly shown that psychopharmacology and psychotherapy work better together than either one does alone. In addition, supportive advice and practical lifestyle changes such as getting enough sleep, getting more household and child care help, minimizing stress, and eating well are important for pregnant and postpartum women. However, there are times when symptoms are severe, disabling, and rooted in biology, making medications the appropriate and necessary treatment.

The fetal brain continues to develop throughout pregnancy and after birth. Because psychotropic medicines affect levels of neurotransmitters or chemical messengers in the brain, there are theoretical concerns that exposure to these medications could interfere with the way that neuronal interconnections and receptors are distributed in the developing fetal brain. This could theoretically result in subtle differences in learning styles, cognitive abilities, or emotional regulation later in life. No antidepressants have been shown to cause any of these effects, but children exposed to psychotropic drugs in utero have not been followed late enough into adulthood to assure that this is not a possibility. The information we do have from studies is considerable but limited, making medication decisions during pregnancy an art and not a science. It is a matter of balancing the known and unknown risks of medications with the severity and risks of the pregnant woman's individual symptoms, history, and life situation. The following example illustrates how these decisions may be made.

Deborah is a thirty-eight-year-old graphic designer with a history of depression who came to my office sixteen weeks pregnant with her first child. She described a long history of depression dating back to her childhood, which was dominated by an unpredictable and violent alcoholic father and a depressed and withdrawn mother. When she was in her twenties, Deborah struggled through years of chronic depression. She felt bleak, empty, and despairing and had trouble finding solace from her emotional pain. She was often tired and irritable and was unable to maintain any romantic relationships or settle on a career path.

> Pregnancy can be accompanied by feelings of apprehension, depression, and anxiety.

> It is crucial during a woman's pregnancy that the stability of her life not be sacrificed, such as her relationship with her partner, her job, and her family. Psychiatric illness can threaten these aspects of a woman's life and affect her future ability to care for her children.

In her late twenties, Deborah finally began seeing a psychiatrist. She began weekly psychotherapy and also tried a variety of different antidepressants. Finally, she started on an antidepressant called Wellbutrin and had a dramatic improvement. Her "veil of darkness" lifted and she felt optimistic, energetic, and able to enjoy life. Relationships seemed to go better, and within a few years she married a long-time acquaintance. Her working life finally felt right, as she was able to put her artistic talents to use as a graphic designer.

Deborah became pregnant and immediately stopped her medication. She did not want to expose her child to any unknown risks. Things went well for the first month, but after about six weeks, she felt herself sinking into a familiar dark and empty hole. She began to fight with her husband and felt hopeless about their relationship. She felt slow and plodding at work and was unable to meet her deadlines. She was not eating or sleeping well, and as she saw her "perfect life" slipping away, she had fantasies about dying. Finally, she came to my office to ask about her options. She said that she was very worried about taking anything during the pregnancy but felt desperate. She wanted to know what the safest and most carefully tested antidepressants might be and wanted help assessing the risks and benefits.

I first explained to her that she had gone a long way in assuring the well-being of her baby by making it through the first trimester drug-free. The first twelve weeks of the pregnancy marks the completion of the fetus's physical development—all limbs, facial features, and major organs are fully formed by this time. Getting through this period drug-free dramatically reduces the possibility that the fetus will have a drug-induced congenital malformation.

In terms of selecting a medication to take later in the pregnancy, Deborah wanted to go with one that was considered the safest and most carefully tested, even if it was not the most optimal medication for her. At the time of Deborah's visit, I explained that two medications seemed the safest according to current data. One was Prozac, for which the results of a number of studies seemed to suggest it caused no increased risk of birth defects, miscarriages, or delivery complications above baseline levels. In addition, a carefully implemented study by a group of researchers in Toronto followed exposed children to preschool age and found that there was no effect on language development, cognitive development, or social development at this age.

The other class of medications that has had a significant number of studies done researching its safety in utero is the tricyclic antidepressants (Pamelor, Norpramin, Elavil, and others). This group of antidepressants was the first to be discovered and manufactured. It has been in use since the 1950s, so there is long-term data on the drugs' safety. Many

> The information we do have from studies is considerable but limited, making medication decisions during pregnancy an art and not a science.

thousands of pregnancies with exposure to tricyclics have been documented and reviewed with no increased risk of congenital malformations noted. In addition, the Toronto study also looked at tricyclic antidepressants and found no effects on language, cognitive, or social development. Since the tricyclics tend to have more side effects for the person taking the drug than Prozac does, the tricyclics are used less frequently these days but certainly are another relatively safe option during pregnancy.

> ✦
>
> **Depression during pregnancy has known risks, and treatment is therefore often indicated.**

In weighing the risks and benefits of taking medications during pregnancy, it is important to bear in mind that depression during pregnancy definitely has known risks, and that treatment is therefore often indicated. In Deborah's case, it was apparent that withholding antidepressant treatment could have resulted in damage to her marriage and to her career. These factors are important to family life, and their erosion could have a great impact on the child's future well-being. Untreated mood disorders during pregnancy have also been linked to premature delivery and low-birth-weight babies. In addition, depression during pregnancy can lead to postpartum depression, which can seriously impair the attachment relationship between mother and child.

Deborah did start on Prozac and noted an improvement in her mood after two weeks. She felt more hopeful about her ability to be a good mother, began to eat better and sleep more, and was able to function better at home and at work. Although she did not feel as good as she had felt on the Wellbutrin, she was comfortable that she was taking a medication that had the greatest number of studies suggesting its safety in pregnancy. Deborah was able to make better use of her psychotherapy, since her symptoms had largely abated, to explore the ways her difficult childhood interfered with her view of herself as an adequate mother.

After Deborah's child was born, her depression recurred even though she continued to take Prozac. This was not unexpected since the postpartum period is by far the most vulnerable time for depression in women. A classic study shows that the risk of psychiatric illness rises dramatically during the first three months postpartum. This is likely due to the dramatic shifts in hormones that occur after birth, most notably a rapid drop in estrogen levels, as well as psychosocial factors. A history of depression or anxiety earlier in life increases the chances a woman will develop postpartum depression.

> ✦
>
> **The decision of whether to treat depression during pregnancy with medication is a personal one that is influenced by many individual factors.**

I added Wellbutrin to the Prozac, and Deborah's mood returned to normal. After her child was one year old, we weaned Deborah off of the Prozac, but she remained on Wellbutrin and continued to do well.

Medication decisions during pregnancy can sometimes be more complicated. Bipolar Disorder, also known as "Manic Depression," probably presents the greatest challenge to treatment during pregnancy. The medications used to treat Bipolar Disorder, a class of drugs called "mood stabilizers," have been shown to slightly increase rates of specific congenital abnormalities above baseline levels. However, the rapid discontinuation of these drugs has been shown not only to increase the risk of having an acute manic or depressive episode, but also to increase the rate of cycling through these episodes for years to come. The dramatic changes in mood, behavior, and mental status can lead to severe disruption of a woman's family, work status, and social relationships. In addition, women with a personal or family history of Bipolar Disorder are at highest risk for postpartum disorders including postpartum psychosis. Postpartum psychosis is a psychiatric emergency that generally requires psychiatric hospitalization to stabilize the mother and assure the safety of the infant. Given the risks of taking medications during pregnancy coupled with the risks of discontinuing medication, treatment decisions are complex and sensitive and require an individualized approach to balancing the risks and benefits for each woman.

The decision of whether to treat depression during pregnancy with medication is a personal one that is influenced by many individual factors. A pregnant woman needs to weigh the potential disruption that depression during pregnancy and the postpartum period can have on herself, her child, and her ability to mother against the risks or uncertainties of taking medications. Working with a clinician who is knowledgeable about medications in pregnancy and can help navigate these decisions in a well-balanced and holistic manner is essential for the health and well-being of women and their families.

—*Lori Kaplowitz, M.D.*

Complementary Treatments for Depression and Anxiety

Margaret called my office with a common request: "I've been on Prozac for years, and I'd like to try to get off it."

Jenny called in with this: "My psychotherapist has recommended that I see a psychiatrist and try medication, but first I'd like an evaluation and to see what other options might be available. I've heard so much about St. John's Wort. What about that?"

I usually tell people that I will be happy to evaluate them, but I can't promise to keep them off traditional psychiatric medications. Many people need these medications to function. That said, there are a number of approaches to optimizing brain functioning in more "natural" ways. Some natural supplements and healing therapies are fine to use along with medications, which is why this type of medicine is called "complementary." Each type of treatment should complement the other to improve the end results.

There are many different types of complementary treatment: nutrition, herbal therapy, acupuncture, bodywork, hormones, and light therapy will be covered here.

The notes highlighted with **Caution:** will also tell you when *not* to use these approaches, especially with psychiatric medications. Of course, you should always consult with your own doctor before beginning any complementary treatment. In addition, not much evidence exists regarding safety of these supplements during pregnancy or lactation, so they are best avoided unless specifically prescribed by a health practitioner who knows you well.

NUTRITION

Vitamins and Minerals Vitamins are important for optimal functioning of the whole body, including the brain. Certain vitamins are essential for production of important neurotransmitters, the body chemicals that help brain cells communicate with one another. In addition, researchers have found that people with depression may especially lack some of the B vitamins. B_{12} deficiency has long been known to cause depression. In one study, women already on antidepressant medication improved just by adding one of the B vitamins, folic acid, to their medication.

I usually recommend that people with depression take a good general multivitamin as well as a B-complex supplement, aiming toward getting the following amounts of supplementation:

- B_1 (thiamine) 1.5–10 mg/day
- B_2 (riboflavin) 1.7–10 mg/day

- B_3 (niacin) 13–19 mg/day (may be toxic in doses above 100 mg/day)
- B_6 (pyridoxine) 10–100 mg/day (may be toxic in doses above 200–500 mg/day)
- B_{12} (cobalamine) 5–50 mcg/day
- Folate (folic acid) 400 mcg–5 gm/day
- Vitamin C (ascorbic acid) 250–1000 mg/day
- Vitamin D 400–800 IU/day (toxic at more than 100,000 IU/day)
- Magnesium 200–400 mg/day

As you can see, the dose ranges are wide, since this is a general guide that may be discussed with your medical provider.

There are also reports that chromium, selenium, and zinc may be helpful in treating depression.

Amino Acids/Protein Amino acids are the building blocks for many parts of the body, including the neurotransmitters. Protein, whether from meat, eggs, beans, tofu, or other dietary sources, is made up of amino acids. By supplementing some of the specific amino acids that the body turns into neurotransmitters, it may be possible to increase the levels of these neurotransmitters and improve symptoms of depression.

Balanced Amino Acid Supplement. How do you know which amino acid to try first? Sometimes, it is not entirely clear. There are a number of chemical reactions in the body that require more than one amino acid to work along with more than one enzyme or vitamin cofactor. A "quick and dirty," and often less expensive, approach is to buy a good general amino acid (protein) supplement powder, and give that a try. The usual dose is a tablespoon mixed into juice or a smoothie, once or twice a day. If you do not feel better and somewhat more energetic within a week or two, then it may be time to try one or more of the following amino acids in progressively higher doses. **Caution:** People taking an MAOI antidepressant (monoamine oxidase inhibitors such as Parnate or Nardil) should *not* take amino acids because of the risk of a hypertensive reaction.

Tyrosine. Tyrosine is converted in the body to norepinephrine and dopamine, both neurotransmitters that may be deficient in depressed brains.
Many antidepressants also work by increasing levels of these chemicals in the brain. Tyrosine may be able to complement the effects of other amino acids, such as 5-hydroxytryptophan (5-HTP), and to help out the antidepressants as well. Doses range from 100 to 500 milligrams (always start low) per day.

> Some natural supplements and healing therapies are fine to use along with medications, which is why this type of medicine is called "complementary." Each type of treatment should complement the other to improve the end results.

Phenylalanine. Phenylalanine may work in a number of different ways to promote healthy brain functioning. It is a precursor to tyrosine. Phenylalanine inhibits the breakdown of endorphins, the naturally occurring "feel-good" chemicals in the brain. It can be converted into phenylethylamine (PEA), a stimulating neurochemical in its own right. PEA (also found in chocolate) has been called the brain's natural amphetamine and creates a feeling of contentment by causing the release of central nervous system dopamine and norepinephrine. Dose ranges for phenylalanine start at 50 milligrams; the usual dose is 100 to 200 milligrams per day. Some people may find these amino acids too stimulating. Those who develop trouble sleeping or get jittery, anxious, or irritable may need to cut back on the dose or stop the supplement.

5-HTP. 5-hydroxytryptophan (5-HTP) may be one of the most effective natural treatments for depression, anxiety, and insomnia. When you take 5-HTP, your body converts it into serotonin; higher serotonin levels can help combat depression. Prozac and the other drugs in its family, the serotonin reuptake inhibitors (SSRIs), also work by raising serotonin levels. Tryptophan, which is a precursor to 5-HTP, received attention as an effective antidepressant and sleep aid prior to 1989. Tryptophan itself is no longer sold in the United States except by prescription, since a contaminated batch in 1989 unfortunately sickened a large number of people with an illness called eosinophilia myalgia syndrome. This was traced to one batch of tryptophan contaminated with a by-product of the production process called "peak X." 5-HTP appears to be safe, although there is some question of peak X having been found in low levels in some brands. The safest thing to do is to look for a brand of 5-HTP that tests for peak X. 5-HTP is usually supplied in 50 milligram tablets. I recommend that adults start by taking one at bedtime and increase up to as many as two tablets three times a day. It is more effective if taken on an empty stomach. **Caution:** 5-HTP is not safe to take along with SSRI antidepressants, as this can result in an overload of serotonin.

SAM-e. SAM-e, or S-adenosylmethionine, is an amino acid critical to the production of serotonin, norepinephrine, and dopamine—all the major neurotransmitters that may be low in depressed people. The theory is that by supplementing with SAM-e you can increase the production of key neurochemicals that help neurons communicate with each other. Take note that for SAM-e to work you also need to have B vitamins present, so I always recommend a B supplement along with the SAM-e. Usually supplied in 200-milligram capsules or tablets, SAM-e can be started at 200 milligrams per day and the dose increased up to as much as 1,200 to 1,600 milligrams per day in the treatment of depression. SAM-e can be used along with antidepressants (not MAOIs) and with other supplements such as vitamins and amino acids and, in fact, may be more effective that way.

Essential Fatty Acids There is substantial evidence that a group of essential fatty acids called the omega-3 fatty acids (named for their molecular structure) are important in maintaining a stable mood. These fatty acids are especially found in fish, and are termed essential because the body cannot manufacture them; they must come from an outside nutritional source. In one epidemiological study in 1998, countries with the highest fish consumption had the lowest rates of depression. Another study indicates that fish oils may be helpful in stabilizing bipolar disorder.

One mechanism of action for the omega-3s appears to be improved cell membrane functioning, as these fatty acids are incorporated into the neuronal cell membrane structure and help it to maintain necessary flexibility. A diet of processed foods often incorporates unhealthy, rigid fats that are then integrated into our cell membranes. By replacing unhealthy fats with healthy omega-3s, we can improve cell membrane flexibility. Omega-3s are largely found in cold-water oily fish (salmon, anchovies, mackerel), flaxseeds, and green, leafy vegetables (spinach, kale). Fish oil supplements are another great omega-3 source.

The omega-3 fatty acids studied for mood stabilization are EPA (eicosapentaenoic acid)

TYPES OF COMPLEMENTARY TREATMENT

+ *Nutritional supplements*
+ *Herbal therapies*
+ *Acupuncture*
+ *Bodywork*
+ *Hormones*
+ *Light therapy*

and DHA (docosahexanoic acid), which can be directly incorporated into cell membranes. While EPA may be the most active component for antidepressant effect, DHA probably also provides some mood stabilization. Both are currently being studied as treatments for depression. A fish oil supplement ideally should be able to provide 1.5 to 10 grams per day of EPA + DHA, often in divided doses. For those who don't like fish, flaxseed oil, in doses of 3 to 5 grams per day, may also be tried, although there is evidence that some people may be genetically unable to convert it into active EPA and DHA in the body. Taking fish oil supplements with meals will increase absorption of the oil, and vitamins E (400–800 IU/day) and C (250–1000 mg/day) should be added as antioxidants. Cod liver or other fish liver oils are not recommended because they contain too much vitamin A and D and can become toxic in high doses.

HERBAL THERAPY

St. John's Wort (**Hypericum perforatum**) St. John's Wort has been in the news a lot in the past few years. First, it received a lot of positive publicity as studies seemed to indicate that it was an effective antidepressant. More recently, a multicenter study in the United States found that St. John's Wort was no better than placebo in treating major depression. (The antidepressant Zoloft didn't perform well in that trial either, although it was used in low doses.) Critics argue that St. John's Wort has never been indicated to treat major (more serious) depression, but does appear effective for mild to moderate depressions. In addition, if an antidepressant that is known to be effective did not perform well, it may indicate that the study was flawed.

Where does that leave us? St. John's Wort seems to have many of the same actions as a number of prescription antidepressants, but it is less potent. St. John's Wort may inhibit reuptake of serotonin, norepinephrine, and dopamine and therefore may be useful in the treatment of milder depression and anxiety. It has few side effects, stomach upset being the most significant. At high doses, sun sensitivity may also be a problem. So, for someone with a mild depression who wants to try an herbal intervention on her own, St. John's Wort may be an appropriate choice. **Caution:** St. John's Wort should *not* be used during pregnancy, as it may induce uterine contractions. It should *not* be used with the SSRIs, as there is a potential for interactions. If you are already on other medication, you *must* check with your doctor before starting St. John's Wort since there is also interaction potential with some types of medicine, including other antidepressants, some types of chemotherapy, and oral contraceptives.

St. John's Wort is usually supplied in 300-milligram or 450-milligram capsules, standardized with a 0.3 percent hypericin concentration. Hypericin appears to be one of the active components of the St. John's Wort preparation; hyperforin may be another one. Daily dose ranges from 900 to 1800 milligrams per day total, usually taken in divided doses two or three times per day. It may take four to six weeks to notice a full effect, just as is true for medically prescribed antidepressants.

Ginkgo Biloba Ginkgo acts as a mild stimulant. It may help augment antidepressant therapy and may alleviate the sexual side effects of SSRIs, such as loss of libido and anorgasmia. Gingko may actually improve memory and learning in normal people; studies have been mixed regarding its efficacy for treating or slowing the progress of Alzheimer's disease. It may be necessary to take ginkgo for six to twelve weeks to achieve a full effect. Its possible mechanisms of action range from its antioxidant activity to an ability to enhance cerebral blood flow. Ginkgo also has some antiplatelet activity, acting as a mild anticoagulant. **Caution:** People taking Coumadin, aspirin, or other anticoagulant medications should not use ginkgo. because of potential bleeding problems. For the same reason, it should be discontinued at least two weeks prior to any surgery.

Look for a preparation that has 24 percent ginkgo-flavonglycosides, or for one that has been standardized in Germany, where ginkgo is widely prescribed, especially for people over the age of fifty. The German standard preparations are called EGb761 and LI1370. Usual starting dose is 60 milligrams twice per day, and the dose can be slowly increased to as high as 400 milligrams per day to treat sexual dysfunction.

> ✦
>
> Kava should be used with caution, in low doses for a limited time.

Kava **(Piper methysticum)** Kava has been used for centuries in the South Pacific to induce feelings of well-being and relaxation, particularly in social situations. In recent years, people in the United States have started using kava to treat anxiety.

Unfortunately, there have been some recent reports from Germany and Switzerland linking kava use with cases of liver failure. The reports of these cases reveal many confounding factors. In a number of cases, people were on other potentially liver-toxic medications or already had actual liver damage associated with alcohol use. Some of the cases have not yet been explained, leaving the question of whether kava is indeed toxic to the liver. Since it seems to have been used safely for so long in the South Pacific, one question is whether the potency of the extracts used in Europe and the United States is in some way responsible.

The Swiss and French governments have banned the sale of kava, and the Food and Drug Administration (FDA) in the United States has issued a warning to doctors and patients. The American Botanical Council, the country's leading nonprofit organization dealing with research and educational issues regarding medicinal plants and herbs, has issued recommendations that include the following:

- Do not use kava on a daily basis for more than four weeks without the advice of a qualified professional. The adverse reactions, so far, are reported with chronic use.
- Do not combine kava with alcohol or with any other drug that is known to affect the liver, including acetaminophen (Tylenol). Anyone who has any liver problems or anyone who is a regular consumer of alcohol should not use kava.
- Discontinue use if symptoms of liver problems (such as jaundice, yellowing of the eyes or skin) occur.
- Inform your health care provider if you are going to use kava so that your liver functions may be monitored.

Before these recent reports, kava appeared to be an effective remedy for anxiety, with few health risks. To put things somewhat into perspective, the incidence of adverse events reported with kava is still lower than with many prescription medicines for anxiety. We must continue to watch as it becomes clearer what effects kava has on the liver. In the meantime, kava should be used with caution, in low doses for a limited time. Usual doses for anxiety are 45 to 70 milligrams of kavalactones (thought to be the active ingredient) three times per day. Kava is sold in preparations containing 30 to 70 percent kavalactones. **Caution:** Kava should never be used with other sedative medications, such as Xanax or Valium, or other members of the benzodiazepine family of anxiety-reducing drugs, since effects can be additive and adverse reactions have been reported.

Valerian **(Valeriana officinalis)** Valerian is used mostly for sleep and sometimes to help with anxiety. As you might guess from its name, it is related to the medication Valium and is a mild sedative. It is available as an extract with 0.8 percent valeric acid, and the usual dose is 150 to 300 milligrams thirty minutes before bedtime. People already on a sleeping medication should avoid taking valerian because of the possibility of oversedation. Under medical care, however, it may be used to help wean people off more potent sleep medication.

> In some people acupuncture can be very helpful in lowering anxiety and getting energy and mood back on track.

ACUPUNCTURE AND BODYWORK

Chinese medicine practitioners have used acupuncture for thousands of years to treat many different illnesses. Through the meticulous placement of very fine needles, acupuncture manipulates the flow of the body's energy or "qi" to promote a state of health and balance. Acupuncture is usually not painful and is often described as deeply relaxing. In some people it can be very helpful in lowering anxiety and getting energy and mood back on track. It may safely and effectively be used along with the other approaches mentioned here. Acupuncture treatments may also be used along with antidepressant or antianxiety medications, and may even help to treat some of the side effects of these medications.

Although some people are uncomfortable being touched, most people also experience massage as relaxing. Massage can help alleviate muscular tension and can lower heart rate, blood pressure, and harmfully high levels of stress hormones such as cortisol. Chronically high cortisol has been linked to the development of depression.

Different types of energy work are often considered a form of bodywork. This is somewhat misleading, since most do not involve actually touching the body, but instead manipulate the energy fields that some believe exist immediately above the body. Reiki and therapeutic touch are probably the most common forms of energy work. Some people find these deeply relaxing; others experience them as energizing. While energy work may not be a sole treatment for major depression, it can be a useful and pleasant adjunctive therapy.

> Women who use excessively high doses of DHEA risk raising their testosterone levels too much.

HORMONES

A *hormone* is any kind of chemical messenger produced by a gland or organ in the body that can affect functioning in various parts of the body. This is not the place for an extensive discussion about hormones, but there are a few things worth mentioning.

Women who are perimenopausal or who suffer from PMS may in fact have a hormone imbalance and may want to see a doctor to check their estrogen and progesterone levels. Depressed women treated with estrogen have responded well in a number of cases studied.

All depressed women should have their thyroid function checked. Thyroid disorder is extremely common in women and is a well-known cause of depression. There is evidence that some people may suffer from a relative inability to transform the most common form of thyroid hormone, T_4, into the most active form of thyroid hormone, T_3. In fact, the chemical form of T_3, called Cytomel, is sometimes added to antidepressants when medication alone has not completely treated a depression.

DHEA, or dehydroepiandrosterone, is a hormone made by the adrenal glands and is a precursor for estrogen and testosterone, as well as other hormones. A number of studies have shown antidepressant response with the use of DHEA. There is some controversy as to appropriate dosing. I favor testing to obtain a baseline blood level, and then supplementing with low doses (5–25 mg/day) if the blood level is low or low normal. Higher doses of DHEA are easily available over the counter, but I think it is unwise to supplement at higher levels without medical supervision. Women who use excessively high doses of DHEA risk raising their testosterone levels too much. This can result in the side effect of virilism, which may include facial hair and lowered voice. **Caution:** Women with a history of estrogen-sensitive breast cancer, or at high risk for developing breast cancer, should probably avoid taking DHEA.

LIGHT THERAPY

Ample evidence now exists for the use of light therapy in the treatment of Seasonal Affective Disorder (SAD). This treatment has become so accepted that it is no longer considered alternative. As a general guideline to treat depression, you should sit in front of a full-spectrum light for approximately twenty to thirty minutes each morning. You can read or do other activities, but you must glance at the light every few seconds during the session.

A device called a dawn simulator has also shown promise. This device attaches to a lamp with a full-spectrum light bulb and is placed at the bedside. You set the timer for the time you want to wake in the morning, just like an alarm clock, and the light gradually increases, becoming brightest at wake-up time. For people who clearly relate their depressions to the darkening winter months, either of these approaches can be a very helpful, nonmedication way to start treatment.

There are many, many other alternative therapies, but those described here appear to be the most useful and scientifically valid. As the use of complementary medicine increases, doctors are learning more about it and working with their patients to achieve the best results in the safest possible manner. Don't forget to mention your use of any complementary therapies to your health care practitioners.

—Laura Kramer, M.D.

RELATED

ENTRIES

Aging and Its Effect on Mood, Memory, the Brain, and Hormones

Anxiety Disorders

Depressive Disorders

Don't forget to mention your use of any complementary therapies to your health care practitioners.

Cognitive Behavioral Therapy

Cognitive behavioral therapy (CBT) is a collaborative effort between client and therapist to understand the problems for which the client has sought help and to make a systematic plan for change. This therapy is not only about talking; it's also about doing.

One of the most important principles of cognitive therapy is that the way we think about ourselves and the world has a profound impact on what we do and how we feel. The meaning we ascribe to events actually determines how we feel about them. It is one thing if someone feels loss and grief when a relationship ends; it is another if she feels depressed, believing the relationship ended because she had nothing to offer and no one could ever love her. Cognitive therapy provides a way to evaluate and change the interpretations of our experience that are faulty and cause emotional distress. It is not just a method of thinking positively, but a way to rethink the way we see things.

Traditional behavior therapy limited itself to working only with behaviors that could be objectively defined and measured. It was expanded to include internal thought processes when Aaron Beck introduced cognitive therapy with his 1976 book, *Cognitive Therapy and the Emotional Disorders*. Unlike some traditional schools of psychotherapy, the source of the client's problems is not attributed to some underlying psychological defect or failure to master developmental stages. Problematic patterns of behavior and thinking are assumed to be acquired according to the same principles of learning that account for all human behavior and thought. Maladaptive patterns are learned and, therefore, can be unlearned.

Beck noticed that his depressed patients had characteristic patterns of negative thinking about themselves, the world, and their future. Depression was a result of the faulty logic they typically used to interpret their experiences. Our ideas about ourselves are formed in the context of important relationships. We learn who we are through our interactions with others, their responses to us, and ours to them. As a result of the meanings we make of these experiences, we develop core beliefs that determine how we perceive the world and ourselves.

Negative experiences can produce core beliefs like "I am unlovable" or "I am incompetent." Often we don't even realize that we hold these deep beliefs, let alone think to question whether they are realistic or helpful. The underlying assumptions we use to guide interpretations of our day-to-day experiences are related to these core beliefs. These give rise to the automatic thoughts that can produce depressed or anxious mood states. The underlying assumption "If I don't pass the exam, it means that I'm a failure as a person" results in the distorted automatic thought "I'm a failure" and a feeling of self-loathing.

To understand how this theory would apply to the treatment of someone with depression, let's consider the example of Jan, a lesbian in her late fifties with Bipolar Disorder (manic depression). Her psychopharmacologist was working on stabilizing her mood. He thought she might benefit from the addition of cognitive behavioral therapy, because of the research suggesting that cognitive therapy combined with medication is more effective than either alone.

When I first met Jan, she cried easily, lacked the energy to do things she used to enjoy, felt hopeless about her future, and, most notably, had very negative thoughts about herself. Like most depressed people, Jan would never dream of criticizing anyone else the way she did herself. She said that she had no friends, that she didn't fit in anywhere, that she was a loser and had nothing to offer. She was convinced that she was a burden to her adult son. She saw a bleak future in which she would always be depressed and alone, imagining herself aging without anyone to help her.

The initial phase of cognitive behavioral therapy is assessment, asking the *what*, *when*, *where*, and *how often* questions about the problem behaviors and thoughts. The focus is on the present, but past history is helpful in understanding how the problems developed. Core beliefs are often learned from our families while we are vulnerable children, but continue to be influenced by other significant relationships and experiences throughout our lives. The client participates by keeping records of self-observations that pertain to the issues central to the therapy—for example, keeping a record of thoughts and feelings or writing a food diary or tracking the frequency of a harmful habit. Apart from collecting information that helps the client and therapist design their plan, self-monitoring has been shown to create changes in the behavior being observed even before there has been an intention to change. Self-monitoring records also allow the client and therapist to track progress.

Jan started by keeping a record of the thoughts she was having when she felt acutely sad or anxious. For some people, the first step is to turn up the volume on the steady stream of internal dialogue and simply listen to what they are saying to themselves when they are feeling painful emotions. Once Jan was able to record the situations, thoughts, and feelings that went along with her low mood, she was in a position to look for patterns in her thinking that might be problematic. Looking at these records, we started to question some of her interpretations of her experiences. She would eventually be able to look for the core beliefs underlying her automatic responses to situations and challenge those as well.

Another area of self-observation had to do with her daily activities. She was not involved in any activities outside her home, and thus had no possibilities for building new connections. Instead of calling her closest friend, she would wait to hear from her because she feared rejection. She was very lonely, but too depressed and fearful to be able to create opportunities for being with others. The lack of energy and inertia that are symptoms of depression also contribute to prolonging it by trapping the person in a prison of social isolation and cutting her or him off from activities that could bring pleasure or a sense of accomplishment.

A woman who has experienced rejection or criticism in important relationships may come to believe that she is unworthy and to predict that her chances of being valued by others are low. In Jan's case, she had learned to see herself through the critical lens of her parents. They disapproved of her rebellious spirit and were emotionally unavailable to her because of their alcoholism. Their lack of regard for her led to the formation of such beliefs as "I'm not loveable," "I don't belong," and "People won't be interested in me."

Later experiences only deepened these convictions. In high school, she won a scholarship to a boarding school, where she found herself to be different from the others in social

> **COMMON COGNITIVE DISTORTIONS FOUND IN AUTOMATIC THINKING**
>
> ☞ *Labeling,* the tendency to call oneself hurtful names
>
> ☞ *Mind reading,* the assumption that you know what other people are thinking
>
> ☞ *All-or-nothing thinking,* the tendency to see things in polarized extremes
>
> ☞ *Fortune telling,* the tendency to predict that things will turn out badly in the future
>
> ☞ *Should statements,* the tendency to impose harsh dictates upon oneself
>
> ☞ *Catastrophizing,* the belief that something will be so awful you won't be able to stand it

class and education. She developed the idea that she was stupid because she was less academically prepared than other students. Her sense of being different was further heightened by a beginning awareness of her sexual orientation during an era when coming-out did not seem like an option. Later, when she finally left an unhappy marriage, her husband was so outraged by the discovery that his wife was a lesbian that he fought for and gained custody of their two children. Along with internalized homophobia, guilt and shame over losing her children created severe self-recrimination. Jan was politically liberal, yet she held the belief that being a lesbian made her a "loser." The diagnosis of a major mental illness made her a "crazy lady" as well.

Jan was slowly able to break this depressive cycle of self-loathing and isolation through a combination of cognitive-restructuring and behavioral homework assignments. Cognitive behavioral therapy assumes that what happens between sessions is as important as what happens in sessions, so homework is an important component. Homework assignments are designed to build skills and create experiences that lead to change.

For Jan, it was crucial that she learn how to recognize and correct her errors in thinking and challenge old beliefs, a process called cognitive restructuring. The client learns the skills to do this through discussion with the therapist, readings, and written exercises. Jan brought her record of thoughts and feelings into the session to use as a jumping-off point for discussion.

One important way to challenge automatic thoughts is to look for the cognitive distortions they contain. *Labeling,* essentially a tendency to call oneself hurtful names, is one of them. This is what Jan is doing when she calls herself a loser or a crazy lady. Other cognitive distortions include *mind reading,* the assumption that you know what other people are thinking ("She thinks I'm doing a lousy job"); *all-or-nothing thinking,* the tendency to see things in polarized extremes ("I'm a complete failure"); *fortune telling,* the tendency to predict that things will turn out badly in the future ("This relationship isn't going to last"); *should statements,* the tendency to impose harsh dictates upon oneself ("I should have known better" or "I shouldn't get angry"); and *catastrophizing,* the belief that something will be so awful you won't be able to stand it ("If this relationship ends, I'll fall apart"). At first, it takes the assistance of the therapist to look for these distortions and to help generate a more accurate interpretation of an event that the client can believe. A depressed person can find it extremely difficult to see that this negative self-evaluation might not be absolutely true.

The cognitive-restructuring work was important as a way to ease Jan's depressed mood, but it was also instrumental in helping her overcome the blocks to engaging more actively in the world. Jan began making daily schedules designed to get her moving. These initial daily schedules were focused on simple things like limiting time spent in bed or taking a short walk. When she found the courage to ask about volunteer work at a local art college, she was sure this would lead to a humiliating failure. Getting out of bed in the morning was nearly impossible, but she got herself to her new job and faced down her fears. This was the first of many steps that would eventually lead to an increased sense of competence and the formation of new friendships.

Change is always hard. The therapist and client take care to design the steps in tolerable increments. The therapist acts as a coach and a cheerleader. The strength of this relationship often provides the energy necessary to take initial risks. Later on, these actions are maintained by the natural rewards that come. A positive self-reinforcing cycle has begun.

The therapeutic relationship in CBT is interactive and collaborative. The therapist acts as a teacher rather than an all-knowing expert. When appropriate, the therapist might use examples from her own experience. The therapist shares hypotheses with the client and enlists her help in testing them out. The therapist and client work together to set goals and design homework. If a client does not do the homework, it signals a need for reassessment. Therapist and client try to look for factors that they had failed to take into account. One assignment builds upon another until the goals are met.

Jan continued to expand the scope of her activities with an ever-increasing understanding of how her patterns of thinking got in the way. In addition to identifying cognitive distortions, she practiced using other strategies to challenge her negative self-talk. When something went wrong, she looked for alternative explanations instead of assuming it meant something negative about her. For example, if her friend hadn't called in a while, Jan would no longer say, "This proves she doesn't care about me." Instead, she considered the possibility that her friend might have been busy or preoccupied with some problem of her own, and then checked it out with her directly. She tried to reevaluate the probabilities she associated with her negative predictions. "If I speak in my book group, people will laugh at me" changes to "I've participated in the discussion there before and no one has ever laughed at me. It's unlikely this will happen."

Taking another viewpoint by asking herself, "What would I say to a friend if she were telling me this?" always yielded a more compassionate way of looking at a situation. She

There are many problems for which cognitive behavioral therapy seems to be particularly useful, including:

- *Mood disorders* (depression, bipolar disorder)

- *Eating disorders* (anorexia, bulimia, obesity)

- *Anxiety disorders* (panic, phobias, post-traumatic stress disorder, obsessive-compulsive disorder)

- *Behavioral medicine* (stress management, insomnia, pain management, smoking cessation)

- *Habit control* (nail biting, procrastination)

questioned whether there was really any evidence to support her negative conclusions and tried to take note of the evidence that supported more positive thoughts. By asking, "Whose voice is this?" she sometimes caught herself repeating the same hurtful things her parents had once said to her. While she still struggles with the same themes whenever she is depressed, the degree to which she believes her negative thoughts has lessened over time.

If depression can be described as a downward spiral, then what Jan put into motion was a gradual upward spiral. The volunteer job she had sought out when she was at her lowest point eventually grew into a paid job. Now she had strong evidence to dispute her claims that people disliked her and thought she was stupid. By joining a woman's group and participating in some of their social events, she decreased her isolation and actively challenged her belief that "lesbians are losers." One thing built upon and energized another. Each positive experience made it more likely that she would take the next step toward her life goals. The structure she has created and the skills she has acquired mean that her low moods never get as low or last as long as before. Jan no longer sees herself as a crazy lady. Ironically, her ability to manage her illness has itself become a source of pride.

CBT has a reputation for being a short-term treatment, but this is not always the case when dealing with longstanding and entrenched patterns of behavior like Jan's. In real life, therapy doesn't always proceed as smoothly as self-help books might suggest. But there are many problems, such as mild depression or a simple phobia or procrastination, which can be resolved with a brief course of therapy.

The application of cognitive and behavioral therapies extends to a broad range of psychological problems, and there are many problems for which cognitive behavioral therapy seems to be particularly useful. Included among these are *mood disorders* (depression, bipolar disorder); *eating disorders* (anorexia, bulimia, obesity); *anxiety disorders* (panic, phobias, post-traumatic stress disorder, obsessive-compulsive disorder); *behavioral medicine* (stress management, insomnia, pain management, smoking cessation); and *habit control* (nail biting, procrastination).

CBT is arguably the treatment of choice for many of these problems, because insight alone is not always enough to produce change. Maladaptive behaviors often persist even when the person understands their psychological causes. The behaviors can seem to take on a life of their own because they have been so continually reinforced. For example, a client with bulimia might understand that she binges whenever she feels alone and might know that the feelings of intense sadness originated in her childhood. What she may not understand is that her inability to stop bingeing is related to the purging that she does afterward. Because purging decreases anxiety about gaining weight, it actually reinforces bingeing and the cycle continues.

The treatment of depression with CBT was illustrated in Jan's story, but the therapy might look somewhat different when applied to another problem. For example, Karen was a woman who sought help for her multiple phobias. A bright, attractive, self-possessed, married woman in her twenties, you would never guess that her life was ruled by irrational fears. Her freedom to move in the world was limited by the need to avoid the things that caused her to have extreme anxiety or panic attacks. The list was long and overwhelming: riding elevators, being in large crowds, being in public buildings, fears of having a serious illness, thunder and lightning storms, using public transportation, driving near parts of the city she deemed unsafe, driving over bridges, and staying alone overnight. The treatment plan would be simple, but challenging. Karen was going to need to expose herself to these feared situations without fleeing. If she were able to stay in these situations and have the experience of her anxiety lessening, she would become progressively less afraid of them.

During the assessment phase, Karen kept an anxiety log. She recorded the situations and thoughts that triggered anxiety, rating the degree of anxiety on a scale of 1 to 10. This gave us a picture not only of the situations in which she was afraid, but also of the internal dialogue that made her afraid. In the process of talking about her life history, Karen came to understand that her exaggerated need to feel in control was related to her father's abandonment of the family when she was a young child. Karen felt it was her job to protect her depressed mother in a world that suddenly felt unsafe. Avoidance of feared situations decreases anxiety in the moment, but, over time, it reinforces the fear. As an adult, her fears had multiplied precisely because she had gone to such great lengths to try to make her world safe.

To begin, Karen chose one category on her list: fear of being in public buildings. She created a hierarchy of scenarios involving going to the bank that ranged from low to medium to high levels of anxiety. Her fear of going to the bank had been caused by the thought "What if there is a man with a gun here?" She would think about being killed in a robbery and her vigilant scanning of the scene for anyone who looked suspicious increased her anxiety. Finally, she concluded it was too dangerous and stopped going altogether. As preparation to begin tackling her hierarchy, Karen learned to use cognitive restructuring to find ways of countering her anxiety-producing thoughts. She also practiced relaxation techniques.

Karen was very anxious about starting this exercise, so we went together to the bank near my office the first few times. First, she went in with me and stayed close to the door, reminding herself that the probability the bank would be robbed was quite low and stopping herself from scanning for suspicious characters, all the while remembering to breathe. The work continued between sessions as homework assignments that we designed together. When she mastered one phobia, she moved on to another on her list, working with it in the same way—elevators, crowds, trains, and so on.

Thunderstorms were particularly challenging. Nature didn't allow for planning her practice sessions. From spring through fall, Karen was on alert, watching the weather report, listening to the radio, and looking at the sky. She would leave work and run home to ride out a storm, panicking in her basement. Again, her work was to challenge the probability she would be struck by lightning, reduce her attention to weather forecasts, practice relaxation, and gradually move herself from the basement to the first floor of her house and beyond. Through determination and hard work, Karen was able to rid herself of all of her phobias. The world opened up to her, and her life changed dramatically.

Eating disorders are another problem area for which CBT interventions are especially helpful. Cognitive distortions usually play a significant role in the development of an eating disorder. The belief that "I am more worthwhile and loveable if I am thin" is, unfortunately, held by many, if not most, women in our culture. Going on a diet is the event that most girls and women cite as the beginning of their eating problems. Anorexia, bulimia, and chronic overeating are all examples of a diet gone seriously wrong.

Beth was a young woman with bulimia who told me that she could be happy if it were somehow possible to live just from the head up. Looking at this attractive woman, it seemed tragic that her body image could be so distorted. Beth's mother was extremely weight and appearance conscious, and she sent the message that Beth needed to be thin to be truly acceptable. Also, Beth was sexually molested by her uncle during her preteen years. Her parents believed and supported her, but her relationship to her own body would never fully recover. Beth was on a chronic diet, but her efforts to restrict her food intake sometimes led to episodes of overeating and a promise to start the diet again the next day. Her fear of gaining weight and disgust with herself after an episode of overeating was so strong that she eventually started to induce vomiting. She also used exercise as a way to purge, going to the gym frequently and feeling terrible guilt if she missed a day. Because the purging reduced her anxiety, it became a powerful reinforcer of the cycle of restrict, binge, and purge.

The way out was to help Beth begin to normalize her eating behavior. She began to keep a food diary and to record the thoughts and feelings associated with episodes of bingeing and purging. Beth now understood that eating too little set her up to binge. She became familiar with the harmful beliefs she held about food and weight. She also saw that bingeing was more likely to happen when she was upset. The eating plan would involve asking her to begin to approximate three normal meals and snacks each day. When she had urges to binge, she tried to identify what was happening and find other ways to manage her feelings. If she did binge, she tried not to purge. It was very difficult for Beth to tolerate feeling full. She needed to tell herself that being full was not the same as being fat and to remind herself of the health problems caused by vomiting. It was sometimes helpful to do something active when she had the urge to binge or purge. If she was able to delay acting upon them, the urges often passed. Beth also needed to stop linking exercise to her eating. We agreed that she would limit herself to a reasonable exercise schedule. The ritual of getting on the scale each morning fueled her obsession about her weight, and she agreed to gradually weigh herself less often.

Over time, her binge episodes became less out of control and she found that her weight did not balloon when she ate a normal diet. She was amazed at what a relief it was to not think so much about what she was eating and when to get to the gym. The shame she felt about hiding her bingeing and purging from people close to her was gone. Most important, she was starting to believe that her self-worth was not defined by how much she weighed.

The treatment experiences of Jan, Karen, and Beth were different, but all were based on the principles of cognitive behavioral therapy. Some clinicians are trained primarily as cognitive behavioral therapists, while others may use some CBT techniques to augment their approach. Professional organizations, such as the Association for the Advancement of Behavior Therapy, and groups for special problem areas, such as the Anxiety Disorders Association of America, can be resources in finding a cognitive behavioral therapist. The client is the consumer and should feel entitled to shop for a therapist. It is important to look for a good match, someone with whom the client feels comfortable and who has had experience working with the problem.

—Susan J. Miller, Psy.D.

Dialectical Behavior Therapy

Dialectical Behavior Therapy (DBT) is a complex blend of the steps to change, derived from behavior therapy, and the steps to acceptance, derived from Zen meditation. This outpatient treatment is delivered in weekly individual therapy sessions coupled with group skills training under a one-year treatment contract that is renewable if desired or recommended. DBT provides access to the therapist via telephone coaching after hours and requires that the therapist be a member of a consultation team that keeps the treatment on track.

Developed by Dr. Marsha Linehan, a professor of psychology at the University of Washington in Seattle, DBT was designed for and tested on women with borderline personality disorder (BPD) who were chronically suicidal and self-injurious. In her study, women randomly assigned to DBT had fewer and less serious episodes of suicidal behavior, were less frequently hospitalized, used drugs and alcohol less, improved their social functioning and anger control, and were more globally improved than those who were given "treatment as usual." DBT has been modified for delivery in different settings: inpatient, partial, day hospital, and residential. Study of its use with people who have a variety of diagnoses (e.g., substance abuse, bulimia, post-traumatic stress disorder) but who have in common dysregulated emotions is ongoing.

DBT TARGETS PERVASIVE EMOTIONAL DYSREGULATION

Patty is a fifty-year-old divorced woman who makes a living providing childcare. One day, Patty is accidentally locked out of the house of a child for whom she is babysitting. Patty handles the situation well: she picks up the toddler at school and they entertain themselves successfully, regularly calling home until the child's mother returns. When Patty arrives back at the house with her charge, the mother is very upset. She had called the house to check in just before going into an important meeting. When she had not been able to reach Patty at the house, she became frightened that Patty was not going to show up. In her fear and anger, she lashes out at Patty, who begins to angrily defend herself and leaves in a huff. As she is driving home, Patty thinks over the incident. She feels hurt ("It's obvious she doesn't know me at all if she thinks I would just not show up!") and angry ("She shouldn't talk to me that way after all the times I've put myself out for her!") at criticism that seems unjust. She is afraid she might lose the job and contact with a child she has grown to love.

Patty tells herself that she is stupid to take the criticism so seriously and commands herself to let it go, but her mind keeps going back to the scene and the shame she felt when the woman screamed at her. As she recalls similar incidents in her life, the shame intensifies. She thinks, "There must be something about me that makes this happen over and over." She thinks about how much therapy she has had, how hard she tries, yet this is still happening and she still doesn't know what is wrong with her or how to fix it. This thinking leads her to despair and thoughts of suicide.

When Patty gets home she feels stirred up and can't focus on anything. She wanders into the kitchen. She takes ice cream out of the freezer and soon she feels out of control, bingeing on large amounts of food, eating mindlessly until her stomach is so full it aches. She goes to the bathroom and vomits over and over. She sits on the floor beside the toilet feeling weak and tearful. The terrible energy she felt before has left her. She feels calmer. In the back of her mind is a sense of disgust at herself, but it is pretty far away. When a friend calls later, Patty doesn't mention the incident with her employer.

Women assigned to DBT had fewer episodes of suicidal behavior, were less frequently hospitalized, used drugs and alcohol less, improved their social functioning and anger control, and were more globally improved than those who were given "treatment as usual."

DBT assumes that Patty, an intensely emotional person, has never learned effective means of regulating her feelings. When stimulated by events in the environment, such as the angry employer, her emotions seize control. Patty is more or less aware that her emotions are taking over, but she has not learned to gain control effectively. She commands herself not to have emotions, punishes herself with shaming thoughts about her inadequacy, reflects upon her past experiences, considers escape from it all by suicide. Ultimately she changes her physiology, and thus her emotional experience, through bingeing and purging. All of Patty's efforts are aimed at getting herself out of emotional pain that she finds intolerable. What she neglects to do is face the problem with her employer, a lack of resolution that leaves her vulnerable to future incidents.

DBT TEACHES NEW SKILLS FOR OLD SITUATIONS

DBT assumes that your current predicament results from a combination of factors. On the one hand is the biological endowment of passion: Some people simply experience emotions, especially painful ones, more intensely than others do. On the other hand is a poor fit between the emotional person and her environment, both in the past and in the present-day. In such an "invalidating environment," emotions, dreams, thoughts, ambitions, perceptions, and other personal experiences are indiscriminately rejected or punished as wrong or invalid ("I'll give you something to cry about!") or as a sign of illness ("Here goes Sarah Bernhardt again!"). Along with either innate passion or an invalidating environment, there is a lack of supportive learning experiences through which you would acquire the ability to regulate your emotions. DBT's intention is to provide that learning opportunity by teaching a package of skills over a year in a skills group. Four modules are taught in sequence: core mindfulness, interpersonal effectiveness, emotion regulation, and distress tolerance.

The first module, mindfulness, or control of the attention, is key to success and is revisited several times over the course of a year of DBT skills training. Emotionally vulnerable people tend to spend a fair amount of time on automatic pilot, floating along, not noticing the increasing sound of the waterfall ahead until they are trapped in its current. When upset, they may have the opposite problem, focusing obsessively on their unhappy state, compelled to get rid of it but not knowing how. Mindfulness practice trains the mind to observe what is going on in oneself or the environment without judgment. Skillful attention allows one to concentrate on what is required in a situation, shifting focus as needed to be effective.

The second module is interpersonal effectiveness, teaching assertiveness to get what you want. This module teaches how to get what you want not only without damaging relationships with other people but also actually improving relationships in the process.

The third module, emotional regulation, teaches how to both experience emotion without escalation or suppression and how to change persistent problematic emotions.

Finally, in the fourth module, distress tolerance teaches you how to bear pain gracefully without doing something that might provide temporary relief from pain but only make matters worse in the long run.

New DBT programs typically begin by offering skills training that one client called "Life 101." To make such training effective, the skills must be made personally relevant to the person and their application to her specific problems demonstrated, rehearsed, and fine-tuned. It's as if the patient were living in a decrepit house with a leaking roof, sagging floors, a flooded basement, broken stairs, exposed wiring, and volcanic plumbing. In skills group, the leader stands up and announces, "Today, we're going to learn all about the screwdriver." While the group, over time, will allow you to add a whole collection of tools to your belt, you need a coach—your individual therapist—to go into the house with you, help you establish a prioritized list of repairs so that the most dangerous problems get taken care of first, and point out how and where that screwdriver might be useful, as opposed to where a hammer might get more desirable results.

DBT IS BEHAVIOR THERAPY

Laura is a thirty-year-old woman who at six was removed from her family home for severe neglect and who has been in and out of psychiatric hospitals for most of her adult life for anorexia nervosa, chronic suicidal tendencies, and self-injury. She comes to her weekly DBT session. The therapist notes that Laura's diary card shows an incident of self-injury—hitting the wall with her fist—in the last week. Making a tape of the session for Laura to take with her, the therapist zeroes in on this critical incident, launching into a behavioral analysis.

> On the one hand is the biological endowment of passion: Some people simply experience emotions, especially painful ones, more intensely than others do. On the other hand is a poor fit between the emotional person and her environment.

She asks when Laura first began to think about hurting herself. Laura replies that she always feels like hurting herself; but then she says that she doesn't know, she just felt like it all of a sudden. Closer questioning ultimately reveals that her urge to slam her fist into the wall first emerged as she was sitting on the back porch of her group home, enjoying some time alone to write in her journal. Another resident, Mary, joined her and began chatting animatedly about the details of her latest therapy session. As the therapist follows closely, asking, "And then what happened?" and "What did you feel then?" Laura describes feeling annoyed but telling herself not to be rude. The therapist points out that annoyance is a normal response to such behavior and asks if Laura tried to explain that she'd like to be alone. Laura reports that she did try, saying something like, "I like to sit out here by myself sometimes." Mary did not get the hint and continued to chat away, which made Laura become more and more angry.

Laura, frightened by the intensity of the emotion and her mind flooded with angry images, became concerned that she might hit Mary. She jumped up, ran inside, and slammed her fist against the living room wall over and over. Her anger evaporated. She then reported the injury to staff, who sent her to the ER. There was no fracture, but she received a prescription for narcotic painkillers. She spent the next couple of days in an opiate haze.

The therapist sums up the analysis by pointing out that fear is a conditioned response to anger for this abused woman. In order to escape this frightening emotion, Laura hit the wall. Going to the hospital allowed her to avoid the conflicted social situation for several hours, therefore strengthening her action as a future behavior. The opiates were an added bonus.

The therapist validates annoyance as a reasonable response, countering Laura's judgment of herself as rude, and points out that if Laura's efforts to assert her wishes had been successful,

> Laura's childhood set the stage for many of her difficulties, but the past can't be changed, and the present can.

the self-injury would never have occurred. Laura recognizes that "doormat behavior"—allowing people to insert themselves despite her real wishes—is pervasive throughout her relational world. They spend some time in the session rehearsing interpersonal effectiveness skills from the DBT skills package, role-playing the interaction and others like it that Laura has had with Mary. Laura makes a commitment to practice these skills during her next conflict with Mary. She'll call for coaching if in the heat of the moment she forgets what she's learned.

DBT is, at heart, a behavior therapy, which means that both therapist and client actively collaborate to solve the client's problems. Laura and her therapist target specific behaviors for Laura to work on, and she keeps a daily record of her target behaviors on a diary card. The card is reviewed to set the agenda for a given session. If she has behaved in a life-threatening manner over the last week, she and the therapist analyze what set off the behavior and what steps—thought, feeling, and action—took her from annoyance to hand-bashing. The primary focus is on the present. Laura's childhood set the stage for many of her difficulties, but the past can't be changed, and the present can. The operating assumption is that these behaviors achieve some present goal of the person. For Laura, self-injury regulates her anger for the moment and allows her to avoid conflict when her skills to handle it are inadequate.

This insight is not enough, however. Laura has to stop doing what she's always done (being a doormat and regulating anger with self-injury) and start doing something new and more effective (using the energy of anger to maintain her limits with skillful interpersonal behavior). In-session treatment might include education about the normal functions of anger to assert self-interest, skills training in respectful self-assertion, cognitive restructuring of her self-invalidating judgments about herself, and exposure to the feared situation of relational conflict through role-play and homework assignments. The success of these interventions and of the therapy will be confirmed when and if incidents of self-injury decrease, as measured on the diary card. If they don't, the client and therapist reevaluate their hypothesis and try again.

Other talking therapies may look a lot more like a heart-to-heart conversation, and the techniques the therapist employs may not be as evident or as intrusive. The client enjoys considerably more control over the agenda and content of the session. A "good" session may generally involve feeling "better" after it's over. DBT can look like that too, but generally after the major problem areas have been brought under control.

Sometimes clients complain that behavior therapy is "impersonal," a description that may result from the technical aspects of behavior therapy other therapies do not share. While to the client feeling suicidal is an extremely personal and private experience, to the therapist, it is a common and familiar one that ultimately yields to techniques of treatment: skills training, cognitive modification, contingency management, and exposure. To the person with appendicitis, her pain and the details of how she got sick are desperately important. To the surgeon, no matter who has an inflamed appendix and what her personal experience is, there is only one proper response.

> While to the client feeling suicidal is an extremely personal and private experience, to the therapist, it is a common and familiar one that ultimately yields to techniques of treatment.

This tension between where the client is and her reasons for being there and where the therapist's expertise says she could be is central to the therapy. Dr. Linehan found it useful to modify standard Cognitive Behavioral Therapy (CBT) by adding validation and accep-tance strategies to balance the push for change. The DBT therapist is trained to provide an atmosphere of liking and acceptance, to search for what makes sense in the client's current behaviors. At the same time, DBT treatment values the changes necessary to create a life worth living. The therapist is very much in control of the session when target behaviors are the focus. She may set the agenda, interrupt, directly block escape from an important topic, and generally hold her client's feet to the fire. No matter what the problem—thoughts of suicide, throwing up lunch, failing to pay bills, or using heroin—the methods are the same: monitoring on a diary card, behavioral analysis, choosing a solution, applying that solution. Rinse and repeat. The specifics of approaches to particular problems—heroin addiction, say, over bulimia—will be derived from the extensive CBT literature on therapies supported by observation and experience.

DBT IS STRUCTURED

Sally, a twenty-seven-year-old woman with borderline personality disorder, arrives for her session twenty minutes late. Her diary card for the last week records suicidal ideation ranging from 0 to 8 on a scale of 0 to 10. She cut herself once and didn't call for coaching until after the incident. She drank three to five beers every day and smoked pot as well. She has been restricting her eating again, usually eating one meal a day, and often purging that. She shoplifted beauty supplies for her hairdressing job but called in sick most days, feeling weak and dizzy from using laxatives to lose weight. She had a fight with her mother over the money Sally owes her parents, and she's worried about making her rent this month.

Even if we assume that all of Sally's behaviors either functioned to regulate emotion or were the consequence of failed emotional regulation, where on earth do we start? DBT responds to multiple problems by establishing an order of importance. The most important class of behaviors is those that are directly life-threatening to oneself or others. Sally's therapist will target the suicidal ideation and cutting; in fact, if the therapist ignores self-injury, the treatment isn't DBT.

The second-most important class is therapy-interfering behavior—things Sally does that interfere with the progress of therapy. Arriving twenty minutes late is a big problem, especially if it happens frequently, and so is failure to call for skills coaching before she cut herself. The session is likely to focus a lot of time on these problems.

The third category, quality-of-life-interfering behaviors, includes Sally's eating disorder, her substance abuse, her chronic debt, her dysfunctional work patterns, and her shoplifting. None of these will kill her right away, but having a life worth living in the face of such chaos and disorganization is pretty hard. Sally and her therapist have come to an agreement about the order of importance of these behaviors, with substance abuse heading the list.

The structure ensures that progress will be made.

This structure serves a number of purposes. First, it keeps the therapy going. Targeting suicide thoughts or attempts ensures that the client will be alive from week to week, a necessary prerequisite for effective therapy. Indeed, the commitment to DBT is a commitment to record suicidal ideation, urges for self-harm, and incidents of self-harm on one's diary card; to agree to functional analysis of all critical incidents; and to make every effort to solve problems using new learned behaviors.

Second, the structure ensures that progress will be made. With multiple problems, it is easy to become distracted and unfocused, putting out fires from week to week without resolving anything overall. Armed with the target hierarchy, the therapist moves into the burning building of Sally's life. First they focus on getting Sally to safety, then they put out the fire, and then they build a flame-retardant life for the future.

Sometimes clients resent this rather rigid structure because they don't want to talk about their self-injury—that was last weekend, and it's painful and embarrassing! Sally wants to talk about the fight she had with her mother this morning. Sally's therapist might point out that Sally will gain control of the agenda when she lets go of suicide as a solution to her problems, creating an incentive toward giving up well-learned but problematic problem-solving techniques. As one client said, "I realized I had to stop cutting myself or we would never get to talk about anything else!"

DBT BALANCES CHANGE WITH ACCEPTANCE

Paul has a history of severe depression. When he notices that he has been a bit gloomy for several days, he tries to ignore it. When that doesn't work, he panics. "Oh, God! It's happening again. I can't go through that again! I'll kill myself first."

Janice has severe bulimia and has not stopped bingeing and purging despite years of therapy. "I know I do this to get rid of how I feel. I'll die if I have those feelings!"

Liz has been treating Amy for some time. Amy has on several occasions stated her intention to stop using crack, a dangerous drug associated with very risky procurement behavior and chaotic life conditions. Amy continues to use crack, and the best explanation she can muster is "I don't know what happened. I just found myself using." Liz tells her team that Amy is lying and just doesn't want to recognize that she is making a choice to use. "She just isn't committed to treatment."

Paul, Janice, and Liz are suffering. They each face a situation fraught with pain and uncertainty, one that stretches the limits of what they know how to handle. Paul might be heading into the valley of depression. Janice feels trapped between behavior that is repellant to her and gradually destroying her life and facing emotion that she is convinced will overwhelm and destroy her. Liz is coming up against the edge of her clinical competence and finds herself attached to someone whose out-of-control behavior may lead to her death.

You may have been told that suffering makes you stronger. These three people may dispute that assertion. In fact, at least two of them are convinced their suffering may destroy them. And it might. If they continue to devote themselves to avoiding pain, Paul or Janice or Amy might die. And Liz may decide she doesn't want to treat addicts anymore, thinking that so many of them are hopeless.

> ✦
>
> Acceptance, that gentle inquiry into what is happening in this moment, is the way beyond suffering.

There is another way: the path of acceptance. Instead of feeling dread at the onset of a depressive period, Paul could think, "Here it is again, my old friend depression. I can't say I'm glad to see him. How is it that he is here again, despite my best efforts?" Or Janice, "I am a very sensitive person with lots of painful feelings. I can find room in my heart for all that I feel." Liz could take Amy at her word—Amy doesn't know why she uses, despite her clear and conscious intention not to—if Liz accepted that to care about someone who is out of control is to risk losing them. How would things be different for them if they chose the path of acceptance? What would happen immediately is a softening, an opening to the situation as it is, not as it might have been if conditions were otherwise. Acceptance, that gentle inquiry into what is happening in this moment, is the way beyond suffering.

Amy is a thirty-year-old nursing student and single mother with almost four years of sobriety from drugs and alcohol. She has a history of more than fifty psychiatric hospitalizations for suicide crises but has not been an inpatient in more than four years. She hasn't hurt herself since she got sober. Cleaning up her room, she comes across the stacks of notebooks in which she has been keeping a journal for years. She flips through some of them dating from the time when her life was consumed with misery. The entries document her hopelessness and despair, her generally failed efforts to resist urges to cut herself, to use drugs, to binge and purge, to shoplift. They describe numerous hospitalizations, therapies, medications, etc. She almost cannot recognize the person writing in those journals, the painful emptiness of that life. These days, she feels connected to her life, filled with friends from AA, work, school, and caring for her child. Life is still hard, but she has a growing confidence that she can meet its challenges or get help when problems overwhelm her. Her son toddles in and snuggles into her lap. Soon she will graduate, get a full-time job, and leave disability behind. She is grateful for the help she has received and proud of her achievements. "I feel like I belong."

> ✦
>
> If therapy is going well, it radiates from the treatment relationship between two people who accept each other as they are at the same time that they work like hell for change.

The practice of acceptance permeates Dialectical Behavior Therapy and serves to balance the relentless focus on change that behavioral techniques bring to the therapy. Acceptance is included in the treatment because of Dr. Linehan's extensive personal experience with the effects of Zen meditation, but DBT also represents an emerging trend in the world of behavior therapy. Acceptance is expressed on the most immediate level of searching for the wisdom in the client's current behavior, seeking out what is valid and functional. You can see its influence in the concept of distress tolerance, where you learn that it is possible to bear pain without resorting to strategies of change and control that work only temporarily at best. If therapy is going well, it radiates from the treatment relationship between two people who accept each other as they are at the same time that they work like hell for change. The dance between these fundamental truths, the wisdom in what is and the need for change, is dialectics. As a wise old analyst once said, "Meet the patient where they are and take them where they don't want to go."

—Elizabeth B. Simpson, M.D.

RELATED ENTRIES

Cognitive Behavioral Therapy

Anxiety Disorders

Depressive Disorders

Women and Trauma

Women and Addictions

Eye Movement Desensitization
and Reprocessing (EMDR)

Although I have always been committed to learning new theories and techniques in order to tailor my work to each individual, when I first started hearing reports about Eye Movement Desensitization and Reprocessing (EMDR) in the early 1990s, I was highly skeptical. How could a therapy in which the therapist waves her hands back and forth in front of her clients' eyes and *voila!* the patient gets better be taken seriously?

My first real knowledge of EMDR came by experiencing it while I was at a five-day women's retreat. We were scheduled to do an exercise that involved sustained deep breathing. I was afraid to do the exercise, as in the past I had found deep breathing to trigger an old traumatic memory: When I had my tonsils out as a three-year-old child, I was separated from my parents and put in a crib with bars on the top so I couldn't climb out.

While talking to the facilitator about my fears and the memories connected to them, I found myself having intense panic sensations that made me feel like I was choking. The facilitator must have seen my intense fear, as she asked me to look up and follow her fingers with my eyes. Although the presence of her fingers felt intrusive, I did as I was told. I felt my heart slow down, my breathing return to normal, and the fear diminish. Afterward, I felt calm, as if an enormous weight had been lifted from my chest.

Generally speaking, EMDR techniques ought to be used only with full preparation and explicit consent. In this case, however, the facilitator knew me well and could see that I was in trouble. While I hesitate to even write about such an unorthodox use of one component of EMDR therapy, the point of mentioning it is that it took this extreme for me to be convinced of EMDR's merits.

The next day, I talked about EMDR at length with the facilitator, who was also a psychologist. What she said was interesting, but it was my own experience, the feeling I had of having let go of fear, that really intrigued me. And my feeling was borne out in the longer term: After the EMDR experience, I was able to do the breathing exercise with no fear, no old memories, and a profound sense of peace. And now I use EMDR as a powerful tool in helping my clients to heal and grow.

So, what is Eye Movement Desensitization and Reprocessing? It is an integrated approach to psychotherapy discovered and named by Dr. Francine Shapiro. EMDR came out of Dr. Shapiro's work with Vietnam veterans suffering from Post-Traumatic Stress Disorder (PTSD). Since the September 11th terrorist attacks, much has been written about PTSD, but when Dr. Shapiro began experimenting, PSTD was understood to be primarily a phe-

THE BASIC EMDR THERAPEUTIC PROTOCOL

- ☞ Therapist and patient discuss patient's personal history
- ☞ Therapist and patient agree on problem areas to be addressed
- ☞ Patient learns visualization and relaxation techniques
- ☞ Patient recalls all aspects of difficult memory(ies) while receiving bilateral stimulation
- ☞ Processing of memories with bilateral stimulation is repeated as necessary
- ☞ Therapist and patient anticipate future difficulties and apply new skills to problem solving

nomenon of war veterans and survivors of rape and violence. The hallmark of PTSD is the experience of reexperiencing the trauma, often through flashbacks and often with gaps in understanding of the event and distorted beliefs. Dr. Shapiro found that asking people to recall their memories while tracking her moving finger with their eyes allowed the patients to rapidly process new information. As they proceeded through the treatment, they came to understand that they were safe in the present and that the trauma was in the past. In essence, EMDR allows the trauma victim to integrate the experience into the ebb and flow of his or her life, the way we do with our memories of more everyday experiences, without overwhelming feelings. But how does tracking eye movement accomplish this?

Traumatic memory is thought to be stored in nonverbal areas of the brain, including the limbic system, which is responsible for emotional arousal. Research by Bessel van der Kolk and others found that successful treatment with EMDR shows through positron emission tomography (PET) scans that there is increased activation in the frontal lobes after EMDR treatment. Because the brain functions in a hierarchy, this increased activity in the cortex of the brain implies that EMDR allows the patient to have increased access to integrative functions and to words. Without language, we lose our inherent ability to name our truths and to tell a story that allows us to "make sense" of what has happened to us.

EMDR has continued to evolve since Dr. Shapiro first began training other clinicians in the early 1990s, but her basic protocol remains the basis of all good EMDR treatment. It has since been discovered that eye movements themselves are not necessary but that any prompt that involves bilateral stimulation, such as alternating pulses, knee taps, or beeps through earphones, is effective. What appears to be essential is both a split in the person's attention between the painful memory and the here-and-now stimulation of both hemispheres of the brain. EMDR appears to help patients reorganize fragmented memories, faulty perceptions, and distorted thoughts. In addition, people who have had successful EMDR experiences have decreased emotional activation, more coherent narratives, and more positive beliefs. Sophisticated research into how EMDR changes the activation of neural networks and how it heals is ongoing.

> EMDR allows the trauma victim to integrate the experience into the ebb and flow of her life, the way we do with our memories of more everyday experiences, without overwhelming feelings.

What happens during EMDR therapy? EMDR descriptions often focus on the bilateral stimulation component. But as developed by Dr. Shapiro, EMDR is a structured therapeutic protocol including distinct phases of which bilateral stimulation is one. The EMDR-trained therapist is still a therapist first. There are many types of therapy, of course, and each therapist will approach and apply the basic steps of EMDR therapy in the context of her own theoretical approach and personal style.

All EMDR therapy begins with the taking of a personal history, which includes gathering information on symptoms, major developmental milestones, and any traumas, large or small. While EMDR is used very successfully with major traumas and losses, it also works well with more minor traumas, such as being made fun of by peers or a history of criticism by family members. EMDR is also now used successfully with problems other than trauma, such as phobias and other anxiety disorders, as well as nonclinical problems, such as fear of public speaking and performance inhibitions. And many clinicians have creatively expanded parts of EMDR to help patients with affect modulation addictions, eating disorders, and learning disabilities. Generally, then, EMDR seems to be quite effective in addressing many areas in one's life where one feels stuck.

> What appears to be essential is both a split in the person's attention between the painful memory and the here-and-now stimulation of both hemispheres of the brain. EMDR appears to help patients reorganize fragmented memories, faulty perceptions, and distorted thoughts.

After the history-taking segment is complete, the therapist and patient agree on problem areas to be addressed. Then the patient is taught visualization techniques that foster a sense of safety and relaxation. One of the best aspects of EMDR is that it is patient-centered: Learning to self-regulate gives the patient the skills needed to return to a calm state if the processing is too intense or if he or she needs to regulate feelings outside the session.

At this point, the patient recalls a difficult memory or series of memories while receiving a form of bilateral stimulation. When negative events happen in our lives, we store the memories of those events as images, thoughts, feelings, and sensations. In order to make the processing of any memory as complete as possible, patients are asked to think of three things: Their most vivid image of the event, the negative belief they have about themselves because of the event, and what they would rather believe. Patients are also asked to describe and rate the intensity of their feelings. Here's an example:

> EMDR is also now used successfully with problems other than trauma, such as phobias and other anxiety disorders, as well as nonclinical problems, such as fear of public speaking.

Tania came to see me at the beginning of her junior year in college. Over the summer she had been in a minor car accident. While not physically hurt, she continued to have nightmares of looking up, seeing the other car running the red light and slamming into her car. She no longer wanted to drive but hated relying on her friends, many of whom thought she was overreacting. Tania's history involved no major trauma and she came from a loving intact family. Her most vivid image of the accident was seeing the car coming toward her and not being able to stop. Her negative thoughts were: "I have no control. I am going to die." Trauma often alters our general beliefs about ourselves; identifying those beliefs as well as more potentially positive beliefs is central to EMDR. Tania's preferred belief was "I can be in control. I survived."

When asked how true that preferred belief felt, Tania laughed, "I know I am alive but I still feel scared." Tania rated the intensity of her discomfort as an eight on a scale of ten and said that she felt it in her heart and in her forearms. I asked her to bring up the picture of the car coming toward her, the belief she had no control and was going to die, and to focus on the sensations in her body. Tania had on earphones and had pulsars that delivered alternating tones and pulses. After a brief interval, I would ask Tania to let me know what she was experiencing. One of the nice aspects of EMDR is that it allows but does not require the patient to divulge details of the traumatic memory to the therapist. Reporting shifts in thoughts, feelings, or sensations is enough to assure that the processing is moving and that the patient is not stuck.

> When negative events happen in our lives, we store the memories of those events as images, thoughts, feelings, and sensations.

Tania quickly moved through the memory with very few sets of stimulation, each lasting less than a minute. For the first few sets she felt as if she were in the car, reexperiencing the impact. She reported that the image began to retreat and after the fifth set, she reported that she felt as if she were watching from above, as if looking at Matchbox cars. After several more sets, she stated with wonder, "I don't know why I thought this was such a big deal. It doesn't bother me anymore. I know I am fine." She reported being able to think about the accident without any panic or discomfort.

Tania's processing was quick and completed in several sessions. While many patients are astonished by how quickly they can let things go, some find the memory linking to older memories. With a good history, the patient and the therapist often choose to work on the earliest linking memory first.

People with multiple traumas and complicated histories often need a great deal of stabilization before trauma processing. Bilateral stimulation can be used to help them learn to use their internal resources and to manage intense feelings. Although EMDR can work at amazing speed with many people, it can involve a much longer and slower process for many others with more complicated histories or issues, as the following case suggests.

Martha is a thirty-five-year-old woman who came to see me, complaining of depression and anxiety that were compromising her ability to function at work. Martha was very successful in her career and was in a good marriage, but she felt as though no one really knew her and how hard it was for her to function. Martha had a history of profound losses, including the death of both her parents while she was in her mid-twenties. Martha and I spent several months focusing on history taking, as well as problem solving her immediate concerns about potentially losing her job. I referred her for antidepressant medication, and we helped worked on steps in her daily life to tackle her depression, including adding exercise, reaching out to

> Trauma often alters our general beliefs about ourselves; identifying those beliefs as well as more potentially positive beliefs is central to EMDR.

friends, and reducing stress. Martha made a lot of progress during the course of which we were able to see how much of her depression and anxiety was related to experiences that she had had growing up, including her sadness at her parents' deaths and her fear of losing people she loved.

It was several months into the therapy before we started using EMDR, again first focusing on current reactions that were causing her to overreact at work. When Martha felt she was functioning better and was less depressed, we agreed to target memories of her parents' deaths. Martha's mother died of complications of open-heart surgery—surgery that she was told was her only chance for survival, that she was afraid to undergo, and that Martha encouraged her mother to have, leaving Martha with profound guilt. Martha always cried when she talked about her mother; a day did not pass when she didn't miss her or feel responsible for her death.

After several painful sessions using EMDR, Martha came to a sense of peace around her mother's death, realizing that she had done all that she could to support her mother choosing a healthier lifestyle for better heart health and perhaps a better outcome from surgery. She accepted that she wasn't responsible for her mother's behavior and although she continued to miss her, she realized that continuing to feel sad couldn't help her mother or change her loss.

Martha's processing of her father's death was longer and more complicated. He was a highly critical and emotionally abusive man. Martha had internalized his critical voice and made it her own. Her work in therapy, with and without EMDR, helped her separate his issues from her own and to develop a kinder and more compassionate view of herself and others. Needless to say, these shifts have also greatly helped Martha function as a more supportive and well-liked manager at work. In this case, EMDR was used at various points in an ongoing therapy.

EMDR is not without controversy. Critics question whether the bilateral stimulation adds any benefit at all, claiming that EMDR is ultimately just a rehash of older therapies. Despite this skepticism, EMDR has been found by the American Psychological Association to be effective in the treatment of PTSD. There has been a great deal of research on EMDR, and it is currently being studied as treatment for a wide range of difficulties. The importance of formal training cannot be overemphasized, as the improper use of EMDR therapy can potentially lead to patients being retraumatized.

My training in EMDR and use of it in my work has given me great pleasure and constant wonder at the resiliency of the human spirit and our capacity to grow and change. While researchers are still trying to discover exactly how, it seems to me that EMDR's effect is to allow us to get out of our own way and to access our own capacity to heal ourselves. As an EMDR-trained clinician, it is a joy to be along for the ride.

—Patricia A. Geller, Ed.D.

Insight-Oriented Psychotherapy

Metaphors that describe insight-oriented therapy never quite capture the whole experience. One patient I know likens the first few sessions of psychotherapy to an intensely intimate conversation with a person she just met on a train. Another says it is like autobiographical writing in which you write whatever comes to you, without editing, going for all the sensuous details of your experience, pressing on to get past what you fear most. Some think of it as a little like falling in—and then out of—a new love in which we face and then must master our wish to be admired, to adore, to come to terms with all of who we are and see others more realistically too. The British analyst Nina Coltart describes therapy as a "slow jettisoning of a lifetime's bathwater": we come to know ourselves, slowly, amazed at how much water must drain away for us to discover both our false selves and our truer and happier selves. As a psychotherapist, I sometimes compare it to learning to ride a bicycle: when it comes right down to it, specific instructions have little to do with the gestalt of cycling.

Maybe the difficulty in describing insight-oriented therapy is that it is one part science, one part art, and a dose of magic too. It is also paradoxical. We think of talk as the means of expression and communication in insight-oriented therapy. But often silence, pregnant pauses, and the therapist's abstinence (so as not to tell the patient what to do or feel) lead to the creation of authentic expression. And it may happen that a patient starts therapy because she needs support, and receives it through the therapist's attention and concern, although the best therapy is shaped by the therapist's ability to challenge the patient.

What is certain is that insight-oriented therapy takes two people working together in a relationship over a period of time. This therapy is distinguished by its emphasis on the use of the therapeutic relationship to come to know oneself by understanding one's internal world and its impact on interpersonal relationships.

WHAT IS INSIGHT-ORIENTED PSYCHOTHERAPY, AND WHAT ARE ITS ORIGINS?

Insight-oriented therapy originated with Freud when he developed the practice of psychoanalysis as a form of treatment that through talk would transform "misery into common unhappiness" and allow the patient to understand the workings of her mind. Although Freud's ideas still shape the practice of insight-oriented therapy, there is a great deal of discussion and controversy among clinicians about what we are all about, what the practice of insight-oriented psychotherapy should be, and to what extent knowledge leads to insight and insight leads to change.

The emphasis on the relationship between therapist and patient, particularly on the patient's hopes, disappointments, and difficulties in the relationship, and the working through of these feelings in order to feel better, is the hallmark of psychoanalytically oriented insight therapy and is one of Freud's major contributions. The use of free association (a process in which a patient talks about whatever comes to mind without attention to any imagined censor) and the patient's resistance to doing just this (talking freely) are traditional mechanisms by which therapist and patient gain access to the unconscious workings of the patient's mind and come to know more about her psychic reality. This reality includes internal conflicts, psychic structures, and interpersonal dynamics that are influenced by the powerful, albeit invisible, force of the unconscious.

Partly because he was self-conscious about looking at and being stared at by patients, Freud pioneered the use of the couch, using it to treat highly symptomatic patients privately. Today psychoanalysis is still distinguished by the use of the couch, but it is just one form of insight-oriented treatment based on psychoanalytic ideas. In psychoanalytic psychotherapy, a patient is seen several times per week, but other forms of psychodynamic therapies involve fewer sessions a week and sometimes focus less intensely on the relationship between therapist and patient. Both psychoanalytic and other types of insight-oriented therapy are practiced with adults, children, families, couples, and groups. These therapies borrow from psychoanalytic thinking a focus on what we feel, how we think, and why we act the way we do. They pay particular attention to our personal history: if and how we reach milestones (going to school, for example, or choosing a partner); major changes and traumas in our lives; our family, work, and social relationships; and the things that bother and stress us. They look for patterns in relationships and feelings and uncover core internal conflicts.

> The emphasis on the relationship between therapist and patient, particularly on the patient's hopes, disappointments, and difficulties in the relationship, and the working through of these feelings in order to feel better, is the hallmark of psychoanalytically oriented insight therapy.

Insight-oriented therapies in which the therapist and patient meet frequently provide an opportunity to closely examine the therapy relationship and what the patient recreates in it. How the patient perceives the therapist and feels perceived by her becomes a window onto understanding how the patient feels about herself and experiences others. Reenactments within the therapy relationship (in which the patient creates or sometimes co-creates with her therapist the same psychological dynamics she experiences outside therapy) are often cultured in a close therapy relationship and allow both patient and therapist to analyze a pattern of relating that they directly experience rather than solely relying on the patient's reports of emotional turmoil or troubling interpersonal difficulties in her life. For instance, if the patient is habitually late for therapy appointments, this behavior can be examined in the here and now—why here and why now—rather than chalked up to, say, particularly bad traffic.

The clinicians who followed Freud saw their role in the relationship and the treatment somewhat differently because they experienced their patients as needing something more from them. They recognized that their patients had a drive to make connections and have satisfying relationships, although many of their patients had problems based on early experiences with their parents that made it difficult for them to do this well. The British School of Object Relations (D. W. Winnicott, W.R.D. Fairbain, et al.) focused on the notion that we internally take in our experience of our parents as "objects." Problems arise when we take in "bad objects"/destructive parents or are unable to take in a sense of our parents/others as "good objects." From this perspective, the therapeutic relationship should provide a holding environment for the patient, with the therapist assuming a nurturing (and, in some cases, almost parental) role, so that the patient can internalize a good object, develop a sense of being lovable, and become capable of loving.

> How the patient perceives the therapist and feels perceived by her becomes a window onto understanding how the patient feels about herself and experiences others.

Self psychologists thought that unempathic parents and/or other early figures in one's life cause (structural) deficits in the self that make it difficult to know or manage one's feelings. The purpose of therapy is thus to develop the patient's capacity to feel authentically. This is accomplished through the therapist's empathy toward the patient's experience of her world, including her experience of the therapist's inevitably incomplete understanding of the patient. The patient's working through of this perceived failure in the therapist helps develop a sense of a thriving, stable self as the patient becomes increasingly cognizant of what she has been missing, what may be provided by another person, and what is to become a part of her self in the future.

In more recent years, feminist thinking, among other influences, has raised important questions about the nature of psychological growth in insight-oriented psychotherapy and the therapist's role in the treatment. Such questions have contributed to the development of a true two-person psychology, with greater mutuality and reciprocity between patient and therapist. This approach puts aside, but not necessarily away, a focus on the therapist's interpretations or provisions (e.g., being a good "object" for the patient) and has opened the door to an understanding of how the relationship between therapist and patient can help both understand the patient's emotional life and its resonance within that relationship. Psychiatrist George Fishman has described this as a nearly invisible process in which both patient and therapist are operating within a mutual, affective attachment.

HOW DOES INSIGHT-ORIENTED THERAPY CREATE CHANGE?

To provide a better understanding of how insight-oriented therapy works, let me describe some of its important components.

Interpretations Interpretations may be thought of as particular narratives that seek to explain why you think, feel, or act the way you do. Interpretations often look to the past to explain what is going on today. Freud saw himself as a scientific observer who by offering an interpretation could bring the patient's repressed material to consciousness. This new

> Interpretations may be thought of as particular narratives that seek to explain why you think, feel, or act the way you do.

awareness could in turn be a catalyst for change. For example, a patient might come to understand more about her unfelt anger toward her brother by appreciating that although she is especially nice to him, she always gets a nasty rash before visiting him. This insight may help to explain some of the difficulties she has in expressing her ambivalence about her brother and ultimately may change how she relates to him.

Traditionally, interpretations have always been the province of the therapist alone. Nowadays, however, some clinicians question the wisdom of this practice, pointing out that interpretations made solely by the therapist may be clumsy, overly intellectual, authoritarian, or even unempathetic. One clinician I spoke with believes that while interpretations can be formulated by either the therapist or the patient, a good interpretation is always the result of a collaboration between the two, embellished and revised throughout the course of therapy. Here is how one analyst described it:

Rachel's mother was hospitalized when Rachel was very young and after that she became her guardian, always watching her mother's shifting moods, afraid that she would leave again. It's difficult for her to separate her feelings from those she is close to, and she experiences this anxiety as though it's about basic survival. She feels she must constantly contain things, but she obviously can't always do it or can't do it in a way that takes care of her too. She had made these connections in therapy, but elaborating the primary experiences, seeing how much they have affected her life, and experiencing this with me, someone she is close to but doesn't need to take care of like her mother, is what's meaningful.

Whereas some clinicians have raised the question of who should do the interpreting, others have gone so far as to ask whether interpretations truly lead to insight or promote change. Some have wondered if even interpretations need to be interpreted!

Defenses and Projections Defenses, understood in a psychological context, are mechanisms that help us cope and manage how we feel. They are absolutely basic to who we are, and no one can do without them. But much insight-oriented therapy focuses on knowing when and why we use them, and changes experienced in therapy are frequently shaped by the discarding of old defenses and the deployment of new ones. Defenses can work adaptively so that we are able to use what we feel on behalf of growth and change, or they can function maladaptively, so that we are working against ourselves, sometimes even self-destructively. We can defend against an uncomfortable feeling by not experiencing it fully, and therefore act without being aware of the feeling, or we can defend against feeling uncomfortably vulnerable by intellectualizing an experience and making it devoid of feeling. Perhaps most often we defend ourselves against the full experience of a feeling by projecting that feeling onto others.

> Perhaps most often we defend ourselves against the full experience of a feeling by projecting that feeling onto others.

In his memoir, *A Secret Life*, Michael Ryan describes coming to terms with his history of sexual abuse by a neighbor. He has difficulty holding down academic positions and is ultimately fired from Princeton because he has sexually abused a female student. At one point, he goes home to confront his mother. He describes understanding his use of psychological defenses and projections:

The way I always expressed my anger towards my mother was through coldness, a steel-plate hardness a hundred inches thick, and a subtle diminishment of her to make her feel stupid (although she isn't.... I took [her] hand in mine [and said], "Mom, no matter what you knew or didn't know I don't blame you for it. I know you wouldn't have hurt me on purpose." ... I didn't want to be angry with her anymore.... I didn't have to blame her anymore for who I am.... For almost thirty years, I blamed [her] for everything I suffered as a child ... because it justified my monstrous behavior. I could do anything as long as it was her fault.... I [needed] to ask her forgiveness for punishing her for almost thirty years.

The Repetition Compulsion The idea that unresolved loss compels us to repeat the very thing we wish to avoid is a significant feature of human nature that insight-oriented therapies seek to treat. This process was first named by Freud, but here I mostly work with the ideas of Paul Russell, a Boston analyst well known for trying to unravel the enigma of this process. The basic idea is this: if we do not come to terms with loss, we repeat aspects of it (feelings, thoughts, behaviors, etc.) until we are able to fully feel and grieve the original loss. When our sense of loss is not fully known to us it nevertheless operates just outside our awareness through these repetitions. In this way, the repetitions (often uncomfortably and confusingly) allow us to hold onto the unknown past until we can understand its meaning. If the repetitions continue unabated, the capacity to feel and to form loving attachments is arrested. When things are working well in therapy, the safety and containment of the therapeutic relationship diminishes the repetitions (because they have functioned in place of the lost relationship).

> ✦
>
> Insight-oriented therapists think that a person's symptoms are important signals that often dramatically (and painfully) herald a need to understand something that at the outset may seem confusing or unbearable.

Michael Ryan ultimately faced his compulsion to repeat sexual abuse while working with a student in his writing class. This student had also been sexually abused and was expressing sexual interest in him. But he didn't approach her sexually—his usual practice—when he saw that, as with him, her trauma "made her believe down to the microbes in her blood cells that her human value equaled her sexual value." Her sexual interest in him, he realized, came out of a "desperation to be healed." And he also recognized that he could show her how much he valued her, as student, writer, and courageous person, by not having sex with her.

WHO IS INSIGHT-ORIENTED THERAPY FOR, AND WHAT PROBLEMS DOES IT ADDRESS?

Psychoanalytic ideas are enough a part of our culture that most people have at least a passing familiarity with Freud's concept of "penis envy" or have read about his treatment of women who displayed "hysterical" symptoms when there was a suspicion of trauma. Most clinicians today have their own sense of how to interpret these ideas and understand what happened. For instance, we no longer believe that "penis envy" means literally "longing for a penis"; feminists appropriated the term to mean a female's envy and justifiable outrage at being denied the goods of our culture that are reserved for men. Even more significantly, the conversation has recently tipped in the direction of appreciating the often unspoken envy that our culture has of women and the effects of this envy.

In fact, feminism has been instrumental in revising Freud's ideas. While Freud was a brilliant, original thinker, his views were understandably limited by the mores of his time. Freud at one point in his career decided that the incestuous tales of his female patients were fantasies while in fact they were often memories of real events that were not deemed possible to recount in proper Victorian society. Current-day feminist historians have reinstated these "fantasies" and the seemingly disembodied memories of many sexual abuse survivors as the results of just that: sexual abuse. Insight-oriented therapy recognizes and honors the prevalence of sexual abuse as a literal phenomenon; at the same time, it continues to pay homage to the centrality of fantasy in the construction of the human mind. Insight-oriented therapists know that sexual abuse occurs, but they are not overly quick to lead their patients to believe that all fantasies are facts. Some fantasies are simply fantasies. But fantasies at times may be as powerful as, if not more powerful than, the literal language in which we live our lives. The goal of good insight-oriented therapy today is to hold both beliefs as possible—tales of sexual abuse may be fact or may be a symbolic representation of a psychological truth.

Some people think that insight-oriented therapy is for anyone and others think of it as being for particular problems or for particular people. The experience of feeling stuck, not being able to establish and maintain satisfying relationships, feeling as if old patterns keep surfacing and getting in the way, and self-esteem issues seem to typify why insight-oriented therapy is sought today. One person I spoke with, Sonia, thought insight-oriented therapy was for people who "suffer from the quality of their life because they don't pursue important things and then face not doing the things they want to do." She explained:

I started insight-oriented therapy not knowing that I needed insight about anything . . . our defenses are very good at not letting us know! Now I know I experience distress. I had struggled with my weight, tried to diet seriously twice, and had gained the weight back. I felt over-stimulated when I began relationships and anxious that I didn't have much to say or talk about. I was aware that I chose people who didn't make it easy for me, but I didn't know what these symptoms were sitting on.

Felice spoke about it in this way:

I went into therapy because I wanted to be in a relationship. Before therapy, when thinking about how my family felt about me, I would tell myself to get over it—that basically I was loved. But it wasn't working because I felt angry inside. It actually got played out in stupid ways –I'd have mood swings and would bang a drawer, for instance. I thought I could make it on my own but I knew I was running away and felt lonely.

THE VALUE OF INSIGHT-ORIENTED PSYCHOTHERAPY

Cultural expectations about the pace of change as well as expectations about the results of therapy contribute to controversy about the value of insight-oriented psychotherapy today. It is now practically a cultural norm that one takes a pill for depression or anxiety and that one can and should get rid of these "abnormal" emotional states as quickly as possible. In fact, most insight-oriented therapists support the use of medication and know from experience that it can be beneficial or even necessary, but they don't consider medication a substitute for therapy. Insight-oriented therapists think that a person's symptoms are important signals that often dramatically (and painfully) herald a need to understand something that at the outset may seem confusing or unbearable.

Changes in training, limits on reimbursement for fees, and an emphasis on shorter-term treatment are some of the challenges that insight-oriented therapists face today. While some fear that insight-oriented therapy is a dying art, it is still available through publicly funded clinics, managed care plans/organizations, and private practitioners. Many people with a wide range of problems still choose insight-oriented therapy today even though shorter or quicker treatments are ubiquitous. Insight-oriented therapists continue to wrestle with ideas about the place of knowledge, empathy, and affective communication as elements in the intricacies of the therapeutic relationship, and how indeed it takes another mind to know oneself.

—*Dale Young, Psy.D., M.P.H.*

Group Psychotherapy with Women

Groups have been used therapeutically since the beginning of time; in churches and synagogues, in Bedouin campgrounds and on the Pleistocene plains, when our ancestors huddled together in caves for warmth and protection, for a feeling of safety. However, the first formally recorded instance of the use of a group expressly for clinical purposes was in 1905, when Joseph Pratt assembled his tubercular patients together to help them cope with the illness by trading tips and keeping company. The first psychotherapeutic use of groups began with Edward Lazell in 1921. Lazell developed an educational group approach, which included the discussion of the ideas of Sigmund Freud and Carl Jung, to help patients coping with psychotic illness, as well as to help patients in clinical settings.

Group psychotherapy has evolved considerably since then, with the addition of psychoeducational groups, self-help groups, encounter groups, and Transcendental Meditation groups, to name a few. These groups are offered in different settings, including hospitals, outpatient clinics, private offices, family service agencies, and correctional institutions. The majority of women, however, will probably experience group psychotherapy within an outpatient mental health setting.

Empirical studies have provided ample evidence for the effectiveness of group psychotherapy in various settings. M. L. Smith and Thomas I. Miller, in a classic study published in 1980, found that group psychotherapy was generally as effective as individual psychotherapy in addressing psychological distress. The psychiatrist Irvin D. Yalom has proposed some interesting theories as to why this is so. He cites universality as being one of the healing variables in group psychotherapy. People often feel their problems make them outcasts, and the sheer act of knowing others share your plight, suggests Yalom, can be healing. For women who are isolated at home with children or struggling under the myths that plague women in general, such intimate sharing of plain truths can be politically and personally powerful.

Women's involvement in group psychotherapy is often preceded by a pregroup individual interview, during which the therapist assesses the appropriateness of the match between the client and the group and describes group structure and guidelines to the client. The various psychological problems addressed in group psychotherapy are similar to those addressed in individual psychotherapy, including depression, anxiety, trauma (i.e., childhood physical and/or sexual abuse, rape, domestic violence, political trauma), chronic mental illness, substance abuse, medical illness, relational issues, sexuality, sexual orientation issues, and issues related to race and ethnicity.

The treatment goals of group and individual psychotherapy often overlap. Yalom, in his classic 1985 book, *The Theory and Practice of Group Psychotherapy,* describes some factors that are unique to group experience, including, as previously mentioned, universality or similarity of experiences among group members. He also discusses the development of social skills and interpersonal learning. Feminists have noted that group psychotherapy is a useful modality of treatment that addresses interpersonal processes valued by women, such as the presence of other women, shared client–therapist experience, and emphasis on relatedness to others.

Because women are often the victims of discrimination, inequality, harassment, and violence, groups provide a safe space for women's exploration of these and other issues. Women's capacity for empathic connection and their ability to build rapport in general can be a source of enormous support for other group members.

PSYCHOTHERAPY GROUPS FOR WOMEN

Psychotherapy groups for women are diverse with respect to areas of focus, treatment approach, and group composition. Some prominent types of group psychotherapy for women include psychodynamic groups addressing relationship difficulties, trauma-informed groups focused on management of personal sense of safety and self-care, groups focused on cross-cultural and immigration issues, cognitive behavioral groups addressing substance abuse, interpersonal groups focused on depression, and integrative groups focused on stress management. The therapist's theoretical approach guides the nature of the focus and process of the group.

Psychodynamic perspectives, in general, emphasize the "centrality of transference" in the group process. Sigmund Freud defined *transference* as the reproduction of images of significant people in one's life, such as parents, siblings, and partners, in the therapeutic relationship. A positive transference develops when the client regards the therapist as an ideal and trustworthy figure, similar to the way the client may have idealized a parent or a favorite relative or friend. A negative transference develops when the client sees the therapist as someone who disappoints or fails to be trustworthy, similar to significant others who have emotionally failed the client. More recently, psychoanalysts have suggested that the patient's transferential responses to the therapist are actually cocreated by both the patient and the therapist, and that the therapist's countertransferential responses to the patient are also cocreated by the therapist and the patient. Psychodynamically oriented group psychotherapy addresses group members' transference responses to the therapist and to other group

> People often feel their problems make them outcasts, and the sheer act of knowing others share your plight can be healing.

members, in order to help members gain insight into their relationships. A major goal of psychodynamic perspectives entails the group members' acquisition of insight and internalization of new realities and experiences.

Cognitive behavioral (CB) group psychotherapy aims to teach group members to manage painful emotional experiences, solve problems more effectively, and address negative thoughts or beliefs about oneself and one's life situation. Some strategies used in these groups include grounding, reattribution, and cognitive restructuring. CB groups for women address negative affect (i.e., guilt, anxiety, shame, self-blame, hopelessness, depression, dissociation, and suicidal feelings), relationship-building skills, and relapse prevention. In contrast to psychodynamic groups, cognitive behavioral groups consist of a highly structured format and regular homework assignments aimed to help group members practice and retain their learning from the group.

> Women's capacity for empathic connection and their ability to build rapport in general can be a source of enormous support for other group members.

Women's groups focused on issues related to *psychological trauma* have developed in more recent years, in light of an increased understanding of the aftermath of trauma on women's sense of safety and relationships. Judith Herman describes a stage model of trauma recovery in her 1992 book, *Trauma and Recovery*. Dr. Herman's model of recovery identified three stages that most trauma survivors move through. Trauma and abuse is often most devastating because of the social isolation and shame a woman develops. Group therapy is a powerful tool in healing, as it can help break this isolation.

Stage one groups focus on safety and self-care. These groups tend to be psychoeducational—they help women learn about the impact of trauma and abuse on their relationships and on their ability to care for themselves. Although stage one groups often do not have women discuss the details of their abuse, they can be powerful: Often the group is the first time a traumatized woman realizes that there are other women who have had similar experiences.

The second stage of recovery has been named remembering and mourning. It is a time of healing that is filled with intense feeling. For many women, it is the first time they have been able to feel what has happened to them, and they may feel great grief and rage. Experiencing these feelings within the context of healthy group relations significantly changes the pattern of isolation. Empathy toward and from other group members as stories are shared begins to decrease the shame. Because of the intensity of affect at this stage of treatment, women should not enter a stage two group unless they have basic self-care needs met (stable home, no current abusive relationships, no self-destructive behaviors, no substance abuse, etc.).

The final stage of treatment has been named reconnection—when the survivor's life is no longer focused on the abuse. At this stage, much of the overwhelming affect has been worked through and the woman is now focused on building a new life. It is a time of establishing safe connections in work, family, and community. Stage three groups can often seem like a basic women's psychotherapy group. At this stage, a woman has integrated her abuse history into her life history, and it no longer stands out in high relief.

In the past decade, psychotherapy groups have developed for women focused on eating disorders, anxiety disorders, self-mutilation, and self-esteem, to name just a few. In each case, women come together to discuss a shared problem and related areas of concern and to provide one another with support in coping with symptoms and encouragement in learning new ways of behaving. These groups tend to focus much less on the group process and interpersonal relationships, and much more on shared support.

> Cognitive behavioral groups consist of a highly structured format and regular homework assignments aimed to help group members practice and retain their learning from the group.

INTERPERSONAL GROUP PSYCHOTHERAPY WITH WOMEN

Unlike the topic-driven groups previously mentioned, general interpersonal group psychotherapy for women is committed not to symptom management or even support, but to open-ended exploration of how the members interact with one another and how those interactions reflect the constraints and choices faced by group members in the outside world. Irvin Yalom, in describing his notion of the "social microcosm," has suggested that the group comes to reflect the interpersonal universe where one lives. As the group proceeds, gradually, each member of the group interacts with other members and the therapist as she interacts with others in her personal social environment. Gender stereotypes play a significant role in defining these interactions and the self-concepts of group members. For instance, in mainstream U.S. culture, women who express their needs for intimacy are often perceived as clinging and demanding, whereas men who withhold expressing their needs for intimacy are seen as independent. The psychotherapy group can serve as means for exploring women's views concerning intimacy and dependency, in the context of understanding general socialization processes.

ETHNIC AND RACIAL DIVERSITY IN GROUP PSYCHOTHERAPY

Ethnic minority women have experienced some conflicts relevant to the decision to join group psychotherapy. Consider the following vignettes:

Julia is a thirty-five-year-old single African American teacher who is coping with anxiety in social situations. She worries about other people's perceptions of her ability to be social and of her attractiveness. She grew up with her brother, cousin, and aunt in a neighborhood with primarily African American residents. Her parents encouraged her to focus on her career, and they focused their energy almost entirely on her and her brother. Julia overheard her parents argue almost daily about their private marital conflicts. Her parents worked in an automobile factory, where they had both experienced significant racism. She maintains a close relationship with her family, and with members of the community where she was raised. She has few friends and has been increasingly sad because of this lack of intimate relationships in her life outside of her family.

> The group comes to reflect the interpersonal universe where one lives.

Julia has worked with a therapist in individual psychotherapy, and she and her therapist have discussed the possibility of Julia joining a group. Some of her concerns about joining a mixed-race, women's group include that her experiences as an African American woman would not be acknowledged, and that she might feel more inhibited about speaking out about her anxiety if her racial background was overlooked. She also worries that other group members might find it strange that she visits her parents and relatives weekly and that her family is highly interdependent. Julia is also concerned about joining a group for African American women because she worries that she might know some of the group members in her social network, in which case her privacy may be violated.

Prema is a forty-four-year-old Indian American computer engineer who is coping with stress related to conflicts with her husband and her twenty-year-old daughter. Prema and her husband were born and raised in India, and both immigrated to the United States as graduate students. They continue to struggle with their distance from their families, who live in India, and trying to raise their daughter with traditional Indian values. They have emphasized the importance of educational achievement and family unity with their daughter. Prema is particularly close to her daughter, who is a college student majoring in engineering. Recently, Prema's daughter disclosed to her that she is a lesbian and is coping with a great deal of anxiety in disclosing her sexual orientation to significant people in her life. Prema has felt overwhelmed by her daughter's coming out to her, despite wanting to support her daughter. Prema has felt increasingly depressed and confused about how to address with her husband their daughter's issues. She worries that her husband will not be able to accept their daughter's coming out.

One of Prema's colleagues, also an Indian American woman, recommended that she seek group psychotherapy to talk about her concerns. Joining a mixed-race group concerns Prema—that group members are unfamiliar with her cultural background and that they would negatively stereotype her as a passive woman in her marriage. Prema also worries that if she joined a group for Indian women, that group members may blame her for her daughter's homosexuality. Prema, in fitting with her cultural background, has been taught throughout her life not to disclose family issues to anyone outside of her family. Consequently, she is also concerned about maintaining the privacy of her family conflicts, in either of these two types of groups.

Both Julia and Prema are concerned about the sensitivity of group members and therapist toward their cultural backgrounds and about privacy. At the same time, they also recognize their need to engage in a group healing process in which they will be able to share their experiences openly and hear others' experiences and ways of coping. Their dilemmas are complicated by a general reluctance in both of their communities to seek help outside of one's immediate and extended family units. At the same time, they both have the encouragement and support of significant people in their lives (i.e., therapist, colleague) to seek help.

A distinguishing feature of the experiences of many ethnic minorities in the mental health system involves prejudice and discrimination. While white Americans may express cautiousness in their participation in group psychotherapy, many ethnic minorities experience a distrust of the nature of these services, in light of historical and ongoing culturally biased treatment approaches. Furthermore, many ethnic minorities feel more vulnerable than white group members in disclosing personal details, partly because they fear that their cultural perspectives will be pathologized or negatively construed. These issues contribute to

> Many ethnic minorities feel more vulnerable than white group members in disclosing personal details, partly because they fear that their cultural perspectives will be pathologized or negatively construed.

FREQUENT CONCERNS IN GROUPS FOR WOMEN OF COLOR

- Bicultural identity
- Emotional expression
- Community expectations of relationships with men
- Family responsibilities
- Mother-daughter relationships

- Spirituality
- Sexual orientation
- Desire to connect with women of similar ethnicity
- Socioeconomic differences

members of the psychotherapy group feeling disrespected, ignored, or marginalized, sometimes experiencing the group dynamic as a reenactment of their position in their world outside the group.

In groups consisting of minority individuals of a similar ethnic/racial background, there tends to be concern about issues of confidentiality with respect to disclosing information to those whom group members interact with in the larger community. Sometimes, group members are in a position to speak more freely about some issues but not others if they are considered taboo topics within their ethnic communities. In the case of groups that consist of white majority participants, issues of culture and race may be ignored entirely, or in some cases, serve to reinforce internalized stereotypes and prejudice toward minority groups and feelings of superiority over these groups. In either case, the group therapist and members face the challenge of addressing both the shared ethnic/racial experiences and the diversity of individual members with respect to other variables such as age, class, religious faith, family background, sexual orientation, skin color, and education.

SPECIFIC GROUPS FOR WOMEN OF COLOR

Women of color in the United States often hold the least amount of social and economic power in our country. One consequence of these sociopolitical realities is the diminished access to culturally competent mental health services for women of color. In recent years, in response to this crisis, several mental health practitioners and researchers have focused on developing group therapeutic interventions with women of diverse ethnic and racial backgrounds. These women's psychotherapy groups have varied with respect to theoretical perspective and areas of focus.

> Immigrant women experiencing psychological distress often feel isolated and alienated from their ethnic communities, due to the stigma of mental illness evident in many ethnic minority communities. For these reasons, groups can provide a sense of connection for women.

Some central themes of exploration in these groups included struggles with bicultural identity, emotional expression, community expectations of relationships with men, family responsibilities, mother–daughter relationships, spirituality, sexual orientation, the desire to connect with other women of similar ethnicity, and socioeconomic differences. Isolation is an increasing problem for many ethnic minority women, and group psychotherapy can be particularly useful in providing a supportive function and in exploring issues such as skin color, body image, and racial identification, which are sometimes difficult to address in cross-racial groups.

One of the most important functions of groups for women of color relates to the discussion of racism. It is of critical importance for many women of color to participate in the exploration of racism and racial trauma in their lives and its impact on their identifications. Immigration is another salient issue relevant to many women of color in the United States. In recent years, groups for immigrant, bilingual, and bicultural women, conducted in English and in members' native languages, have addressed various unique processes. In particular, the number of groups with women of Latino and Asian descent has been increasing. Immigrant women experiencing psychological distress often feel isolated and alienated from their ethnic communities, due to the stigma of mental illness evident in many ethnic minority communities. For these reasons, groups can provide a sense of connection for women. The supportive connection with members of one's family and ethnic group is particularly important for women whose ethnic identifications rely on a more collective sense of self.

Group psychotherapy has been an increasing source of psychological support for women over the past several decades in the United States. They provide some key benefits not accessible through individual psychotherapy, including the opportunity to explore both the commonality and the diversity of experiences and to address significant relational difficulties via the examination of group dynamics. Group psychotherapy can also reach larger numbers of women across socioeconomic backgrounds who are in need of professional help for coping with psychological distress, as groups are often less expensive than individual psychotherapy. Furthermore, regardless of the theoretical perspective guiding the group psychotherapy, groups provide a supportive function for the individual's healing.

—*Pratyusha Tummala-Narra, Ph.D., and Lauren Slater, Ed.D.*

RELATED ENTRIES

Cognitive Behavioral Therapy

Depressive Disorders

Domestic Violence

How to Find and Choose a Therapist

Post-Traumatic Stress Disorder

Racism and Mental Health

Sexual Abuse and Rape

How to Find and Choose a Therapist

Many people find it much harder to decide to see a therapist for psychological pain than see a medical doctor for physical pain. Our emotions seem to feel much more intimate to many of us than our bodies do. Perhaps our culture still holds a stigma regarding psychiatric care, or perhaps exposing one's vulnerability is part and parcel to asking for help, especially when it comes to emotional suffering. Whatever the reason, it is difficult to go out there and get help.

The fact that it is hard to make the decision to get help, and then to open yourself up to a professional, makes it even more important that you make a good choice with regards to whom that professional will be. When I meet clients for the first time, I always ask them to pay attention to how it feels to be with me and to notice, despite the fact that I am a total stranger, whether or not they feel comfortable with me (or can imagine feeling comfortable with me once they get used to the whole idea of therapy). Psychotherapy research has shown that the match between therapist and client is critical to the success of the treatment. But before you learn how to know whether you are well matched, you need to know about how to find a therapist in the first place.

A personal recommendation is the best way to find a therapist. Ask people you are close to whether they know of anybody, and if not, whether they know anybody who might know someone. For example, if your friend has a therapist he likes and finds helpful, ask him to request several names of other providers that his therapist knows and trusts.

If you plan on using your health insurance, it is a good idea to speak to a representative beforehand to discover what your benefits are. Make sure the insurance agent is clear and that you understand because it can be confusing. For example, some insurance companies will only pay for you to see a provider (therapist) that is part of their plan or on their "panel of providers." If this is the case, they will send you a list of names. Other companies will allow you to go "out of network," but if you do, they may only pay a percentage of the costs. In that case, you might have to pay the therapist yourself and then submit the paid invoice to your insurance company, which would then reimburse you for part of the cost. And if you get a list of names from your health insurance company, ask that friend of yours with the great therapist to inquire whether his therapist might know of and recommend anyone who is on the list.

Other questions you might have for your insurance company include: How many sessions does my policy cover? What kind of information is the therapist required to provide the company? Who has access to such information? Is there a copayment required? And am I allowed to see a provider that is not in the company's network?

Whether you locate names of therapists from people you know and trust or whether you locate names from a phone book, your insurance company, or an ad in the newspaper, it is always a good idea to interview a few of them to see who you feel most comfortable with despite the discomfort you might feel of going and talking to a stranger about yourself. When you do talk with a potential therapist, pay attention to your experience. And always remember, the therapist is working for you.

> Our emotions seem to feel much more intimate to many of us than our bodies do.

Before the session, think about important questions you might have. For example, what are the therapist's qualifications? How strongly do you feel about the therapist's type of qualifications—do you want to see a psychologist, psychiatrist, social worker? (The following list will help you understand the differences.) Does it matter which type? In addition, do you want to know what the therapist's theoretical stance is; that is, what does the therapist believe will be of use to you? How does he or she believe that treatment works? What is the therapist's underlying philosophy? Pay attention to whether the therapist uses language that you can understand and relate to. If you get confused or something the therapist says raises further questions, ask them. Is the gender of the therapist important to you? Do you want a therapist who asks a lot of questions and talks a lot or a therapist who primarily listens? All of these questions will help you to determine whether the therapist is a good match for you. If you are not sure, give it a couple of sessions, and if it doesn't feel right, then stop and try someone else. Trust yourself.

All of this is the basis for what I mean by a good "match" between therapist and client, but let's go into even more detail. Finding a match is not an obvious science. Most likely, no one factor is going to determine who will be the best therapist for you. As I said before, it is important for you to pay attention to how comfortable you are. Your next questions might be: "So, I like this therapist, I can imagine being comfortable with her/him, but how do I know that she/he is competent? How do I know I have chosen a good therapist?" Thinking about the four following questions may enable you to further determine whether you have found a match:

Has someone recommended this therapist to me?

Having someone you know direct you to someone he or she knows and trusts may allay some of the anxieties related to opening up to a professional. In other words, it is always helpful to go to a known entity rather than to just start out cold.

What are the issues I am struggling with? Is there any evidence that a certain kind of treatment approach might be best for these issues?

Research on psychotherapy has shown that certain disorders are best helped by certain treatment approaches, while other disorders or issues have been found to be successfully treated by number of different approaches. Ask each therapist you interview how he or she might approach a particular issue/disorder; although a therapist may not primarily identify herself as a "cognitive behavioral therapist," she may have the appropriate training and expertise necessary to provide cognitive behavioral treatment. It is the therapist's ethical responsibility to refer you to an appropriate provider

QUESTIONS FOR YOUR INSURANCE COMPANY

+ *How many sessions does my policy cover?*

+ *What kind of information is the therapist required to provide the company?*

+ *Who has access to such information?*

+ *Is a copayment required?*

+ *Am I allowed to see a provider who is not in the company's network?*

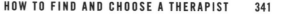

should he or she not be competent to provide the best treatment for you; however, having a sense of what might be most helpful to you will enable you to make a more educated decision. Reading through this book and making notes of issues that you relate to and what their recommended treatment options are will help you get a sense of what treatments you want your therapist to be skilled in.

IMPORTANT QUESTIONS FOR
THERAPISTS AND YOURSELF

+ *What are the therapist's*
qualifications?

+ *What is the therapist's*
theoretical stance?

+ *How does he or she believe*
that treatment works?

+ *Does the therapist use language*
you can understand and relate to?

+ *Is the gender of the therapist*
important to you?

+ *Are you comfortable with*
the therapist?

What is the educational background of the therapist? What does that mean and is it important to me?

Deciphering what all the letters following a therapist's name mean in terms of education and training can be confusing. The following list describes some of the more common initials and what they mean, but keep in mind that there are variations between different schools and programs and that requirements change over time. The various degrees are listed according to the amount of time required to complete the associated training, starting with the highest number of years; the list does not reflect an opinion regarding the value of the types of education.

M.D. These "doctors of medicine" are also known as psychiatrists. Psychiatrists are required to go to medical school and complete the additional training necessary for a specialization in psychiatric medicine. Psychiatrists can prescribe medication and often work as both "psychotherapists" and "psychopharmacologists."

Ph.D. This "doctor of philosophy" degree may be in either clinical, counseling, or school psychology. Licensed therapists who hold this degree are called psychologists. Programs usually take five to seven years to complete and require extensive course work and hands-on clinical training both "pre-doc" and "post-doc" (before and after graduation).

Ed.D. This degree designation refers to a "doctor of education." The length of education and clinical practice is similar to the Ph.D., but the focus of the course work differs.

Psy.D. This is a "doctor of psychology" degree. Licensed therapists who hold this degree are also called psychologists. Programs usually take four to seven years to complete and require intensive course work and hands-on clinical training both pre- and post-doc. The Psy.D. degree is usually less focused on research than Ph.D. programs and was developed as a "professional" degree.

LICSW Translated, this means "licensed independent clinical social worker." Those therapists whose names are followed by LICSW have obtained a master's degree in social work. Programs usually take two to three years and require both intensive coursework and hands-on clinical training.

M.A. There are numerous "masters of arts" degrees, including (but not limited to) counseling psychology, school psychology, expressive therapy (such as art, dance, and music therapies), and clinical psychology. Master's programs usually take two to three years to complete and require both coursework and hands-on clinical training.

As stated earlier, there are many variations of degrees and programs out there. If you are interested in the type and length of training that your potential therapist has had, it is perfectly okay to ask for the general landscape of his or her education, experience, and training. This may or may not be a contributing factor in deciding which therapist is the best match for you. There are good and not-so-good therapists who hold any given degree, so even if the therapist's education is important to you, you will still need to pay attention to the other factors that determine a good fit.

What is my style of communication and with what kinds of personalities am I most comfortable?

We wind up back where we started: focusing on the importance of style of communication, level of warmth, and so forth. Can you imagine feeling comfortable? Do you want to talk to this person? This does require you to have a sense about what feels right or wrong to you, and sometimes that is challenging. Sometimes, new clients I have seen have found it helpful to use what I call the "four-session frame": give it four sessions before making a commitment to the treatment. This can be helpful because it frames a period of exploration. It can be difficult to remember all the questions you may have for a potential therapist in the first one or even two sessions. In addition, it allows the client to get a sense or a feel over the course of several sessions. This can help clarify not only what the hopes and expectations of the client are going in, but also how they compare to what the reality looks and feels like. The fourth session can focus on how it is or is not what the client wanted/expected/hoped for—useful in itself, but this also allows the client to see how the therapist responds (or doesn't) to these issues or concerns. Clearly, you may not want to employ the four-session frame with numerous therapists as it would quickly add up in both time and money, but it may be useful if you are just not sure and want to give yourself the time to explore. You could narrow your choices and try the four-session frame with the top two therapists that meet your other criteria.

Ultimately, if it doesn't feel right, if it feels off in some way, trust yourself. Try someone else.

As you begin the process of seeking out a therapist, use these questions as a guide; however, you probably also have other questions that were not raised here that are important to you. Think about what those are and ask them. Knowing what is important to you in choosing a therapist will enable you to make the very best choice.

—Jennifer Coon-Wallman, Psy.D.

RELATED ENTRIES

Cognitive Behavioral Therapy

Dialectical Behavior Therapy

EMDR

Group Psychotherapy with Women

Insight-Oriented Psychotherapy

What to Expect from Ethical Psychotherapy

The psychotherapeutic relationship is complex: Each practitioner of each approach represents a unique understanding of how to help clients live a healthier, better, more fulfilling life. Yet, there are some identifiable elements common to effective treatment that are helpful for the consumer of psychotherapy to understand. You also need to be aware of the various risks in the psychotherapeutic relationship in order to understand what constitutes an ethical and appropriate psychotherapeutic experience.

THE NEED FOR PSYCHOTHERAPY

Mental health is fundamental to health, according to Dr. David Satcher, in the first U.S. Department of Health and Human Services Surgeon General's report ever to focus exclusively on mental health. Good mental health is the basis for successful involvement in family, community, and society, allowing for healthy thinking, communication, learning, resilience, and positive self-esteem. One in five Americans experience mental health problems, which, if untreated, can result in major problems for the individual, his or her family, workplace, and community. Yet the majority of people with diagnosable disorders do not receive treatment! There is a range of effective treatments for most mental disorders and the surgeon general made a clear recommendation that anyone who has or thinks he or she has mental health symptoms should seek help.

As a consumer of mental health services, you will approach treatment options with more confidence if you understand more about effective, ethical psychotherapy. There are virtually hundreds of different approaches to counseling and psychotherapy. Despite the approach, there are certain common factors that are important across almost all therapeutic modalities and approaches.

WHAT DO THERAPISTS DO?

Psychologists, clinical social workers, and other counselors help people to be emotionally healthy and lead fulfilled lives by promoting skills, attitudes, and knowledge to help find solutions to life problems. Some mental health professionals conduct studies to understand how people think, feel, and act. That information then helps other professionals to more effectively treat consumers of mental health. Mental health professionals use tests and/or interviews to diagnose problems and provide psychotherapy for psychological disorders. They use a variety of therapeutic approaches to help people alleviate distress; resolve crises;

strengthen interpersonal relationships to engage in effective career, work, and family experiences; increase their ability to be effective; and to help improve their well-being. Practitioners also promote skills, attitudes, and behaviors to help prevent disorders throughout life. Mental health professionals provide services to individuals, couples, families, and groups from organizations and systems.

THE THERAPEUTIC ALLIANCE AND THE ETHICS OF CARE

A good therapeutic relationship is related to positive outcomes across various counseling strategies and methods, according to research on effective therapy outcomes. A positive alliance reported by the client appears to be the strongest predictor of outcome.

What promotes a positive alliance between patient and therapist? Nel Noddings, author and professor of child education at Stanford, and Carol Gilligan, author and psychologist, propose the importance of being caring in relationships with others. Karen Kitchener, author of *Foundations of Ethical Practice, Research, and Teaching in Psychology*, suggests that others have labeled this concept as "compassion," and that acting out of care or compassion means acting out of regard for the patient's welfare rather than simply responding to fixed rules and principles. The caring therapist feels the patient's pain and sees the situation through the patient's eyes, but simultaneously does not give up responsibilities for ethical decision making.

One controversy suggests that patients whose therapists take this caring approach to its extreme could become dependent, disempowered and may idealize relationships in which there is no mutual responsibility. However, others propose that a therapist who cares for the patient as a full human being also sets limits, says no, and is strict in judgment but from a more supportive and compassionate stance.

Most research indicates that your therapist should create and facilitate a trusting relationship in which you perceive care, and that this is one of the most critical activities a therapist does. In *Ethics in Psychotherapy and Counseling*, written by Ken Pope and myself, we suggest that because clients place their trust in professionals, it is critical that caring about the client's well-being should be a defining characteristic of the professional. Therapists must acknowledge the reality and importance of the individuals whose lives they affect by their professional actions. The client should feel the therapist's compassion for the client as an individual and should feel that the climate for ethical behavior and a positive alliance are enhanced by this caring approach.

The nature of the psychotherapeutic relationship involves an inherent power differential, even among those therapists who work toward a relatively egalitarian relationship. The therapist's professional status and powers are justified within a context of caring about the client's well-being—that is, whether these powers will ultimately benefit or harm the client.

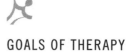

GOALS OF THERAPY

+ *Alleviate distress*

+ *Resolve crises*

+ *Strengthen interpersonal relationships*

+ *Increase one's ability to be effective*

+ *Improve well-being*

+ *Promote skills, attitudes, and behaviors that help prevent disorders*

> Good mental health is the basis for successful involvement in family, community, and society, allowing for healthy thinking, communication, learning, resilience, and positive self-esteem.

BARRIERS TO THE THERAPEUTIC ALLIANCE

You, the therapy consumer, do not have to simply defer to your therapist's suggestions. The therapy patient should feel comfortable expressing to her psychotherapist negative reactions to treatment. Concealing negative reactions, automatically deferring to the coun-

BASIC PRINCIPLES OF
ETHICAL THERAPY

+ *Nonmaleficence*

+ *Beneficence*

+ *Justice*

+ *Autonomy*

+ *Fidelity*

selor's suggestions, and failing to communicate irritation with and mistrust of the counselor can interfere with the development of a genuine alliance. Your therapist should create opportunities for you to express your reaction by checking frequently regarding your feelings about the therapy; this way, the counselor can intervene before a difficult situation reaches a crisis point. The ethical therapist follows several basic principles to help develop and maintain a fundamental climate of respect and care in the therapeutic relationship.

MORAL PRINCIPLES

Karen Kitchener and others propose that moral education be part of the training and education of all therapists. Therapists need to understand the underlying moral principles of ethics codes, practice laws, and other requirements and guidelines so that they can think in complex ways about how one makes decisions in ethical work. The five ethical principles that Kitchener suggests include nonmaleficence (do no harm); beneficence (do good); respect for justice; autonomy; and fidelity. They serve as the foundation for ethical decision making in psychology, including establishment of policy. These broad principles were initially proposed by Beauchamp and Childress as principles of biomedical ethics and are often used in society to establish policy, such as in the court system. As a consumer of psychotherapy, it may help to understand these principles that therapists use as guides when faced with ethical decision making.

Nonmaleficence Nonmaleficence is a concept that finds its roots in the history of medicine and that means "above all, do no harm." All therapists have a responsibility to know what behaviors, attitudes, and so forth have potential to do harm. Specific principles in the therapist code of ethics that evolve from this general principle include not violating an individual's civil rights, guarding against the misuse of assessment results, competence, and avoiding dual relationships. Maintaining competence by improving skills through continuing education and other activities is a major responsibility of all therapists. Therapists are expected to provide services to clients only within the boundaries of their competence.

Beneficence Beneficence involves the contribution to the health and welfare of those with whom we work. The profession of mental health is based upon the dedication to use knowledge to promote human welfare and to promote positive growth. Mental health professionals are considered members of the so-called helping professions, reflecting this obligation.

> Your therapist should create and facilitate a trusting relationship in which you perceive care; this is one of the most critical activities a therapist does.

Justice In its broadest sense, justice means "fairness." This includes dealing with others as one would like to be dealt with oneself, behaving toward others in an impartial manner, and treating others equally. Fairness is the basis for the ethical value that we provide services for little or no financial reimbursement to those who cannot otherwise afford services. It is also the foundation for the requirement that we be concerned with equal treatment for all individuals, according to Karen Kitchener. An ethical therapist asks, for example, "Am I less vigilant, less focused, or less on time for the 'sliding scale' client?" Every therapy patient should expect the same treatment as any other patient, regardless of the fee she is paying.

Autonomy The autonomous person has the responsibility for her own behavior and decision making, has freedom of choice, and is at liberty to choose her own course of action. Autonomy implies a freedom to do what you want to do, as long as it does not interfere with similar freedoms of others. Respect for autonomy is the moral principle embedded in political institutions, the law, and in psychology. For example, the concepts of unconditional worth and tolerance for individual differences both imply a respect for clients' rights to make their own decisions.

Mutual respect, a basic element to the therapeutic bond for most therapists, implies a relationship between autonomous individuals. The principle of autonomy is also the foundation of confidentiality and right to privacy. The right to privacy follows from the assumption that autonomous individuals have the right to make autonomous decisions about their own lives and the information relevant to it. It is a respect for the fact that individuals have the power and skills to decide for themselves.

> The client should feel the therapist's compassion for the client as an individual and should feel that the climate for ethical behavior and a positive alliance are enhanced by this caring approach.

Fidelity Fidelity involves questions of faithfulness, loyalty, and promise keeping. These are issues basic to trust, and fidelity is especially vital to all human relationships. The relationship between therapist and client is dependent on honest communication and the assumption that the contract on which the relationship was initiated obliges both parties to fulfill certain functions. The rule of maintaining confidentiality, in addition to stemming from the broad principle of autonomy, also is based on this moral principle.

ELEMENTS INVOLVED IN THE CHANGE PROCESS

Effective therapy involves the right combination of support as well as challenge, which varies from person to person. Attitude or behavior change is often required in order for an individual, family, or group to improve the quality of life. Therefore, the "fit" between therapist and client must be such that you are able to perceive support from the therapist in the form of care and in the context of trust and that the challenge is experienced as motivating, not overwhelming. Your psychotherapist should be aware of his or her own cultural orientation, as well as know your background and have some understanding about different cultural, gender, social class, religious, ability, and sexual orientation groups. Psychotherapists should be able to work as effectively as possible with those different from themselves. In addition, psychotherapists are encouraged to consider matching counseling interventions to needs. In other words, your problems and treatment goals should influence the suitability of the counselor's choice of interventions.

> The relationship between therapist and client is dependent on honest communication and the assumption that the contract on which the relationship was initiated obliges both parties to fulfill certain functions.

You will expect to feel better as a result of psychotherapy. While that is certainly a long-term goal, increased awareness, exploring sources of trauma, realizing the errors one has engaged in life, and so on often result in experiencing pain. Pain is often simply a cue that change is necessary.

With the belief that human beings have an innate propensity for development and growth, the psychotherapist's job is to remove obstacles for growth. The self-actualizing forces in each person then does the rest of the job. Obstacles to growth can consist of negative attitudes, lack of skills, faulty thinking or belief systems, and historical events that keep one "stuck" in negative patterns of thinking, feeling, and behaving.

BASIC RISKS IN THE THERAPEUTIC RELATIONSHIP

There are some areas in which ethical violations frequently occur in the therapeutic relationship and of which any psychotherapy consumer should be aware.

Sexual Violations Perhaps the area that causes most harm and that, unfortunately, happens most frequently is the area of sexual violations. Avoiding sexual intimacies with clients is one of the oldest ethical mandates in the health care professions and is very clear in all mental health ethics codes and practice laws. Sexual violations by psychotherapists result in a variety of symptoms reflecting harm to clients, including ambivalence, guilt, emptiness and isolation, sexual confusion, impaired ability to trust, confused roles and boundaries, emotional liability, suppressed rage, increased suicidal risk, and cognitive dysfunction, according to research by Ken Pope. The fact that the majority of perpetrators are male therapists and the majority of victims are female clients reflects an oppressive exploitation of women in the therapist–client relationship similar to that in society in general.

Multiple Relationships and Other Boundary Issues Boundary setting has evolved as an important strategy in applying the ethical proscription for therapists to "do no harm" to clients. Because the needs of the psychotherapist could potentially get in the way of the therapy, the mental health professions have established guidelines, often referred to as "boundaries," that are designed to minimize the opportunity for therapists to use their patients for their own needs and gratification. The therapist is especially responsible for distinguishing the therapeutic relationship from previous harmful relationships.

Some psychotherapists work best by maintaining fairly strict rules. However, for other therapists, many "gray areas" exist in regard to behavior with clients. If you feel that your therapist is crossing boundaries with which you are uncomfortable, you may need to find another therapist who does not work in that "gray area." Or perhaps the therapist you have chosen is very strict in adhering to boundaries and you would prefer the style of someone more flexible. In either case, you should bring up your concerns to your therapist, and together you can decide if the approach can be altered to meet your needs within the therapist's style of working. If not, it is important to find a new therapist with whom you can be more comfortable.

> Your problems and treatment goals should influence the counselor's choice of interventions.

Special attention to how we distance our clients is an important goal for therapists working from a feminist/multicultural perspective. It is especially true for clients of color, most of whom have experienced distancing in their lives in the form of discrimination. Some forms of therapeutic boundary setting may actually make you feel a distance, disconnection, and oppression that are not conducive to a good therapeutic relationship.

SELF-DISCLOSURE

Feminist therapists were among the first to challenge the proscription against self-disclosure. The Feminist Therapy Code of Ethics (1990) provides guidelines to therapist disclosure in the context of the power differential. With the well-being of clients as the overriding principle, the guideline states: "A feminist therapist discloses information [about her- or himself] to the client which facilitates the therapeutic process. The therapist is responsible for using self-disclosure with purpose and discretion in the interest of the client." From a feminist perspective in general, the issue is to acknowledge the real and genuine aspects of the human interaction in psychotherapy—the therapist is also a person with life experiences that may relate to the patient's problems.

Psychodynamic approaches tend to focus more on the symbolic transaction, in which the therapist puts aside his or her own feelings and contributions to the interaction and assumes that all issues that evolve in therapy revolve around the client. In the feminist approach, it is also important not to deny various aspects of the symbolic transactions, including the power differential between therapist and client, because doing so is a failure to take responsibility for the roles that clients inevitably put therapists in by virtue of the therapist's position. No matter how genuine and real aspects of the human part of the therapeutic interaction are, the therapist still has the responsibility to maintain knowledge and to promote competent interventions that "do no harm" in working with clients. So, self-disclosures must be in the service of the client and not designed to meet the therapist's needs.

However, used appropriately, self-disclosure can be a powerful way for a therapist to increase her or his mutuality and connection with you as client. Information is a form of power. The therapist who makes herself visible in the relationship allows you to have more power in the relationship than you would have with a less-forthcoming therapist. Therapist self-disclosure also serves the function of allowing you, the client, to reciprocate empathy.

However, what is therapeutically self-disclosing for one person may not be for another. Mistakes can happen, even with the most ethical therapist, and unless the mistake was seriously exploitative, the relationship should be able to recover and move on. Again, it is important for the client to be forthcoming in the type of relationship she feels comfortable with, and, so, if self-disclosure by the therapist is not comfortable for the client, she should discuss this with the therapist or find another therapist with a different approach.

EFFECTS OF SEXUAL VIOLATIONS BY PSYCHOTHERAPISTS

+ *Ambivalence*
+ *Guilt*
+ *Emptiness and isolation*
+ *Sexual confusion*
+ *Impaired ability to trust*
+ *Confused roles and boundaries*
+ *Emotional liability*
+ *Suppressed rage*
+ *Increased suicide risk*
+ *Cognitive dysfunction*

ASKING QUESTIONS

When a client asks questions, how the therapist responds is related to the issue of self-disclosure. Some therapists work from models in which the question is to be processed and analyzed. Some would answer a question with a question; however, others believe that in certain contexts, this may be perceived as hostile. For example, when scheduling a session for the following week, I indicate that I will be out of town at our usual time, and you ask, "Are you going on vacation or business?" If I responded from a traditional boundary-setting mode, I might respond with a question myself: "Why do you ask? What meaning does that have for you?" This kind of approach could be disconnecting to the relationship. My personal approach is to answer the question within an appropriate realm for the therapist (nonprivate), and then, to process any significance. Perhaps this is a subtle difference, but I think it is a powerful one: One approach fails to gratify the client, and perhaps elicits anxiety or shame for asking the question. The other promotes connection, relating with the client on a real, authentic, genuine level, but can also explore the need/anxiety/symbolic issue behind the question. When the relationship is based on warmth, safety, mutuality, and respect, it allows for deeper and deeper recycling through issues.

RECEIVING GIFTS

The context of gift giving and receiving is crucial. Generally, therapists discourage clients from giving them gifts simply because clients pay for the therapist's services. Receiving expensive gifts from clients can be exploitive, can promote the client to feel unworthy unless she gives continuously, or it can simply be a healthy expression of care on the part of the client. The psychotherapist will find it important to understand the goals, motivations, and expectations when a client gives a gift.

NONSEXUAL TOUCH AND OTHER EXPRESSIONS OF CARE

Practitioners are encouraged to avoid problems with ethical violations by mental health liability insurance companies, who develop "risk management strategies." Some of those specifically exhort psychotherapists not to touch or hug clients.

A therapist will carefully consider the nature of the relationship, the client's personal history, the client's current mental status, the likelihood of nonsexual touch having an adverse impact on the client, and a clear theoretical rationale. What does a hug mean to this client in regard to power and mutuality? Who feels the need to hug—the therapist or the client? Some clients have experienced numerous boundary violations in their lives and either are uncomfortable with touch or must control it to feel safe. A therapist's use of nonsexual touch must take all of these things into consideration.

And, yes, boundary issues are different for women therapists than for men therapists and male and female patients. Some challenges to the boundaries may be appropriate challenges for women therapists, but not necessarily for men therapists.

> No matter how genuine and real aspects of the human part of the therapeutic interaction are, the therapist still has the responsibility to maintain knowledge and to promote competent interventions that "do no harm" in working with clients.

OVERLAPPING RELATIONSHIPS, MULTIPLE RELATIONSHIPS

Not all dual- or multiple-role relationships are avoidable or unethical. However, most practitioners choose to avoid relating to clients in other contexts outside of therapy. In our book about ethics, Ken Pope and I discuss how dual relationships tend to erode and distort the professional nature of the therapeutic relationship, which is secured within a reliable set of boundaries upon which both therapist and client can depend. Even after therapy termination, the therapeutic relationship does not end, as it is the therapist's continued responsibility to maintain confidentiality, to release notes, to testify in court if necessary, and so forth.

Problems with dual relationships are typically explained by role theory. Social roles contain inherent expectations about how a person in a particular role is to behave as well as the rights and obligations that pertain to that role. Role conflicts arise when the expectations attached to one role call for behavior that is incompatible with that of another role.

However, encounters outside of therapy may be unavoidable when the lives of multicultural and feminist therapists overlap with those of the people they serve. One colleague described a dilemma in which a therapist discovered that the new board she had joined included a client who was also a new member of the board. She suggested that decision making in arriving at a solution to that dilemma involved exploration with the client and with colleagues of the key issues involved. The solution at which one therapist arrives may be different from that of another therapist and may be different with the same therapist after time and experience. There are several risks related to dual relationships, which my coauthor Pope and I identified in our book: First, dual relationships can erode and distort the professional nature of the therapeutic relationship; if the therapist is also the patient's friend, landlord, employer, the crucial nature of the therapeutic relationship is compromised. Second, dual relationships can create conflicts of interest and compromise the type of investment necessary for sound professional judgment. Third, dual relationships can affect the cognitive processes that research has shown to play in the beneficial effects of therapy (internalization of the therapist's voice). Fourth, because of the power differential inherent in the roles of therapist and client, the patient cannot enter into any other kind of relationship with therapist on an equal footing. Psychotherapists know secrets and other intensely private information. Fifth, the fundamental nature of psychotherapy would be changed if therapy were to become a place to encounter potential lovers, friends, business partners, social networks. Sixth, testimony and reports in courts and other forums would be compromised, given the fact that the therapist had an additional role (friend, business partner, etc.).

> ✦
> Even after therapy termination, the therapeutic relationship does not end.

BARTERING

Bartering is generally not advisable, and exchange for services is especially problematic since doing so inherently creates a dual relationship—in order for the client to provide a service to the therapist, the two must engage in a relationship outside of the therapy forum. However, in rural areas, mental health practitioners are often challenged with the expectations of exchange for goods. One of the problems with bartering is that expectations of both parties in both roles may be difficult to meet or may conflict directly.

When an ethical therapist applies boundaries, it is with respect and care not to elicit shame in our clients. Traumatized people are easily shamed, and clients can often feel "I'm the bad one." Since therapists recognize that mutuality and respect in their behaviors with clients is core to client's empowerment, they are always careful to apply boundaries with that in mind.

CONFIDENTIALITY AND LIMITS

Confidentiality is a cornerstone to effective psychotherapy. Psychotherapists are obligated by law and by their professional ethics to maintain confidentiality of the psychotherapy content, unless the consumer of psychotherapy services requests release of records. To release records, psychotherapists are encouraged to obtain a client's written consent to release information from his or her records, even when that information is provided directly to the client. Most therapists try to ensure that the client understands the implication of releasing the information. If oral consent to release information is provided in an emergency, psychotherapists will document the details.

There are various limits to confidentiality, and as a client you should be informed of these limits. When a client is harming others such as abusing a child, therapists have a legal responsibility in every state in the United States to break confidentiality; otherwise, the therapist faces criminal charges for not reporting the child abuse.

If a client is evaluated to be a danger to self or others, if the client is a victim of abuse (and if the client is a minor, elderly, or disabled), then the psychotherapist is required to report or prevent danger, which often means that confidentiality is limited. Various states have different requirements—for example, in some states, if the client divulges information about sexual abuse by another mental health professional, the therapist must report it. Also, limits of confidentiality exist if the client files suit against the therapist for breach of duty, or if a court order requires disclosure.

INFORMED CONSENT

Related to the issue of confidentiality is the issue of informed consent. The primary moral principle underlying the obligation to obtain informed consent from a client involves the promotion of autonomy. Any procedure performed on or on behalf of a patient without his or her consent diminishes the patient's autonomy or capacity to act in a free and self-determining manner. Therefore, giving the person an opportunity to make a choice emphasizes his or her autonomy.

Information provided during the consent process differs according to the professional service, whether it be an assessment, psychotherapy, forensic evaluation, and so forth. In our book on ethics, Ken Pope and I suggest to therapists that they try to make sure that clients understand the following questions, whether through provision of information on a form, or on an ongoing basis:

- Do you understand who is providing the service, the clinician's qualifications, and whether supervision is involved?
- Do you understand the reason for the initial session (self-initiated, court- or physician-referred)?
- Do you understand the nature, extent, and possible consequences of the services the clinician is offering? Do you understand the degree to which there may be alternatives to the services provided by the clinician?
- Do you understand actual or potential limitations to the services (e.g., a managed care plan's limitation of four to six sessions unless a major mental illness diagnosis is given)? Do you understand how services may be terminated?
- Do you understand fee policies and procedures, including information about missed or canceled appointments, use of collection fee services, and so forth?
- Do you understand policies and procedures concerning access to the clinician, to those providing coverage for the clinician, and to emergency services? For example, under what conditions, if any, will a therapist be available by phone between sessions?
- Do you understand limits to confidentiality in situations involving partner, family, or group psychotherapy? Do you understand the conditions under which the clinician might be required to disclose information to an insurance company, utilization reviewers, the police, child protective services, or the courts?

RECORD-KEEPING GUIDELINES

Most mental health professionals are required to keep records, but few strict guidelines exist regarding the structure of such records. Psychotherapy notes will minimally include identifying data, dates of services, types of services, fees, any assessment, plan for intervention, consultation, summary reports and/or testing reports, supporting data, and any release of information obtained. I also document any unusual struggles and dilemmas that surface during the therapeutic process.

Notes for psychotherapy groups and family and relationship therapy might also be kept. Although largely unavoidable, complications regarding confidentiality can occur when the information of various family members is kept in one record. For example, one person may request release of records, but another family member may choose for the notes to not be released. Group therapy notes are typically kept per individual, rather than as notes for the group as a whole. State law requirements or the guidelines from the various mental health professionals may vary.

The Freedom of Information Act means that as a client, you legally have access to your records. Various options are provided by therapists to review records, including reviewing notes in a session(s) for therapeutic benefit or the provision of a summary. Ultimately, if a client chooses to have her notes, she can do so in most states. Some state practice laws require that psychotherapists not release notes if they are judged to be potentially harmful to clients.

The minimum requirements for length of time to keep records vary from state to state, and mental health professionals are encouraged to abide by the strictest requirements of their state, their ethics codes, agency requirements, or other guidelines. Psychotherapists are discouraged from refusing to release records on the basis of client failure to pay bills.

> Confidentiality is a cornerstone to effective psychotherapy. Psychotherapists are obligated by law and by their professional ethics to maintain confidentiality of the psychotherapy content, unless the consumer of psychotherapy services requests release of records.

Psychotherapists are encouraged to make arrangements for storage of records when leaving their practice and/or in case of disability or death. Arrangements should be made so that, in the case of death, someone knows how to access information about current clients and notify them. With clients' permission, some psychologists make reciprocal arrangements with colleagues to exchange lists of patients' names, phone numbers, and information about their treatment. In case of death or incapacitation, the designated therapist would notify patients/clients and serve as a referral person or "bridge therapist" for continuation of care and to deal with the death or incapacitation of the original therapist. Some arrangement is typically made for a notice to be placed in the newspaper to inform clients, present and former, of the therapist's death or inability to practice, letting them know who holds their records.

INSURANCE FEE PROBLEMS

Insurance fraud is a major area of violation and includes such activities as billing insurance for services delivered by others; billing insurance for missed sessions; waiving copayments (in most states, psychotherapists may waive copayments on an individual basis, but not as a rule, and there may be a requirement to inform the third party); billing couple, family, or group sessions as individual; falsifying diagnostic categories to fit reimbursement criteria; changing the date of the onset of the client's episode or the beginning of therapy to fit third-party reimbursement criteria; and trying to prevent denial of services based on preexisting conditions.

Often, well-meaning therapists try to provide financial relief by, in effect, colluding with a client to violate the client's contract with the insurance company. While therapists, like most medical professionals, are continuously frustrated by insurance companies and managed care, an ethical therapist will not engage in fraud and will feel that violating this ethic communicates lack of respect for the role of honesty and fidelity in relationships.

TERMINATING THERAPY

Ethical standards and guidelines in most mental health professions suggest that psychotherapists must terminate therapy when it becomes reasonably clear that the client no longer needs the service. When appropriate, therapists provide referrals to other providers. In addition, psychotherapists may terminate therapy when threatened or otherwise endangered by the client or another person with whom the client has a relationship. Most psychotherapists prefer to discuss and review the psychotherapy experience with the client; doing so allows for closure, an important aspect of the therapeutic experience.

—*Melba J. T. Vasquez, Ph.D., ABPP*

Questions to Ask a Psychiatrist

Maneuvering through a mental health system can be confusing and time-consuming at best, enraging and unhelpful at worst. Most women do not know the inner workings of the system, yet some basic knowledge of the system can be crucial to getting good care.

There are many "players" involved in mental health. Different people within the system may be performing similar roles but with vastly different levels of training and experience, as outlined in the chapter on how to choose a therapist. Within this system, only a psychiatrist or a licensed nurse practitioner can prescribe psychiatric medications. Psychiatrists and nurses have advanced medical training and may therefore be in a better position to consider organic causes for psychiatric symptoms. For example, depression may be caused from chronic stress, but the symptoms typical of depression may also be caused by an underactive thyroid gland, chronic alcohol use, or even anemia.

Over the last decade, the psychiatrist's role within the mental health team has been marginalized. Because psychiatrists' fees are usually higher than other mental health practitioners, many health plans have limited their usage. A referral to a psychiatrist is routinely made when medications are needed to treat a psychiatric illness or when the clinical picture is confusing or complicated by medical problems. Once a tentative diagnosis is made and treatment recommendations are agreed upon, the treatment itself may be implemented by other members of the treatment team, often a social worker or a psychologist. The psychiatrist may stay involved as part of the team to continue to assess the progress and to prescribe medications as necessary.

If you are referred to a psychiatrist by a friend, physician, or therapist, you may feel quite vulnerable, scared, or even angry. Entering into the relationship can be easier if you have an idea of what to expect and what to ask. The information that can be helpful to you may be broken down into three broad categories:

1. Information about the psychiatrist–client relationship.
2. Information about your diagnosis and prognosis.
3. Information about the treatment of your illness.

INFORMATION ABOUT THE RELATIONSHIP

Physicians hold a place of prominence and respect in most Western cultures. There are some physicians still practicing who were trained in an earlier, more patriarchal medical system. If you meet with one, you will recognize his or her relational style immediately —the doctor carries the power in the relationship and expects the patient to follow the treatment recommendations with little questioning. For many clients, this model can feel disrespectful. Although you should still feel free to ask questions of this kind of doctor, if this style does not feel comfortable to you, find another psychiatrist. Most recently, trained doctors have moved away from this model and now recognize that the client needs to be a full, active partner in the healing relationship.

You may want to screen a psychiatrist over the phone before you commit to an initial appointment. Before talking with a psychiatrist, you may want to think about what your needs will be in this relationship. Your needs may include the ability for the psychiatrist to communicate effectively with you and to be occasionally available outside of office appointments for emergency phone calls.

The following questions may help you choose a psychiatrist.

> Before talking with a psychiatrist, you may want to think about what your needs will be in this relationship.

What is the psychiatrist's training and specialty?

Psychiatrists are trained to perform a number of different tasks, ranging from medication management to cognitive behavioral therapy. However, most psychiatrists have a more narrow area of expertise. Research into the brain and behavior is expanding rapidly; it is impossible for a psychiatrist to have up-to-date information about all the different areas of psychiatry. For example, if a psychiatrist is training to become a psychoanalyst (a special kind of therapy), he or she may not have had the time to read all the research literature for prescribing new atypical antipsychotics to clients with schizophrenia. The bottom line is that you want to see someone who has general knowledge about what you may be dealing with. An analogy that may help is that you would not want to see a surgeon who specializes in heart transplants for pain in your knee.

> It is important that you start your relationship with a psychiatrist feeling empowered and feeling that the psychiatrist is firmly on your side. Remember that whatever the psychiatrist's education and training, you have hired him or her to work for you.

What is the psychiatrist's relational style?

Some psychiatrists are more reserved, not talking a lot and waiting for you to tell them what is going on. Some clients feel this is off-putting; some feel it is freeing. Other psychiatrists will be more probing and directive in their questioning. Some psychiatrists spend time specifically on the symptoms you are experiencing, while others try to understand your symptoms within the context of your life. Ask whether the psychiatrist is talkative, directive, quiet, and so forth. This way, you will know what to expect in the relationship when you sit down for your first meeting.

What is the psychiatrist's availability?

Many people are referred to a psychiatrist by a therapist or counselor strictly for a medication evaluation. If this is the case for you, you should ask whether the psychiatrist will be available to collaborate with your treatment team as your treatment progresses. It is reasonable to expect the psychiatrist to have regular contact with your therapist, particularly during times of medication change or an increase in your symptoms.

What are the parameters of the meetings?
Where will you meet, for how long, and how often?

Always ask about the psychiatrist's fee and whether he or she accepts your insurance coverage, if you have it. Find out the psychiatrist's policy about missed or cancelled appointments. Most psychiatrists will not bill for occasional contact between appointments, but you should ask. If the contact is frequent and the time spent lengthy, typically the psychiatrist may bill you or the insurance company for this.

It is important that you start your relationship with a psychiatrist feeling empowered and feeling that the psychiatrist is firmly on your side. Remember that whatever the psychiatrist's education and training, you have hired him or her to work for you.

INFORMATION ABOUT DIAGNOSIS AND PROGNOSIS

Initial Psychiatric Consultation Your initial visit or two with a psychiatrist are likely to be longer than the follow-up visits—anywhere from forty-five to ninety minutes. Before a psychiatrist can recommend medication for you, she must have a working diagnosis of what she is trying to treat. Some people feel a diagnosis can be objectifying and uncomfortable; others find comfort in having a "name" for what they are feeling. Initially, the psychiatrist may ask you many difficult emotional questions about your personal life, your friends, and family members, all in a short amount of time. The psychiatrist has to get so much information quickly it may feel as though she is not getting the full impact of your story or is skimming over the painful details. If it feels too hard to open up to a new person relatively quickly, consider bringing a trusted friend or family member along to help support you emotionally.

Most psychiatrists will follow a medical model interview during the initial consultation with questions that cover the following areas:

Presenting Symptoms. For example, if you are being evaluated for depression, the questions will focus on stressors in your life and also on physical effects of the depression such as changes in sleep, appetite, energy, concentration, focus, and sexual drive. If you are feeling frightened that someone is after you, follow-up questions would be designed to differentiate a psychosis from some other problem. You may be asked, for example, whether you hear voices inside or outside your head or whether you have suffered from a history of violence in any relationships in your life.

Past Psychiatric History. This would include any contacts you have had with the mental health system from childhood until the present. If you have taken psychiatric medications in the past, it would be helpful for you to bring the name and dosage of the drugs you were prescribed.

An initial psychiatric consultation will typically cover the following areas:

- *Presenting symptoms*
- *Past psychiatric history*
- *Past medical history*
- *Family history*
- *Social history*
- *Mental status exam*
- *Diagnosis*

> Some people feel a diagnosis can be objectifying and uncomfortable; others find comfort in having a "name" for what they are feeling.

You may be able to get a list of all previous medications from your pharmacy. Knowledge of recreational drug use, including the use of alcohol, is essential to any accurate assessment. Regular use of many recreational drugs (i.e., marijuana, cocaine, alcohol) can cause symptoms that mimic mental illness, particularly depression and anxiety. If you are taking any prescribed medications, there may be interactions between that medication and the recreational drugs you are using that are causing the symptoms.

> A psychiatrist should ask detailed questions about your menstrual history, particularly if it has been irregular or problematic.

Past Medical History. This category includes any illnesses or surgeries you have had. This information may be used to help determine the cause of your current symptoms or to help make a decision about drugs your body can tolerate. A psychiatrist should ask detailed questions about your menstrual history, particularly if it has been irregular or problematic. You may want to let the psychiatrist know whether your symptoms seem to be worse at any time during your menstrual cycle.

Family History. The psychiatrist will want to know whether there is any history of mental illness in your family in any known biological relative, including close relatives who may no longer be alive. A few psychiatric illnesses, for example Bipolar Disorder, have a strong genetic component and can be passed from generation to generation. If there is a mental illness in the family, it important to know whether the relative received any medication treatment for this illness. If a family member has a similar diagnosis and responds well to a medication, then others in the family with the same diagnosis may also have a positive response to the same medication.

Social History. Social history covers a very broad set of questions designed to assess the quality of the relationships in your life. The questions are about your family of origin, social supports, work, and school history. This part also includes questions about violence in your life.

> Never stay with a psychiatrist who does not listen, who does not take your complaints seriously, who is chronically unavailable, or who seems abusive in any way.

Mental Status Exam. This part of the initial interview can often be confusing to clients. To a psychiatrist, the mental status exam is the equivalent of the physical exam to a primary care physician. This exam includes questions about mood, feelings, how your thoughts are working (i.e., are they speedy, slowed down, unusually bizarre), whether you have hallucinations. also, this part includes questions about whether you have had thoughts of hurting yourself or others. Many mental illnesses, including depression, Bipolar Disorder, and schizophrenia, carry a significant risk of suicide. It is essential that the psychiatrist assess the safety of anyone who walks into his or her office.

Diagnosis. Toward the end of the initial evaluation—which may take one, two, or more sessions—a psychiatrist should be able to offer a tentative diagnosis. It is the psychiatrist's job to provide you with as much information as you need about the working diagnosis and the prognosis of the illness.

INFORMATION ABOUT THE TREATMENT OF THE ILLNESS

During the initial evaluation, be clear about the level of information you would like about your diagnosis. You should feel free to discuss the illness in great depth, even if it means returning for another session in the near future to address the nature of the treatment plan. In this collaborative relationship, it is the psychiatrist's job to educate you about the current knowledge within the field—he or she should provide you with enough information so that you are satisfied with the proposed treatment plan.

Since most psychiatric encounters end with a prescription for a psychotropic medication, you will want to get as much information as possible about the various medication options. For example, anxiety may be treated with either a daily dose of a selective serotonin reuptake inhibitor (SSRI) like Zoloft, or it may be effectively treated with a benzodiazepine, like Klonopin, taken on an as-needed basis. Certainly, information about potential risks and benefits of any medication should be outlined in detail.

Your psychiatrist should also be able to refer you to outside resources for support and information when needed. For example, if you have been diagnosed with Bipolar Disorder, your psychiatrist may refer you to MDDA (Manic-Depressive and Depressive Association), a group that provides support and information for individuals with mood disorders and their families and friends.

For most people, seeing a psychiatrist for the first time can be intimidating, perhaps even disempowering. But remember, knowledge is power. The more information you can get about the relationship ahead of time, the less uncertainty you face during the initial encounter. Never stay with a psychiatrist who does not listen, who does not take your complaints seriously, who is chronically unavailable, or who seems abusive in any way. Strive to find a psychiatrist with whom you are comfortable and who is comfortable answering any questions you ask.

—*Amy Elizabeth Banks, M.D.*

RELATED ENTRIES

Antidepressants

Antianxiety Medications

Antipsychotic Medications

Medication in Pregnancy

Mood Stabilizers

Polypharmacy

PART FOUR

Life Enhancements

The Importance of Exercise and Physical Activity for Women

The benefits of physical activity and exercise are well known. They include reducing the risk of chronic illnesses such as heart disease, diabetes, and hypertension, as well as lowering stress, increasing self-esteem, elevating mood, and improving body image. Therapists frequently prescribe exercise programs for their clients, particularly for those who are depressed, as physical activity has been shown to improve mood states and reduce anxiety. Inactivity, on the other hand, is as great a risk factor for illness as is smoking cigarettes. Yet most people will admit that they're not as physically active as they should be and that they feel they should exercise more than they currently do.

It is estimated that fewer than 10 percent of the adult American population meets even the minimal exercise guidelines recommended by the U.S. surgeon general. Women's levels of physical activity are lower than men's at any age, but the comparison gets even worse as women get older. Almost 60 percent of women in the United States are sedentary, and that percentage is reported to be even higher for ethnic minorities. The toll that this inactivity takes can be measured by the relatively high rates of heart disease, hypertension, diabetes, osteoporosis, and obesity among middle-aged and older women. When the risks of depression, anxiety, low self-esteem, and negative body image (problems that affect women at higher rates than men) are taken into account, one can only wonder why the benefits of an active lifestyle aren't enough to convince all women to be physically active.

A quick historical analysis shows that most females, especially those who attended school before Title IX (making exclusion on the basis of sex illegal in schools) came into effect in 1979 or before its full implementation in 1988, were not encouraged, if not actively discouraged, from participating in sports. In the not-too-distant past, exercise was considered to be "unfeminine" and unnecessary (in some cultural groups, this belief still persists). Few opportunities existed for girls, much less women, to be involved in the organized sports activities that were encouraged and readily available for boys and men.

This means that many adult women today, especially those over the age of forty, did not grow up playing team sports or being physically active, are unaccustomed to it, and do not necessarily expect it to be fun and enjoyable. When these (now) middle-aged women were growing up, gym class, or "P.E.," was a requirement that you endured, not enjoyed. Often it consisted of tedious calisthenics or exercises rather than fun and games. Exercise was another unpleasant thing you were supposed to do, almost like eating your full allotment of vegetables or keeping your nails clean. It's no wonder, then, that despite evidence that physical activity is not difficult to begin or to maintain, many adult women are not physically active.

The primary barriers to beginning and maintaining an exercise program are an initial lack of interest and the perception that exercise is neither fun nor enjoyable—that it is, in fact, time-consuming and painful. Since lack of exercise primarily hurts oneself, many women who have other family and job demands find it easy to place it last on their list of priorities.

There are also social and psychological barriers for women to begin exercising. Many women are self-conscious about their body image and weight. They may be anxious about wearing the right clothing or having the proper equipment. They may think they need to join an expensive health club if they're self-conscious about exercising outside or concerned about their safety. Many women simply don't know how to start or maintain a consistent regimen of exercise that could be an enjoyable rather than a painful experience.

> In the not-too-distant past, exercise was considered to be "unfeminine" and unnecessary.

Feminist psychotherapists have commented that exercise on a consistent basis is relevant to many of the goals of feminist therapy. Not only does exercise improve a woman's physical and mental health, it builds self-confidence and self-esteem, aids in stress reduction, and makes one stronger overall. Research has demonstrated that girls and women who are physically fit and who engage regularly in sports have better cardiovascular fitness, maintain an ideal weight, build muscular strength, and have greater stamina and increased energy. These women report more positive mood states, including having feelings of euphoria and a sustained sense of well-being during and after exercise, as well as an enhanced sense of self-confidence and positive body image. In short, they feel better about themselves and feel good about their own efforts to maintain their physical fitness, giving them an increased sense of self-control. Psychologist Joan Chrisler argues that enhanced fitness and strength contribute to independence and well-being, as women find they can do more things for themselves such as carry heavier loads, have greater stamina and endurance, and become less dependent on others to help them. Self-strengthening seems to reinforce self-efficacy —the belief that you are able to do what you would like to do. And it reawakens what almost every child feels when playing—joy in movement.

I coach girls and women in running programs for beginners, and I've found that the sense of mastery that each runner feels in achieving a goal to successfully complete a three-mile or 10K run or even a full marathon cannot be underestimated. When women experience what it is like to stay with a reasonable exercise program, when they see and feel its benefits over time, their sense of mastery is often applicable to other parts of their life as well.

> Exercise on a consistent basis is relevant to many of the goals of feminist therapy.

Participating in physical activities that are group- or program-based also allows women to taste the camaraderie within a group working together toward a common goal. Boys and men have had lifelong opportunities to work together as part of sports teams. In the past, women who exercised tended to be isolated, as there were fewer opportunities for team or group programs. Most girls today have had opportunities to participate on neighborhood soccer teams and, largely due to Title IX, have been exposed to a variety of sports activities in schools. And middle-aged women have been signing up, in greater numbers than their male counterparts, to participate in structured group programs. Often, these exercise programs are sponsored by charities and provide training programs, coaching, and social events at participants can get into shape together while raising money from sponsorship for a social cause, such as completing a twenty-mile hike to help victims of domestic violence, or a five-mile run for juvenile diabetes research, a two-day bike ride for AIDS research, or a three-day walk for breast cancer research. Many participants report that after they achieve their goal, exercise has become either an enjoyable habit or even a positive addiction in their lives, and they continue to pursue their physical activities on their own or with the other "team" members from their programs.

BEGINNING AN EXERCISE PROGRAM

Beginning and maintaining an exercise program are the two most difficult aspects of improved physical fitness. Statistically, almost half of those who begin exercising on their own quit within six months, and only about 25 percent of Americans exercise consistently enough to achieve physical benefits. The charities-based training programs do provide many of the necessary elements that help beginners to continue: a doable structured schedule, weekly face-to-face training sessions, a goal event about six months in the future, trainers, and social support. But these programs are available for only a small number of "privileged" participants. What about the great majority of women who do not have the time or means to spend on a structured program? What can the average woman do to increase her physical fitness and achieve some of the benefits of exercise?

Girls and women who are physically fit report more positive mood states as well as an enhanced sense of self-confidence and positive body image.

First, she can begin with the idea that any exercise and movement is useful and that she does not have to belong to a gym, participate in a program, or learn new skills to be fit. *Any* activity is better than none, so a woman who is busy can increase her fitness by walking briskly whenever and wherever possible in her daily routine. This can include walking up and down stairs in the time it would take to stand and wait for elevators, parking one's car in the first available space on the outskirts of a parking lot and walking briskly to the store, walking around the airport rather than sitting and waiting for a flight, or even walking around soccer or baseball fields while watching one's children's games.

Since women with children are least likely to exercise, they can be innovative in figuring out ways to exercise when children are at home with them, including doing aerobic exercise while watching a fitness videotape, running on a treadmill, taking small children for walks in strollers, and doing physical activities together with older children such as biking, walking, jogging, specific exercises, hiking, and any activity that can be done together as a family.

While certainly better than nothing at all, leaving exercise to chance or to when the weather is good and the children are cooperative is not enough to achieve the benefits of physical fitness. Many physicians counsel their women patients to work toward 120 minutes of aerobic exercise per week because this is a minimum amount to achieve cardiovascular benefits and should be doable for most women. If broken down into three to four segments, the minimum amount of thirty to forty minutes of exercise several times a week should be manageable and still enough to reap physical benefits.

✦

120 minutes of aerobic exercise per week is a minimum amount to achieve cardiovascular benefits.

Novice exercisers who are unaccustomed to the demands of physical activity often feel concern or panic when they experience the symptoms of exercise—many of which are identical to stress responses or symptoms of stress and panic, such as sweating, a pounding heart, breathlessness, muscular tension, or exhaustion. While new exercise programs should only gradually increase these symptoms, novices should know that such responses are normal. Experienced exercisers become habituated to the pounding of the heart, and sometimes even the nausea associated with pushing oneself to the limit, and are not unduly concerned when they engage in vigorous activity.

Most coaches will tell you that a structured program in which the amount of exercise is prescribed on a weekly basis is essential for consistent progress. All a woman has to do is follow the schedule (thirty minutes of fast walking or jogging or swimming, or aerobic dance every other day), but there should also be specific instructions about what to do should disruptions, such as pouring rain, a bad cold, business trips and vacations, illness, a sprained ankle or any other injury, and a sick child or parent, occur. Often it is when one's routine is disrupted that an exercise program falls by the wayside. Good exercise programs, though, generally try to account for such disruptions by allowing for a missed workout here or there or by offering alternatives to keep the momentum and program alive.

Two other important factors in starting and maintaining a steady exercise regimen are social support and companionship. Many programs and even therapists note that women who exercise together in pairs or in small groups are far more likely to continue than those who do it on their own. An exercise companion can serve as a woman's primary reinforcement when she initially begins to exercise until the exercise itself becomes enjoyable and she reaches a level of mastery at which she feels confident doing it on her own. Social support and companionship need not be physical—they can be virtual. Even women who exercise alone consistently but who belong to an Internet running discussion group comprising virtual running partners who e-mail each other daily about their runs, problems, and successes find they are far more likely to adhere to their programs because they know that others are waiting to hear about their progress.

✦

Women who exercise together in pairs or in small groups are far more likely to continue than those who do it on their own.

The most difficult part of becoming an active person is beginning an exercise program and finding activities and companions that you enjoy. Once a habitual routine of exercise is developed and you gain a sense of mastery and accomplishment, finding pleasure in doing the activity and reaping the benefits, you'll be more likely to make it a consistent part of your lifestyle. During consistent aerobic exercise, such as running, the body produces its own endorphins (naturally occurring stress and pain relievers), which create feelings of calmness and pleasure. For consistent exercisers, there is less need for external secondary reinforcement such as weight loss or lowered heart rate, as exercise becomes pleasurable in and of itself.

A PERSONAL STORY

I have been a recreational runner for the past twenty years, running consistently and with enjoyment. But I did not always exercise or run. In fact, I disliked running throughout high school and college even though I played a variety of team sports. Once I was on my own, without the structure of school or a team, physical exercise seemed to be an unwanted chore in an already full day. There was no focus to my exercise and I slowly slipped out of shape while pursuing my studies and career.

One spring many years ago, I went to watch the Boston Marathon with a friend. I thought that I would be there for about an hour. The crowds and the excitement grew as the lead runners arrived, and the stream of runners swelled and just kept on coming. I stood transfixed. I had never seen an athletic event so inspiring and exciting. Runner after runner responded to the crowd's cheers and chants while straining to the finish. I stood and yelled myself hoarse for several hours long after my friend had left. When all the shouting was over, I walked the four miles back to my apartment, marveling that ordinary-looking people could run 26.2 miles without stopping. The next day, still awed by what I'd seen, I ran one very slow and painful mile. I decided I would one day try to be part of that gallant parade on Commonwealth Avenue, streaming down to the finish line. It was the day after the Boston Marathon, the day that I became a runner.

> I walked the four miles back to my apartment, marveling that ordinary-looking people could run 26.2 miles without stopping.

I became a runner because I had a focus and a goal. The benefits of consistent running included more energy and better health, but these benefits were incidental to my goal of finishing a marathon. Over a period of two years, I went from running five miles a week to running almost fifty miles a week. Running daily became as routine as brushing my teeth, and I grew to love my training runs, even as my longer runs were challenging and exhausting. Two years after starting to run, I crossed the finish line of my first marathon. I was thrilled, but I knew it was not my ultimate goal. I knew I still had a long, long way to go to run a qualifying time for the Boston Marathon. But now I had become hooked on running and on the ways that running helped me to alleviate stress and improve my health. I continued to run on a daily basis as my marathon times dropped steadily but slowly. It took a long time, but I never lost sight of my goal. Fourteen years after watching that first marathon and thousands of miles later, I finally achieved my qualifying time for the Boston Marathon.

When the day of the marathon finally arrived, I was ready. I could hardly believe that I was standing at the start line of the Boston Marathon. As we prepared to run, tears welled up in my eyes, and my chest felt tight. I closed my eyes. A kid of twenty-three had set this goal, and now a woman of thirty-eight was fulfilling her dream.

> When I made the final turn onto Boylston Street and saw the finish line, my spirit was soaring.

The gun went off, and the running began. What a joy it was to move. It was everything I imagined—the crowds, the cheering, the excitement. I ran faster than I had planned, but I didn't try to hold myself back. After all, this was my marathon, and my celebration. I was fueled on fifteen years of dreams and training. I savored every minute, slapped every little hand that was offered, and smiled and thanked all the spectators and volunteers I could. I ran hard the whole race and gave it everything I had because I was so excited. When I made the final turn onto Boylston Street and saw the finish line, my spirit was soaring. I had never run this strong and felt this exhilarated at the end of a marathon. My time was 3:20, an impossible dream for an ordinary runner like me. After I finished, I walked back to my home along the course, three miles away, and cheered for all the runners still streaming in. I marveled at their grit and determination as the shadows lengthened and the temperatures dropped. Marathoners all, we were running and living our dreams.

The Boston Marathon made a runner and a marathoner out of me, a runner of ordinary ability but extraordinary determination. It was my challenge and my dream, and it pushed me to run a time I would never have imagined possible. It taught me that we can perform beyond our abilities if we target a goal, believe in ourselves, and allow our spirits to soar.

—*Connie S. Chan, Ph.D.*

Stress Management for Women

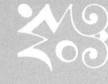

Women have a unique familiarity with stress. For many women, stress begins before they get out of bed. Imagine for a moment being awakened from a deep (and well-deserved) sleep by a four-year-old wanting breakfast. You get up (while your partner—if you have one—is still sleeping) and go to the kitchen to prepare breakfast and pack lunches for your family. By now, it's time to get everyone dressed for the day, and you are challenged with everything from looking for your child's lost sneakers to assisting your partner with selecting a clothes ensemble. Before you go to work, you probably have the responsibility of dropping off the kids, checking homework before the bus comes, and maybe even taking out the garbage. By the time you go to the office for the 8:30 A.M. meeting with an important client, you're exhausted!

While the presence of life stress for many women is a commonly shared experience, knowledge about the positive and negative components of stress often eludes us. Some basic knowledge about stress will lead you to a conceptual understanding of its positive and negative components. The rationale here is that if we, as women, understand ourselves and stress processes better, perhaps we can apply that knowledge to creating healthier, more productive choices for ourselves.

WHAT IS STRESS?

First, our discussion of stress must begin with a definition of what stress is and what it is not. There is also a need to discriminate between stress, stressors, stress reactions, and strain. *Stress* is the general concept of describing an internal or external "load" on the human system. A *stressor*, then, is a specific issue or challenge (external or internal) from which the "load" is derived. A *stress reaction* is the individual's reaction to a given stressor (whether it is physiological, behavioral, emotional, or cognitive). Furthermore, a stress reaction may be described as a responsive state of arousal that is characterized by physiological, emotional, and cognitive/perceptual components.

Within this context, experiencing stress is not solely a "bad" thing. Surely, it beats the alternative: a lack of arousal—or death! Consequently, the presence of a certain amount of stress is necessary and fulfills a basic human need for arousal and stimulation. Key studies in psychology have linked the need for arousal and stimulation to infant depression/death and brain development as well as to motivational factors in adults. Thus, when stress occurs within the context of the ordinary human arousal necessary to accomplish daily activities, it is a "good" thing. The presence of stress is even better when it serves a motivational function and creates within us a positive, exhilarating, and challenging experience that can lead to higher levels of performance. This level of increased performance caused by motivational stress is known as "eustress."

Strain, on the other hand, is the prolonged impact of the stressor on the system that can create overload, fatigue, and precursors to illness. Generally, when people refer to stress they are really talking about strain or "stress overload." Stress overload is a serious problem. Some reports have suggested that between 75 and 90 percent of all visits to primary care physicians are for stress-related complaints or disorders. Stress overload has been linked to many of the leading causes of death such as heart disease, cancer, lung ailments, accidents, cirrhosis, and suicide. It is also estimated 1 million workers are absent on an average workday because of stress-related complaints. Finally, a three-year study conducted by a large corporation showed that 60 percent of employee absences were due to psychological problems such as stress overload.

Consequently, it is the circumstance of experiencing stress overload that can lead to conditions of inadequate levels of functioning known as "distress." Most women can readily identify states of distress because they are often preceded by incidents of failure, threat, embarrassment, disappointment, and other negative experiences.

> Stress overload is a serious problem. Some reports have suggested that between 75 and 90 percent of all visits to primary care physicians are for stress-related complaints or disorders.

WHAT ARE SOME SIGNS AND SYMPTOMS OF STRESS OVERLOAD?

Each woman not only has a unique vulnerability to stress responses, but each person also has a unique and specific way in which she responds to stress. Each woman may exhibit unique symptoms and vulnerabilities in reactions to stress depending on factors such as her unique biological makeup, genetics, environmental situations, social support, and even the way she goes about making an interpretation of circumstances (whether she tends to be an optimist or a pessimist). Consequently, the signs of stress may vary among individuals to include symptoms that are physiological, emotional, or cognitive/perceptual in nature.

PHYSIOLOGICAL SIGNS AND SYMPTOMS OF STRESS

The physical symptoms of stress are first experienced through a gland called the hypothalamus, which produces at least nine different hormones that communicate to other glands in your body either a need for arousal or rest. These systems work together to orchestrate a heightened state of arousal as a physiological reaction to stress and are your body's way of getting you prepared for a "flight-or-fight" experience that is designed to preserve life. Studies have shown that women who are chronically exposed to daily experiences of the

EMOTIONAL SIGNS AND SYMPTOMS OF STRESS

- Irritability
- Angry outbursts
- Hostility
- Depression

- Increased jealousy
- Restlessness
- Withdrawal
- Anxiousness

- Diminished initiative
- Feelings of unreality or overalertness
- Reduction of personal involvement with others
- Lack of interest in previously enjoyable activities

COGNITIVE AND PERCEPTUAL SIGNS OF STRESS

- Forgetfulness
- Blocking
- Blurred vision
- Errors in judging distance
- Diminished or exaggerated fantasy life
- Reduced reactivity, productivity, and concentration
- Lack of attention to detail
- Preoccupation with or orientation to the past

- Decreased psychomotor reactivity and coordination
- Attention deficits
- Disorganization of thought
- Negative evaluation of self and future
- Negative self-esteem
- Perception of lack of control, or need for too much control

physical symptoms of stress (anxiety, racing heartbeat, digestive problems, increased blood flow, tensed muscles, elevated levels of hormones), run greater risks of experiencing health problems, particularly infection risk and hypertension.

Some of the key physical signs and symptoms of stress include, but are not limited to, increased heart rate, elevated blood pressure, sweaty palms, tightness of the chest, neck, jaws, and back muscles. Other physiological symptoms include headaches, diarrhea, constipation, difficulty urinating, trembling, twitching, stuttering, and speech difficulties. Finally, some women complain that when they experience stress, they have symptoms of nausea, vomiting, sleep disturbances/insomnia, changes in eating habits, fatigue, shallow breathing, dryness of the mouth or throat, cold hands, itching, and chronic pain.

EMOTIONAL SIGNS AND SYMPTOMS OF STRESS

While some women report that they experience emotional signs and symptoms of stress such as irritability, outbursts of anger, hostility, and depression, others report symptoms such as increased jealousy, restlessness, withdrawal, anxiousness, diminished initiative, feelings of unreality or overalertness, reduction of personal involvement with others, and lack of interest in previously enjoyable activities. Finally, some women describe that they experience emotional symptoms of stress that include an increased tendency to cry, being critical of others, self-deprecation, nightmares, impatience, decreased perception of positive outcomes, narrowed focus, obsessive rumination, reduced self-esteem, and less positive reactions to events.

> Each woman not only has a unique vulnerability to stress responses, but each person also has a unique and specific way in which she responds to stress.

Women who are placed in conditions of prolonged, insidious stress (such as conditions associated with sexual discrimination, unemployment, violence/abuse, harassment, etc., in the workplace) may report experiencing symptoms of what is known as the General Adaptation Syndrome (GAS). Women who experience the GAS have also experienced prolonged periods of overexposure to arousal/stress, followed by a period of resistance and a period that is finally concluded by an experience of "exhaustion." A woman who reaches the exhaustion or "burnout" phase may feel that she has been emotionally drained or beaten and may also feel that she must "give up." Her emotional reaction of "letting go," "fleeing," or "giving up" may involve characteristics of "survivor's guilt" because she may perceive that her choice to either abandon a cause or become physically removed from the environment leaves other women (potential victims) vulnerable.

COGNITIVE/PERCEPTUAL SIGNS AND SYMPTOMS OF STRESS

The cognitive/perceptual signs and symptoms of stress are usually the ones that may be first noticed by others. These symptoms include forgetfulness, blocking, blurred vision, errors in judging distance, diminished or exaggerated fantasy life, as well as reduced reactivity, productivity, and concentration. Other symptoms of cognitive/perceptual disturbances include a lack of attention to detail, a preoccupation with or orientation to the past, and decreased psychomotor reactivity and coordination. Some women report attention deficits, disorganization of thought, negative self-esteem, a decrease of meaning in life, as well as a negative evaluation of themselves, the future, and the situation. Finally, some women may notice that when they are under stress they perceive that they lack control or have a need for too much control.

When stress reaches the level at which it negatively impacts a woman's ability to attend to details or concentrate, her risks of underperforming or getting into accidents are increased. Some statistics state that 60 to 80 percent of work-related accidents are due to stress.

> Some statistics state that 60 to 80 percent of work-related accidents are due to stress.

WHAT ARE SOME STRESS FACTORS UNIQUE TO WOMEN?

Women experience some stress-related factors that appear to be more prevalent among them. For example, women tend to be more vulnerable to stress-induced illnesses, and their vulnerability can be traced back not only to familial biology and genetic predispositions, but also to women's socialization. From early childhood, girls are socialized to inevitably take on the roles and responsibilities of caretakers. Additionally, because of power differentials in terms of gender, women are often not well positioned in relationships (whether work-related or personal) to have as much control of their environment as men have. One researcher has examined the stressful nature of gender stereotypes and its impact on the task performance among females. This concept, known as *stereotyped threat*, implies that if we think that people hold unfair or unrealistic expectations of us, we may experience levels of stress that detract from (rather than motivate) our ability to perform optimally.

> The concept *stereotyped threat* implies that if we think that people hold unfair or unrealistic expectations of us, we may experience levels of stress that detract from (rather than motivate) our ability to perform optimally.

For women of diverse sexual orientations, ethnicity, or immigrant status, the challenges are even greater. Studies have shown that women of minority groups are at even greater risks for stress-related health problems such as hypertension or other types of cardiovascular diseases. Several studies have demonstrated that risk factors are compounded among these groups because of the multiple social, physical, and economic disparities that exist for women of color in terms of access to resources and services when needed. One study among women who were overextended looked at coping strategies in which women were given a choice of seeking support, letting some tasks go, or working harder. The study revealed that the majority of the women chose to "work harder" rather than to ask for help or to let things go.

WHAT ARE SOME WAYS OF COPING WITH STRESS?

Women who are exposed to high levels of stress could benefit from stress management training. One of the primary benefits of stress management training is that it teaches women to recognize and respond to early warning signs of overload and burnout.

Most experts believe that in order to optimally cope with stress you must learn to reduce the stressors in your life while learning to increase your coping skills to handle the stress that you do experience. Below are some tips on coping with stress by reducing it or managing it:

Share, share, share! This strategy focuses on your need to share the responsibilities (at work or at home) by either delegating or negotiating them. It also refers to your need to talk about the stress that you are experiencing.

Plan regular leisure-time activities. Create time for yourself each day that allows you to get away from routine chores and responsibilities. Women sometimes believe that leisure time must be "earned" after their work is done. But since "a woman's work is never done," we may never be entitled to get any rest! The best strategy is to realize that planning routine "downtime" is just as important as planning any daily activity.

> One of the primary benefits of stress management training is that it teaches women to recognize and respond to early warning signs of overload and burnout.

Just say "no." Give yourself permission to be assertive with employers, friends, and family members when they request that you assume extra responsibilities. It is also helpful to say "no" right away rather than saying, "I'll think about it." If you really want to do something, but know that it is an added burden, give yourself permission to provide an alternate solution such as sharing the job with someone else.

Set realistic daily goals that fit the way you live. Set reasonable daily priorities so that you don't overcommit by trying to do everything in one day. Also, notice when you have more energy during the day and when you begin to run out of gas. Plan more difficult and demanding tasks for those times when you have the most energy and reserve the less demanding tasks for your lowest energy times.

Change your mind. One of the most powerful stress management strategies is to engage in a positive self-talk. If you tend to see the "thorns" and not the roses, perhaps you need to reframe the way that you look at yourself and the world around you. Begin by drawing a vertical line down the middle of a sheet of paper. On the left side of the line, jot down three or four negative thoughts that you may have, then on the right side of the vertical line, write a rebuttal statement.

Remember that "multitasking" is "multitaxing." Combining too many activities can leave you feeling worn out, fragmented, and unbalanced. The key to managing this type of strain is to slow down and remember that just because you *can* do three or four tasks at one time doesn't mean that you *have to*!

Identify your sources of stress. If you feel stressed all of the time, it may be because you haven't reduced or eliminated the key sources of stress in your life. One way to identify key stressors is to analyze your daily activities to try to figure who or what is playing a role in creating stress for you. Sometimes key stressors come from seeing everything as a "priority." Rarely is everything urgent or something that has to be done today. Ask yourself if this is the best use of your time right now. Also, sources of stress may come from the types of people we put in our lives. Author Verna C. Simmons suggests that you divide the people in your lives into four categories: *Adders* (those who add value and support to your life), *Subtractors* (those who take, but rarely give), *Dividers* (those who create discord and chaos), and *Multipliers* (those who not only add value but create opportunities for you).

Learn relaxation techniques. There are several methods of relaxation that you can easily learn and apply just about anywhere. While all of these techniques are best applied while in a quiet place, some of them can be used whether you're standing in a long line or sitting in a traffic jam.

- *Progressive relaxation.* Progressive relaxation is a whole-body relaxation method. It is not wise to try this while in traffic! To utilize this technique, you must first loosen any tight clothing, close your eyes, and take several deep breaths. Uncross your legs and arms and let your hands rest on your lap. Begin by tightening your feet and toes and then relaxing them. Repeat this pattern of tensing and relaxing your muscles by progressively moving upward on your body, addressing areas of legs, thighs, hips and buttocks, stomach, back, hands, arms and shoulders and concluding with neck, face, and jaw muscles. Hold and study the tension that you feel throughout each point, then let go as you breathe out deeply.
- *Move your body.* Regular exercise, simple stretching, swinging your arms, walking around, or shrugging your shoulders can lead to muscle relaxation. Moving your body is a technique that you can use all day long and in just about any setting. Before you know it, you will notice that moving leads to increased energy.
- *Learn deep breathing.* Shortness of breath is a common symptom of stress. When you learn to control your breathing, you reduce the internal physical cues associated with your "flight-or-fight" response. To use this method, you simply take a deep breath through your nose with your mouth closed. Then, exhale very slowly through your mouth (with your lips pursed). Try to make sure that you spend twice as much time exhaling as you spent inhaling. Also make sure that you breathe deeply from your abdomen. Some people find it helpful to place a hand on their stomach to assure that the abdomen goes out and in with each breath. Breathing deeply increases the blood flow, slows down your heart rate, and lowers your blood pressure.

Although women have a unique familiarity with stress, we are capable of reducing the sources of stress and managing the stress that exists in our lives in order to regain a sense of power, energy, hope, and control that will restore balance to body, mind, and spirit.

—*BraVada Garrett-Akinsanya, Ph.D.*

Play

My friend Annie surprised herself a couple of weeks ago: she went sledding with her husband and kids, and she had fun.

"I laughed my head off," she reported. "I couldn't believe how great it was. I never do stuff like that." The experience thrilled her, made her feel alive, and yet, when her family considered going again the following weekend, she was glad that the weather turned rotten.

For Annie, play is alluring; it means freedom, flight. At the same time, it is a dangerous thing, something to be avoided. What is it about play that so threatens her—and is she alone in her ambivalence? Or are there women just like her who cannot, or will not, let themselves play?

Play does not refer only to playful activities per se—a sledding expedition, a game of softball, the staging of a practical joke—but rather to a particular state of mind that one can bring to any enterprise. Play is an attitude of openness and experimentation; it is a willingness to test hypotheses, to fail, to discover; to fly down a slope and land with snow in your face, laughing. It can happen when two musicians get together and jam; the melodies twist and turn, the notes are a string of surprises. It can happen in the kitchen, pots on the stove, the countertop a mess, the world reduced to a place of sizzle and scent. It can happen at the office, if we are lucky, when we hunker down and go deep into work, losing track of the sun's path through the sky. When we enter what psychologist Mihaly Czikszentmihaly calls "flow," when the process that occupies us becomes its own reward, we are at play.

Play magically combines what is earnest with what is fun. Players engage in their chosen activity with intent, but at the same time with a kind of impish refusal to take matters too seriously: the painter at her easel mixes and dabs her colors with focus and concentration, yet she knows that when all is said and done, this is just paint, and the surface before her just a canvas, one of many. She knows that the brush stroke she is considering might well be awful, and so what? There is risk involved, and she is comfortable with that. Above all, play is the embrace of possibility, the enthusiastic exploration of the "if."

We become immersed when we are at play, lost in thought or function. Sometimes, writers do not feel their fingertips hitting the keys. Sometimes, cross-country skiers do not feel their bodies straining into the wind. There is no "me" and then "the writing"; there is no "me" and then "the trails." Annie said she "laughed her head off": she was a disembodied creature, pure spirit sailing fast down a hill. Somehow, the self and the world are fused in an indeterminate middle ground. Psychologist D. W. Winnicott, who made a career out of observing people at play, describes this region as a zone where life is lived "in the exciting interweave of subjectivity and objective observation . . . an area that is intermediate between the inner reality of the individual and the shared reality of the world that is external to individuals."

Women, it would seem, by a combination of nature and nurture, are ideally suited to, in Winnicott's words, the "formless experience" of play. We understand this lack of structure; it inheres within us. Feminist psychologist Dorothy Dinnerstein argues that girls grow up comfortable with the kind of experimentation that play invites, the kind of permeability of self that it requires. Boys, she says, in order to define themselves as autonomous individuals, must pull away from their mothers so as to distinguish the budding male self from the female; they must create clear boundaries. As a result, they have a tendency to develop into rigid men, prone toward distance rather than engagement, toward compartmentalization, toward being cut off. Girls, on the other hand, do not require this kind of separation. The boundaries between a girl and her mother are diffuse; the two, sometimes, are one. The girl grows with and through her mother. She is flexible, porous, and, in a sense, more playful.

> Play is the embrace of possibility, the enthusiastic exploration of the "if."

And we hear often enough that women are more open than men, so much more comfortable with possibility. We are more interested in process than in product. We entertain options. We are multitasking experts. We fuse the personal with the professional: we cannot help ourselves. We are passionate. Our bodies are soft and curvy; we gush fluids without even trying. Like water, we envelop and we yield. *We flow*.

We should be naturals; we should be mistresses of play. But instead of pursuing play, we struggle with it. We see it as indulgent, a luxury we cannot afford. We are reluctant to set aside our obligations in favor of ourselves and our interests (however concealed they might be, these interests do exist). There is vacuuming to be done, groceries to be bought. Excuses can so easily be made. Often, it is the boyfriends and the brothers who play hoops while we sit on the sidelines or climb the Stairmaster to nowhere at the gym, slaves to discipline. Often, it is the husband who rolls around on the floor with the dog or the kids, who retreats from the stream of everyday life to a project in the basement, finding pleasure and solace not in the finished piece but in the tinkering. And if we happen to be upstairs at the same time cooking dinner, and if, for a moment or two, we forget that we are stirring and chopping for a purpose, do we not often enough feel, mixed in with the shock and the pleasure, some small measure of guilt?

Writer Diane Ackerman explains that play creates an almost magical setting in which "selves can be revised." Players test their limits, challenge their own assumptions, and learn new ways to do and to be. But doesn't "revision" of self imply that there is a stable self with which to work? In order to enter into the experimental space of play—to sojourn into strange territory where outcomes are a question mark—one must have a solid launching point, a strong enough sense of identity and purpose to tolerate all the unknowns that play courts.

This dynamic is most vividly depicted in babies who are just beginning to develop autonomy. They cruise across the kitchen floor to grab a bright blue ball; they squeeze a stuffed cow to make it moo. But after each accomplishment, each discovery of their own ability, they turn back to the adult who cares for them, the adult from whom they have not yet separated, and who, therefore, represents a more fixed self. It is a kind of check-in, a confirmation that "home base" still exists for them, no matter how they alter the planet or their understanding of themselves.

On the other hand, if there is no trusted home base, forays into the world of play become difficult. A few years ago I took in a dog from the shelter. She had survived an awful first six months of abuse, the play just beaten right out of her. I could see her trying to frolic with my other dogs when they charged into the woods to chase a scent or bounded down the trail for the delight of movement itself. After a tentative trot in their direction, she returned to my side. She lacked the confidence that if she launched toward discovery, I would remain for her. The prospect of losing oneself is terrifying when one has no faith in the reunion.

Perhaps this is where women are lacking as well. For us, fixed selves are hard to come by. Women, much more than men, suffer from low self-esteem; we typically report more intense self-criticism and problems with self-confidence. Under these circumstances, the permeability of self that Dinnerstein praises turns into a deficit. It can leave us shattered, without a core. We are a collection of fragments and gaps.

Feminist psychologist Kim Chernin, in her analysis of the epidemic of eating disorders among women, suggests that women have "a problem of identity, of not knowing who or what one is or might wish to become." This problem is only compounded by the seemingly limitless options now before us; women are "still deeply confused . . . about what it means to be a woman in the modern world." Chernin was writing over fifteen years ago, but her observations ring true even now. And in reference to the woman-as-man fashions of the 1980s, she asks, "Will we . . . simply dress and shape ourselves like men . . . and thereby avoid the years of experimentation, struggle, trial, and effort necessarily involved in this immense task of creating ourselves?" Could Chernin not, with these words, also be describing the qualities and purposes of play?

When we are missing that self to spring off from and return to, play becomes not a joy but a threat. It becomes, in a sense, too real, and it puts too much at stake. Without an identity that sits beyond the project at hand, waiting with generosity and patience, we see the chaos play necessitates as a reflection of our own internal state, proof of the disorder of identity we experience, on whatever level, in our day-to-day lives. Play no longer occupies a realm that, in Ackerman's words, is "exempt from life's customs, methods, and decrees," but a place that reflects and amplifies our worst fears about ourselves: we are uncreative, clumsy, stupid, a mess.

And let's imagine, for a moment, that we all did in fact have strong selves, clear ideas of who we were and where we were going. Let's imagine that we were comfortable putting our responsibilities on the back burner for a while. Would the world sanction our play? The male painter stationed on the side of the highway painting poppies, oblivious to the traffic whizzing by, is an artist; a woman doing the same is regarded as just a little dotty. A female Jim Carrey, looking foolish—completely foolish—is inconceivable, her face and body morphing before our eyes in the service of a good laugh. For every tame Carol Burnett, there are ten Richard Pryors—foul-mouthed, brilliant, bringing the audience to its knees.

The exuberance often associated with play, the abandon that play at its best demands, are considered unbecoming on women. We are not supposed to lose control; we are not supposed to lose ourselves in a moment. It is bad for us to get in the habit of granting ourselves such pleasure. Ackerman describes play as "rapturous" and "ecstatic," but culture precludes us from rapture and ecstasy, unless we are in the domain of sexuality or reli-

> ✦
>
> Play has so much, after all, to teach us. "We may think of play as optional," Ackerman writes, "a casual activity. But play is fundamental to evolution."

RELATED
ENTRIES

*The Importance
of Exercise and
Physical Activity
for Women*

*Women and
Spirituality*

gion—and in either case we are considered, at the very least, a bit strange. Our repertoire is severely limited.

Can we become players despite the odds? Maybe, instead of cowering, we can. Maybe we can rebel with play, harness it to instruct us and help us grow. Maybe we can find the courage—somewhere—to believe that responsibility can wait until we finish this draft of a poem, that we deserve the exuberance and joy a sled ride gives us, that we are not the mistakes we make at the pottery wheel.

Play has so much, after all, to teach us. "We may think of play as optional," Ackerman writes, "a casual activity. But play is fundamental to evolution." She notes that in animals it "invites problem-solving," it helps creatures hone their survival skills, it does nothing short of preparing them for life. Winnicott says that "on the basis of playing is built the whole of man's experiential existence." Someday, perhaps, woman's too.

—Deb Abramson

Women and Spirituality

The Very Reverend Margarita Martinez is the first female bishop of the Lutheran Synod in the Caribbean. She has, she says, been called to this work and led on this path, grateful that a part of her mission is to open a closed door through which other women may walk. The door has been closed for a very long time.

Women have been said to be the carriers of a culture. Women have also been known as the spiritual sex, oriented more to the metaphysical than the practical world. Yet, spiritual leaders remain traditionally male. In pagan times, gods as well as goddesses were worshiped; however, there was always a senior god, more powerful than the rest. And he was male, such as Zeus the Greek supreme god who reigned from the top of Mount Olympus, and his Roman equivalent, Jupiter.

With the advancement of human knowledge, the refinement of culture, and the modernization of belief in "one true god," this spiritual masculinity became even more apparent. Whether it is God or Allah, Jah or Buddha, the image of a spiritual leader has continued to be male. This belief pattern that fosters the male domination of the realm of the spiritual by definition creates a barrier between a woman and her divine self, thwarting her search for truly spiritually powerful role models.

Spirituality and religion are not used interchangeably. *Publishers Weekly* editor Lavonne Neff suggests that spirituality makes the connection between theology, which focuses on the divine, and psychology, which focuses on the human—spirituality is that interface between the human experience and the divine presence.

Times continue to change, values continue to shift, and women have made strides in assuming more traditionally male roles in domestic, business, and spiritual aspects of their lives. This empowerment has resulted in a dramatic increase in women's manifestations of their own spirituality.

More role models like Bishop Margarita Martinez have risen to prominence. "Father/Mother" God is now a frequent reference within women's groups and within literature. In these seemingly insignificant changes lay the breakdown of these barriers —women are now more able to manifest their inherent spirituality.

Despite these changes, the relationship of women to spirituality is still a very complex one. Women may be perceived as more capable of spiritual understanding; however, few men are yet comfortable with a woman as their most senior spiritual leader, falling back on old stereotypes of male domination of the spiritual realm. Spirituality, then, is nonsectarian, but speaks to the nonsecular aspects of our daily life, as shaped by our beliefs. More significantly, individuals turn to spiritual practices to address a whole host of problems, from stress management to self-empowerment. This clearly points to the importance of women needing to have the spiritual door wide open for them.

In early adolescence, independent spiritual development is minimal. Young adolescents who are involved in spiritual activities tend to reflect the beliefs that they have been taught by their parents. However, as they shift from parent focus to peer influence, adolescents begin experimenting with different ways of life and testing their belief systems.

> Spirituality is that interface between the human experience and the divine presence.

Particularly important for defining oneself and establishing one's authority are to define and establish what one's beliefs are and will be. A major challenge of traversing adolescence for young girls is the difficulty in maintaining their own sense of self and empowerment in the face of powerful societal and even physical pulls to the contrary. The importance of helping young girls to resist the loss of their identity before it is truly formed is well documented.

Even classic fairy tales can provoke the negative consequence of prohibiting the development of a young girl's voice and accelerating a loss of self in pursuit of beauty, boys, and being nice—the bread-and-butter characteristics of most fairy tales. The role that spirituality can play is to provide, in an age-appropriate manner such as a peer-group format, an opportunity to empower girls to challenge those images and expectations that silence their voices and promote demeaning stereotypes. By making them aware of these hidden stereotypes, they can also become aware of their own spirituality filling an essential role in their identity development.

Young adult women tend to have little time for reflection or conscious spiritual development as they confront the challenge of managing the multiple roles and priorities of career and family life. From the boardroom to the Little League field to the bedroom and everywhere in between, women at this stage of life can easily become overcommitted to meeting the expectations of others. If its importance to the individual is preserved, spirituality can, for women at this stage of life, help to maintain balance.

With the increase in the more New Age approaches to spirituality has come a greater focus on the development of the self. However, researchers such as Harold G. Koenig, associate professor of medicine and psychiatry at Duke University in North Carolina, suggest that the power of religion, especially among women, is the power of community. Hence, participation in group-focused spiritual development activities can be an important element in assisting the young woman in maintaining the balance between her secular life and her continued spiritual growth.

> Spirituality can provide an opportunity to empower girls to challenge those images and expectations that silence their voices and promote demeaning stereotypes.

For the midlife woman, the challenges change significantly. The potential for satisfaction and a sense of accomplishment is great with many midlife women at the peak of their careers, still healthy, and no longer subject to the frantic questioning of youth. However, women in this age bracket are also often caught between caring for slightly older but not yet emancipated children on the one end and aging parents on the other. Women of this age group also face major life challenges, any one of which, or even more so in combination, can lead to significant levels of discontent. The aging process can cause shifting self-identity—disability, premature aging, concern about her ability to fulfill all that is expected of her in her multiple roles, and concern about the aging of her own caretakers can cause enormous fears for a woman's future. Spirituality at this time can help the midlife woman maintain stability and reward her with quiet competence.

Another major source of midlife discontent for a woman is difficult relationships, primarily but not exclusively with her spouse. Some women sense that this is their last opportunity to give up an incompatible relationship and finally live the life that they had hoped for. The obstacles to do this at this stage of life, however, are huge—the economic factor alone is often a powerful deterrent as is the statistic that a divorced middle-aged woman has a high probability of remaining single the rest of her life. Other issues include identity confusion and loss and grieving. Women at this age are moving into the time when losses—parents, perhaps older siblings—become a regular part of life. Developing her spiritual needs helps a woman grieve, mourn, and take time to deal with these feelings rather than deny their impact or minimize their importance; this is an essential element of a woman's psychological well-being.

> A positive relationship with one's higher power and the development of one's spiritual center can lead to a renewed sense of meaning and purpose when one starts to feel that one's life is over.

These and other issues all appear to be handled with a minimum of psychological distress in women who have a more stable spiritual center and identity. Research has shown that women who were more connected to a spiritual group were consistently found to have better resilience, a more positive outlook, and a sense that they could overcome life's adversities with the aid of their higher power. With all of these challenges, the major changes taking place at this time of life and the shifts in one's basic identity can cause a woman to lose her "self." However, a positive relationship with one's higher power and the development of one's spiritual center can lead to a renewed sense of meaning and purpose when one starts to feel that one's life is over.

For the older woman, issues of identity and competence appear to give way to purpose and the ongoing need for social connectedness. A study of older women, found that the social aspects of spirituality and religion were most closely correlated with life satisfaction. This research distinguished between inner-directed spirituality, such as meditation, and the more socially based spirituality of group practice, church, and other organized spiritual activities. Although the researchers referenced past studies that had indicated a stronger linkage between intrinsic spirituality and well-being, their findings indicated that participation in religious activities played a key role in a woman's ability to be more resilient and maintain a sense of meaning in her life.

> Ultimately, the goal, aim, and purpose of developing one's spirituality as a woman is to engage in the learning process of a well-lived life.

SPIRITUALITY AND IDENTITY

An interesting theme that runs throughout all of the life stages described in the previous section is the importance of spirituality in assisting in the identity process. At each stage, a strong spiritual base is seen as a major factor in a woman's success with coping skills and self-management, whether it is in development, maintenance, modification, or acceptance of identity. The second equally powerful theme to emerge is not just the need for strong spiritual personal identity but that group-based spiritual activity has been found to be most

**RELATED
ENTRIES**

*Growth in
Connection*

Play

beneficial for women, from adolescents to mature women. Women's socialization tends to be more oriented toward interaction, with cooperation rather than competition the preferred method of play and problem solving. However, a deeper significance is that true spiritual development cannot be separated into internal-based or external-oriented spiritual development. Rather it calls on the individual to develop both the self and her connectedness, concern for, and ability to reach out to her fellow woman. At each stage of life, a connection with one's essence can inform and enhance life experience, build resilience, and bring meaning and centeredness to daily activity.

Ultimately, the goal, aim, and purpose of developing one's spirituality as a woman is to engage in the learning process of a well-lived life.

SPECIAL CONSIDERATIONS: CULTURE AND GENDER IDENTITY

In every culture, spirituality and religion are intertwined and play a major role in manifesting the belief systems that define the essence of the culture. Many of the traditional healing practices reflect the deep connection with the particular culture; for example, the Latino's understanding of the spirit world through Espiritism. In each instance, there is a great respect for those in the afterlife, as well as ancestral and natural forces unseen but present within life itself. For women from cultures where Espiritism, shamanism, or Voudoun are practiced, their role as spiritual healers or simply as the wise "Auntie" or "Grandmother" to whom everyone comes for advice and counsel is an important manifestation of their role as "carriers of the culture."

We can reasonably conclude that spirituality is a key to the manifestation of a woman's highest and best self, allowing her to tap into and bring forth that essential aspect of well–being—her purpose in life.

—*G. Rita Dudley-Grant, Ph.D., M.P.H., ABPP, and Jessica Henderson Daniel, Ph.D., ABPP*

Suggested Reading

ADDICTIONS

Denning, Patt. 2000. *Practicing Harm Reduction Psychotherapy*. New York: Guilford Press.

Kasl, Charlotte. 1989. *Women, Sex, and Addiction: A Search for Love and Power*. New York: Harper & Row.

Kaufman, Edward. 1994. *Psychotherapy of Addicted Persons*. New York: Guilford Press.

Peele, Stanton. 1986. *The Meaning of Addiction*. Lexington, Mass.: Lexington Books.

Peele, Stanton, and Archie Brodsky. 1975. *Love and Addiction*. New York: Taplinger.

Van der Kolk, Bessel A. 1987. *Psychological Trauma*. Washington, D.C.: American Psychiatric Press, Inc.

Online Resources

Alcoholics Anonymous: www.alcoholics-anonymous.org

Alcohol and Other Drug Addiction Services: www.alcohol-drug-treatment.net

Charlotte Kasl Email: empower16@aol.com

National Institute of Mental Health: www.nimh.nih.gov

SMART Recovery: www.smartrecovery.net

Stanton Peele Addiction Website: www.peele.net

Women for Sobriety: www.womenforsobriety.org

ADOPTION

Brodzinsky, David M., and Marshall D. Schechter. 1990. *The Psychology of Adoption*. New York: Oxford University Press.

Brodzinsky, David M., Marshall D. Schechter, and Robin Manantz Henig. 1992. *Being Adopted: The Lifelong Search for Self*. New York: Doubleday.

Lifton, B. J. 1994. *Journey of the Adopted Self: A Quest for Wholeness*. New York: Basic Books.

Simon, R. J., H. Altstein, and M. S. Melli. 1994. *The Case for Transracial Adoption*. Washington, D.C.: The American University Press.

Resources

Boston Korean Adoptees: members.aol.com/boskoradoptees

Global Overseas Adoptee Link (GOAL), Seoul, Korea: www.goal.or.kr

Minnesota Adopted Koreans: P.O. Box 141191, Minneapolis, MN 55414

Open Door Society: www.odsma.org

AGING

Browne, C. V. 1998. *Women, Feminism, and Aging*. New York: Springer.

Cummings, E., and W. E. Henry. 1961. *Growing Old: The Process of Disengagement*. New York: Basic Books.

Erikson, Erik H. 1963. *Childhood and Society*. New York: Norton.

———. 1964. "Inner and Outer Space: Reflections on Womanhood." *Daedalus* 93, 582–606.

Garner, J. D., and S. O. Mercer. 2001. *Women As They Age*. Binghamton, N.Y.: Haworth Press.

Hatch, L. R. 2000. *Beyond Gender Differences: Adaptation to Aging in Life Course Perspective*. Amityville, N.Y.: Baywood.

Rubin, Lillian. 1979. *Women of a Certain Age*. New York: Harper & Row.

Trotman, F. K., and C. L. Brody. 2002. *Psychotherapy with Older Women: Cross-Cultural, Family, and End-of-Life Issues*. New York: Springer.

Unger, Rhoda K. 2001. *Handbook of the Psychology of Women and Gender*. New York: Wiley.

ALTERNATIVE TREATMENTS

Baumel, Syd. 2000. *Dealing with Depression Naturally*. Los Angeles: Keats Publishing.

Dillard, James, and Terra Ziporyn. 1998. *Alternative Medicine for Dummies*. Foster City, Calif.: IDG Books Worldwide, Inc.

Murray, Michael T. 1996. *Natural Alternatives to Prozac*. New York: William Morrow and Co.

Murray, Michael T., and Joseph Pizzorno. 1998. *Encyclopedia of Natural Medicine*. Rocklin, Calif.: Prima Publishing.

Norden, Michael J. 1995. *Beyond Prozac*. New York: HarperCollins.

ANGER

Brown, L. M. 2003. *Girlfighting: Betrayal and Rejection Among Girls*. New York: New York University Press.

———. 1998. *Raising Their Voices: The Politics of Girls' Anger*. Cambridge, Mass.: Harvard University Press.

Brown, L. M., and Carol Gilligan. 1992. *Meeting at the Crossroads: Women's Psychology and Girls' Development*. Cambridge, Mass.: Harvard University Press.

Jack, D. C. 2001. *Behind the Mask: Creativity and Destruction in Women's Aggression*. Cambridge, Mass.: Harvard University Press.

———. 1991. *Silencing the Self: Women and Depression*. Cambridge, Mass.: Harvard University Press.

ANXIETY

Bourne, Edmund J. 2000. *The Anxiety and Phobia Workbook*. Oakland, Calif.: New Harbinger Publications.

Burns, David D. 1999. *The Feeling Good Handbook*. New York: Plume.

Slater, Lauren. 1999. *Prozac Diary*. New York: Penguin USA.

BODY IMAGE

Chernin, Kim. 1981. *The Obsession: Reflections on the Tyranny of Slenderness*. New York: HarperCollins.

Edut, Ophira. 1998. *Body Outlaws: Young Women Write about Body Image and Identity*. Seattle: Seal Press.

Hesse-Biber, Sharlene. 1997. *Am I Thin Enough Yet? The Cult of Thinness and the Commercialization of Identity*. New York: Oxford University Press.

Phillips, Katherine A. 1996. *The Broken Mirror: Understanding and Treating Body Dysmorphic Disorder*. New York: Oxford University Press.

Thompson, Becky W. 1994. *A Hunger So Wide and So Deep: American Women Speak Out on Eating Problems*. Minneapolis: University of Minnesota Press.

Stunkard, A. J., T. Sorenson, and F. Schulsinger. "Use of the Danish Adoption Register for the Study of Obesity and Thinness." 1983. In *The Genetics of Neurological and Psychiatric Disorders*. Ed. S. S. Kety, L. P. Rowland, R. L. Sidman, and S. W. Matthysse. New York: Raven Press.

Wolf, Naomi. 1991. *The Beauty Myth: How Images of Beauty Are Used Against Women*. New York: Anchor Books.

Online Resources

National Eating Disorders Association: www.nationaleatingdisorders.org

Anorexia Nervosa and Related Eating Disorders, Inc. (ANRED): www.anred.com

Body Image and Eating Disorder Referral and Information Center: www.edreferral.com

CHILD ABUSE

Dale, Peter. 1999. *Adults Abused As Children: Experiences of Counseling and Psychotherapy*. Thousand Oaks, Calif.: Sage Publications.

Miller, A. 2001. *The Truth Will Set You Free: Overcoming Emotional Blindness and Finding Your True Adult Self*. New York: Basic Books.

Pelzer, D. J. 2000. *A Man Named Dave: A Story of Triumph and Forgiveness*. Rockland, Mass.: Wheeler Publications.

Rhodes, Richard. 2000. *A Hole in the World: An American Boyhood*. Lawrence: University Press of Kansas.

Schwarz-Kenney, B. M., M. McCauley, and M. A. Epstein. 2000. *Child Abuse: A Global View*. Westport, Conn.: Greenwood Press.

Tower, C. C. 1988. *Secret Scars: A Guide for Survivors of Child Abuse*. New York: Penguin Press.

CHILDLESSNESS

Alden, Paulette Bates. 1998. *Crossing the Moon*. New York: Penguin Books.

Bartlett, Jane. 1994. *Will You Be a Mother? Women Who Choose to Say No*. New York: New York University Press.

Casey, Terri. 1998. *Pride and Joy: The Lives and Passions of Women Without Children*. Hillsboro, Ore.: Beyond Words Publishing.

Ireland, Mardi S. 1993. *Reconceiving Women: Separating Motherhood from Female Identity*. New York: Guilford Press.

Lafayette, Leslie. 1995. *Why Don't You Have Kids? Living a Full Life Without Parenthood*. New York: Kensington Books.

Lisle, Laurie. 1999. *Without Child: Challenging the Stigma of Childlessness*. New York: Routledge.

May, Elaine Tyler. 1997. *Barren in the Promised Land: Childless Americans and the Pursuit of Happiness*. Cambridge, Mass.: Harvard University Press.

Peacock, Molly. 1998. *Paradise, Piece by Piece*. New York: Riverhead Books.

Ratner, Rochelle. 2000. *Bearing Life: Women's Writings on Childlessness*. New York: Feminist Press.

CHRONIC ILLNESS

Kleinman, A. 1988. *The Illness Narrative: Suffering, Healing, and the Human Condition*. New York: Basic Books.

Miller, J. B., and I. P. Stiver. 1997. *The Healing Connection: How Women Form Relationships in Therapy and in Life*. Boston: Beacon Press.

Reid-Cunningham, M., D. Snyder-Grant, K. Stein, E. Taylor, and B. Halen. 1999. *Women with Chronic Illness: Overcoming Disconnection*. Works in Progress No. 80. Wellesley, Mass.: Stone Center Working Paper Series.

COGNITIVE BEHAVIORAL TREATMENT

Babior, S., and C. Goldman. 1990. *Overcoming Panic Attacks: Strategies to Free Yourself from the Anxiety Trap*. Duluth, Minn.: Pfeifer-Hamilton.

Beck, A. T. 1976. *Cognitive Therapy and the Emotional Disorders*. New York: International Universities Press.

Beck, A. T., A. J. Rush, B. F. Shaw, and G. Emery. 1979. *Cognitive Therapy of Depression*. New York: Guilford Press.

Bourne, E. J. 2001. *The Anxiety and Phobia Workbook*. 3rd ed. Oakland, Calif.: New Harbinger Publications.

Burns, D. D. 1980. *Feeling Good: The New Mood Therapy*. New York: William Morrow.

———. 1999. *The Feeling Good Handbook*. Rev. ed. New York: Plume.

Davis, M., E. R. Eshelman, and M. McKay. 2000. *The Relaxation and Stress Reduction Workbook*. 5th ed. Oakland, Calif.: New Harbinger Publications.

Fairburn, C. 1995. *Overcoming Binge Eating*. Rev. ed. New York: Guilford Press.

Foa, E. B., and R. Wilson. 2001. *Stop Obsessing: How to Overcome Your Obsessions and Compulsions* Rev. ed. New York: Bantam Books.

Greenberger, D., and C. Padesky. 1995. *Mind Over Mood: Change How You Feel by Changing the Way You Think*. New York: Guilford Press.

McKay, M., M. Davis, and P. Fanning. 1998. *Thoughts and Feelings: Taking Control of Your Mood and Your Life*. 2nd ed. Oakland, Calif.: New Harbinger Publications.

Nash, J. 1999. *Binge No More: Your Guide to Overcoming Disordered Eating*. Oakland, Calif.: New Harbinger Publications.

Zuercher-White, E. 1998. *An End to Panic: Breakthrough Techniques for Overcoming Panic Disorder*. 2nd ed. Oakland. Calif.: New Harbinger Publications.

DEBILITATING ILLNESSES

Miller, J. B., and I. P. Stiver. 1997. *The Healing Connection: How Women Form Relationships in Therapy and in Life*. Boston: Beacon Press.

Ornish, D. 1998. *Love and Survival: The Scientific Basis for the Healing Power of Intimacy*. New York: HarperCollins.

DEPRESSION

Jamison, Kay Redfield. 1997. *An Unquiet Mind*. New York: Random House.

Manning, Martha. 1996. *Undercurrents: A Life Beneath the Surface*. San Francisco: HarperSanFrancisco.

Smith, Jeffrey. 2001. *Where the Roots Reach for Water: A Personal and Narrative History of Melancholia*. New York: North Point Press.

Solomon, Andrew. 2002. *The Noonday Demon: An Atlas of Depression*. Carmichael, Calif.: Touchstone Books.

Styron, William. 1992. *Darkness Visible: A Memoir of Madness*. New York: Vintage Books.

DIALECTICAL BEHAVIOR THERAPY

Ekman, P., and R. Davidson. 1994. *The Nature of Emotion: Fundamental Questions*. New York: Oxford University Press.

Gendlin, E. 1996. *Focusing Oriented Psychotherapy*. New York: Guilford Press.

Greenberg, L., and S. Paivio. 1997. *Working with Emotions in Psychotherapy*. New York: Guilford Press.

Hayes, S., K. Strosahl, and K. Wilson. 1999. *Acceptance and Commitment Therapy*. New York: Guilford Press.

Kennedy-Moore, E., and J. Watson. 1999. *Expressing Emotion*. New York: Guilford Press.

Linehan, M. 1993. *Cognitive-Behavioral Treatment of Borderline Personality Disorder*. New York: Guilford Press.

———. 1993. *Skills Training Manual for Treating Borderline Personality Disorder*. New York: Guilford Press.

Panksepp, J. 1998. *Affective Neuroscience: The Foundations of Human and Animal Emotions*. New York: Oxford University Press.

Segal, Z., J. Williams, and J. Teasdale. 2002. *Mindfulness-Based Cognitive Therapy for Depression*. New York: Guilford Press.

DIVORCE

Fisher, Bruce, Robert E. Alberti, and Virginia M. Satir. 1999. *Rebuilding: When Your Relationship Ends*. New York: Impact Publishers, Inc.

Ford, Debbie. 2001. *Spiritual Divorce: Divorce as a Catalyst for an Extraordinary Life*. New York: HarperCollins.

Hetherington, E. Mavis, and John Kelly. 2002. *For Better or For Worse: Divorce Reconsidered*. New York: W. W. Norton & Company.

Krantzler, Mel, and Patricia B. Krantzler. 1999. *The New Creative Divorce: How to Create a Happier, More Rewarding Life During and After Your Divorce*. New York: Adams Media Corporation.

Neuman, M. Gary, and Patricia Romanowski. 1999. *Helping Your Kids Cope with Divorce the Sandcastles Way*. New York: Random House.

Rice, Joy K., and David G. Rice. 1986. *Living through Divorce: A Developmental Approach to Divorce Therapy*. New York: Guilford Press.

DOMESTIC VIOLENCE

Bancroft, Lundy. 2002. *Why Does He Do That? Inside the Minds of Angry and Controlling Men*. New York: Putnam.

Gondolf, Edward. 1997. *Assessing Woman Battering in Mental Health Services*. Thousand Oaks, Calif.: Sage Publications.

Jones, Anne, and Susan Schechter. 1993. *When Love Goes Wrong: What to Do When You Can't Do Anything Right*. New York: HarperPerennial.

Nicarthy, Ginny. 1986. *Getting Free: You Can End Abuse and Take Back Your Life*. Seattle: Seal Press.

EATING DISORDERS

Fairburn, Christopher, and Terence G. Wilson. 1993. *Binge Eating: Nature, Assessment, and Treatment*. New York: Guilford Press.

Garner, David, and Paul Garfinkel. 1997. *Handbook of Treatment for Eating Disorders*. New York: Guilford Press.

Johnson, C. 1991. *Psychodynamic Treatment of Anorexia Nervosa and Bulimia*. New York: Guilford Press.

Jordan, J., A. Kaplan, J. B. Miller, I. P. Stiver, and J. Surrey. 1991. *Women's Growth in Connection*. New York: Guilford Press.

Kaplan, Allan S., and Paul Garfinkel. 1993. *Medical Issues and Eating Disorders: The Interface*. New York: Brunner/Mazel.

Keys, A., J. Brozek, A. Henschel, O. Mickelsen, and H. L. Taylor. 1950. *The Biology of Human Starvation*. Minneapolis: University of Minnesota Press.

Miller, J. B., and I. P. Stiver. 1997. *The Healing Connection: How Women Form Relationships in Therapy and in Life*. Boston: Beacon Press.

Thompson, J. Kevin. 1996. *Body Image, Eating Disorders, and Obesity*. Washington, D.C.: American Psychological Association Press.

Zerbe, K. J. 1993. *The Body Betrayed: Women, Eating Disorders, and Treatment*. Washington, D.C.: American Psychiatric Press.

EMDR

Grand, D. 2001. *Emotional Healing at Warp Speed: The Power of EMDR*. New York: Harmony Books.

Lovett, J. 1999. *Small Wonders: Healing Childhood Trauma with EMDR*. New York: The Free Press.

Parnell, L. 1999. *EMDR in the Treatment of Adults Abused as Children*. New York: Norton.

Shapiro, F., and M. Forrest. 1997. *EMDR*. New York: Basic Books.

Online Resources

EMDR Institute, Inc.: www.emdr.com

EMDR International Association: www.emdria.org

ETHICS

Brabeck, M. M. 2000. *Practicing Feminist Ethics in Psychology*. Washington, D.C.: American Psychological Association.

Brown, L. S. 1994. *Subversive Dialogues: Theory in Feminist Therapy*. New York: Basic Books.

Gilligan, C. 1982. *In a Different Voice: Psychological Theory and Women's Development*. Cambridge, Mass.: Harvard University Press.

Lerman, H., and N. Porter. 1990. *Feminist Ethics in Psychotherapy*. New York: Springer.

Lerner, G. 1993. *The Creation of Feminist Consciousness*. New York: Oxford University Press.

Lorde, A. 1984. *Sister Outsider*. New York: Crossing Press.

Noddings, Nel. 1984. *Caring: A Feminine Approach to Ethics and Moral Education*. Berkeley: University of California Press.

Pope, K. S., and M.J.T. Vasquez. 1998. *Ethics in Psychotherapy and Counseling: A Practical Guide*. 2nd ed. San Francisco: Jossey-Bass.

Worell, Judith, and Norine G. Johnson. 1997. *Shaping the Future of Feminist Psychology: Education, Research,*

and Practice. Washington, D.C.: American Psychological Association.

Worell, Judith, and Pamela Remer. 1992. *Feminist Perspectives in Therapy: An Empowerment Model for Women*. New York: John Wiley and Sons.

EXERCISE

Gerrish, Michael. 1999. *When Working Out Isn't Working Out: A Mind/Body Guide to Conquering Fitness Obstacles*. New York: Griffin Trade Paperback.

Goldberg, Linn, and Diane Elliot. 2000. *The Healing Power of Exercise: Your Guide to Treating Diabetes, Depression, Heart Disease, High Blood Pressure, Arthritis, and More*. New York: John Wiley and Sons.

Hays, Kate. 2002. *Move Your Body, Tone Your Mood: The Workout Therapy Book*. Oakland, Calif.: New Harbinger Publications.

Leith, Larry M. 1998. *Exercising Your Way to Better Mental Health: Combat Stress, Fight Depression, and Improve Your Overall Mood and Self-Concept with These Simple Exercises*. Morgantown, W.V.: Fitness Information Technology.

GRIEF

Bowlby, John. 2000. *Loss: Sadness and Depression*. New York: Basic Books.

Doty, Mark. 1996. *Heaven's Coast: A Memoir*. New York: HarperCollins.

Freud, Sigmund. 1976. "Mourning and Melancholia." In *The Complete Psychological Works*. Vol. 14, edited by J. Strachey. New York: Norton.

Kubler-Ross, Elisabeth. 1997. *On Death and Dying*. New York: Simon & Schuster.

Lewis, C. S. 1961. *A Grief Observed*. San Francisco: Harper San Francisco.

Rando, Therese. 1991. *How to Go on Living When Someone You Love Dies*. New York: Bantam Books.

Raphael, Beverly. 1983. *The Anatomy of Bereavement*. New York: Basic Books.

Online Resources

Compassionate Friends: www.compassionatefriends.org
NPO helping families cope with the death of a child.

Death and Dying: www.death-dying.com
Resources at this site include a chat room, message boards, and links to articles, newsletters, and related sites for grief and bereavement.

GriefNet: rivendell.org
Online grief support groups supervised by a clinical psychologist.

State University of New York University at Buffalo Counseling Center: Coping with Death and Dying: www.ub-counseling.buffalo.edu/deathgrief.shtml
Informational site targeted at college students discussing phases of bereavement with suggestions on coping with death.

GROUP THERAPY

Herman, Judith. 1997. *Trauma and Recovery*. New York: Basic Books.

Yalom, Irvin D. 1995. *The Theory and Practice of Group Psychotherapy*. New York: Basic Books.

INFERTILITY

Benson, H., and M. Klipper. 1976. *The Relaxation Response*. New York: Avon.

Benson, H., E. M. Stuart, and Staff of the Mind/Body Medical Institute. 1992. *The Wellness Book: The Comprehensive Guide to Maintaining Health and Treating Stress-Related Illness*. New York: Carol Publishing.

Burns, David. 1999. *The Feeling Good Handbook*. New York: Plume.

Ceballo, Rosario. 1999. "The Only Black Woman Walking the Face of the Earth Who Cannot Have a Baby." In *Women's Untold Stories*, edited by M. Romero and A. Stewart. New York: Routledge.

Domar, A., and H. Dreher. 1996. *Healing Mind Healthy Woman: Using the Mind-Body Connection to Manage Stress and Take Control of Your Life*. New York: Henry Holt and Company.

Griel, Arthur. 1991. *Not Yet Pregnant: Infertile Couples in Contemporary America*. New Brunswick and London: Rutgers University Press.

Mullens, Anne. 1990. *Missed Conceptions: Overcoming Infertility*. Scarborough, Ontario: McGraw-Hill.

Salzer, Linda P. 1991. *Surviving Infertility: A Compassionate Guide Through the Emotional Crisis of Infertility*. New York: HarperPerennial.

MEDICATIONS IN PREGNANCY

Stotland, N. L., and D. E Stewart. 2001. *Psychological Aspects of Women's Health Care*. Washington, D.C.: American Psychiatric Press.

MENOPAUSE

Ford, Gillian. 1993. *What's Wrong with My Hormones?* Newcastle, Calif.: Desmond Ford Publications.

Northrup, C. 2001. *The Wisdom of Menopause: Creating Physical and Emotional Health and Healing During the Change*. New York: Bantam Doubleday Dell Publishing.

Oliver, M. 1986. *Dreamwork*. New York: The Atlantic Monthly Press.

Weed, S. 1992. *Menopausal Years, the Wise Woman Way*. Woodstock, N.Y.: Ash Tree Publishing.

MOTHERHOOD

Benkov, L. 1994. *Reinventing the Family: The Emerging Story of Lesbian and Gay Parents*. New York: Crown.

Garcia Coll, C., J. L. Surrey, and K. Weingarten. 1995. *Mothering Against the Odds: Diverse Voices of Contemporary Mothers*. New York: Guilford Press.

Grossman, F. K., L. S. Eichler, and S. A. Winickoff. 1980. *Pregnancy, Birth, and Parenthood*. San Francisco: Jossey-Bass.

Josselson, Ruthellen. 1996. *Revising Herself: The Story of Women's Identity from College to Midlife*. New York: Oxford University Press.

Lamott, Anne. 1993. *Operating Instructions: A Journal of My Son's First Year*. New York: Fawcett Columbine Book.

Lederman, R. P. 1984. *Psychosocial Adaptation in Pregnancy*. New York: Prentice-Hall.

Leifer, M. 1980. *Psychological Aspects of Motherhood*. New York: Praeger.

Mercer, R. T. 1995. *Becoming a Mother: Research on Maternal Identity from Rubin to the Present*. New York: Springer.

———. 1986. *First-Time Motherhood: Experiences from Teens to Forties*. New York: Springer.

Stern, D. N., N. Bruschweiler-Stern, and A. Freeland. 1998. *The Birth of a Mother: How the Motherhood Experience Changes You Forever*. New York: Basic Books.

POST-TRAUMATIC STRESS DISORDER

Herman, J. 1992. *Trauma and Recovery*. New York: Basic Books.

Jordan, J., A. Kaplan, J. B. Miller, I. P. Stiver, and J. Surrey. 1991. *Women's Growth in Connection*. New York: Guilford Press.

Miller, J. B. 1988. *Connections, Disconnections, and Violations*. Works in Progress No. 52. Wellesley, Mass.: Stone Center Working Paper Series.

RAPE

Warshaw, R. 1994. *I Never Called It Rape*. New York: Harper Perennial.

RELATIONSHIPS

Brehm, S., R. Miller, D. Perlman, and S. Campbell. 2002. *Intimate Relationships*. Boston: McGraw-Hill.

Fehr, B. 1996. *Friendship Processes*. Thousand Oaks, Calif.: Sage Publications.

Hatfield, E., and R. Rapson. 1996. *Love and Sex: Cross-Cultural Perspectives*. Boston: Allyn and Bacon.

Hendrick, C., and S. S. Hendrick. 2000. *Close Relationships: A Sourcebook*. Thousand Oaks, Calif.: Sage Publications.

O'Conner, P. 1992. *Friendships between Women*. New York: Guilford Press.

Steil, J. 1997. *Marital Equality: Its Relationship to the Well-Being of Husbands and Wives*. Thousand Oaks, Calif.: Sage Publications.

Weinstock, J. S., and E. Rothblum. 1996. *Lesbian Friendships: For Ourselves and Each Other*. New York: New York University Press.

Winstead, B. A., V. J. Derlega, and S. Rose. 1997. *Gender and Close Relationships*. Thousand Oaks, Calif.: Sage Publications.

Wood, J. 1996. *Gendered Relationships*. Mountain View, Calif.: Mayfield Publishing Company.

SEXUALITY

Berman, Jennifer, and Laura Berman. 2001. *For Women Only: A Revolutionary Guide to Overcoming Sexual Dysfunction and Reclaiming Your Sex Life*. New York: Henry Holt.

Kaschak, Ellyn, and Leonore Tiefer. 2001. *A New View of Women's Sexual Problems*. Binghamton, N.Y.: Haworth Press.

STRESS REDUCTION

Bach, George R., and Ronald M. Deutsch. 1985. *Stop! You're Driving Me Crazy*. New York: Berkley Books.

Bost, Brent W. 2001. *The Hurried Woman Syndrome: Healing for the 50 Million Women Who Suffer*. New York: Vantage Press.

Carlson, Richard. 1998. *Don't Sweat the Small Stuff at Work: Simple Ways to Minimize Stress and Conflict While Bringing Out the Best in Yourself and Others*. New York: Hyperion Press.

Cook, Suzan D. Johnson. 1998. *Too Blessed to Be Stressed: Words of Wisdom for Women on the Move*. Nashville, Tenn.: Thomas Nelson.

Davis, Martha, Matthew McKay, and Elizabeth Robbins Eshelman. 2000. *The Relaxation and Stress Reduction Workbook*. Oakland, Calif.: New Harbinger Publications.

Jeffers, Susan. 1988. *Feel the Fear and Do It Anyway*. New York: Fawcett Books.

Schulz, Mona Lisa, and C. Northrup. 1999. *Awakening Intuition: Using Your Mind-Body Network for Insight and Healing*. New York: Three Rivers Press.

Weekes, Claire. 1991. *Hope and Help for Your Nerves*. New York: Signet.

TRAUMA

Freyd, Jennifer J. 1996. *Betrayal Trauma: The Logic of Forgetting Abuse*. Cambridge, Mass.: Harvard University Press.

Herman, Judith L. 1992. *Trauma and Recovery*. New York: Basic Books.

Janoff-Bulman, Ronnie. 1992. *Shattered Assumptions: Toward a New Psychology of Trauma*. New York: Free Press.

Contributors

Deb Abramson has had work appear in numerous publications, including *The New York Times Magazine, Self,* and *The Sun*. She received a 1999 Pushcart Prize nomination and an honorable mention in *Best American Essays 2002*. She is the author of *Shadow Girl: A Memoir of Attachment* and lives in Vermont with her family.

Nancy Lynn Baker, Ph.D., ABPP, is a diplomate in forensic psychology and works as a clinical and consulting psychologist. She has extensive experience evaluating and treating individuals who have experienced trauma.

Amy Elizabeth Banks, M.D., is Medical Director for Mental Health at the Fenway Community Health Center; on the faculty at the Jean Baker Miller Training Institute, Wellesley College; and an instructor in psychiatry at Harvard Medical School. Her private practice in Lexington, Massachusetts, specializes in the relational-cultural treatment of trauma survivors.

Susan A. Basow, Ph.D., is Charles A. Dana Professor of Psychology at Lafayette College. She is also the author of *Gender: Stereotypes and Roles* as well as numerous journal articles.

Nadine Boughton, M.A., holds a degree in expressive therapy from Lesley University and is a writer, educator, and psychotherapist in private practice. Her poetry has been published in *Open Mind*, a HarperCollins anthology of women's writing.

Ellen Braaten, Ph.D., is on the faculty at Harvard Medical School and is a staff psychologist at Massachusetts General Hospital. She is the co-author of *Straight Talk about Psychological Testing for Kids*.

Laura S. Brown, Ph.D., ABPP, is a professor of psychology at Argosy University and has a private practice in psychology. She is the 1997 winner of the Sarah Haley Award for her clinical work in the field of trauma from the International Society for Traumatic Stress Studies.

Lyn Mikel Brown, Ed.D., is an associate professor of education and human development and the director of Women's, Gender, and Sexuality Studies at Colby College. She is the author of *Raising Their Voices: The Politics of Girls' Anger* and *Girlfighting: Betrayal and Rejection Among Girls*.

Thema Bryant-Davis, Ph.D., directs SHARE, a sexual harassment/assault counseling program at Princeton University. She is also an American Psychological Association representative to the United Nations. Dr. Bryant-Davis is the author of *Mangos and Manna: Poetry for the Body and Soul*.

Silvia Sara Canetto, Ph.D., is a professor of psychology at Colorado State University. She has edited several books, including *Women and Suicidal Behavior* and *Teaching Diversity: Challenges, Complexities, Identity, and Integrity*.

Nell Casey is the editor of *Unholy Ghost: Writers on Depression*.

Connie S. Chan, Ph.D., is a professor in the College of Public and Community Service at the University of Massachusetts–Boston. A clinical psychologist, she is the author of *If It Runs in the Family: At Risk for Depression*. She is an avid runner and marathoner who coaches and advises athletes on motivation and performance.

Allyson Cherkasky, Ph.D., is a psychologist in the Women's Health Center at the Cambridge Health Alliance and a clinical instructor of psychology at Harvard Medical School. She also works at Newton-Wellesley Behavioral Medicine and Eating Disorders and in private practice.

Dana L. Comstock, Ph.D., is a professor of counseling at St. Mary's University. She integrates relational-cultural theory into her writing and teaching. She is also a therapist in private practice specializing in prenatal and perinatal loss and trauma.

Jennifer Coon-Wallman, Psy.D., is a psychotherapist and art therapist in private practice in Lexington, Massachusetts. She is also an adjunct professor at Lesley University in the master's degree program for expressive therapy.

Jessica Henderson Daniel, Ph.D., ABPP, is a past president of the Society for the Psychology of Women, a Division of the American Psychological Association. She is director of Training in Psychology and associate director of the LEAH Training Program in Adolescent Medicine, both at the Children's Hospital, Boston. Her faculty appointment is in the Department of Psychiatry, Harvard Medical School.

Priscilla Dass-Brailsford, Ed.D., is an assistant professor in the Division of Counseling and Psychology at Lesley University.

Kathryn Davis, B.A., LICSW, holds a degree in psychology from the University of Denver and an MSSW from Columbia University. After completing five years of AIDS social work in the Bronx, she served as the clinical director at a teen emergency assessment unit in Watertown, Massachusetts. Most recently, she's been the clinical director at Aftercare Services, a community-based outpatient mental health and substance abuse program.

Kunya S. Desjardins, Ph.D., is an assistant dean of Counseling and Support Services at the Massachusetts Institute of Technology.

Lisa Dierbeck, who lives in Brooklyn, is the author of *One Pill Makes You Smaller,* a novel about growing up in the 1970s. Twice nominated for a Pushcart Prize, her work has been published in numerous literary journals and anthologies. She is a frequent contributor to *Barron's* and *The New York Times Book Review.*

G. Rita Dudley-Grant, Ph.D., M.P.H., ABPP, is a diplomate in clinical psychology and the director of Program Development for Virgin Islands Behavioral Services in St. Croix, USVI. She is the co-editor of *Psychology and Buddhism: From Individual to Global Community* and has worked and published on spiritual development and psychological well-being for many years.

Mark N. Friedman, D.O., is a neurologist and internist who specializes in neurohormonal disorders and is the director of the NeuroEndocrine Wellness (NEW) Center in Orlando, Florida. His work has been published in various academic journals and textbooks and has appeared in *Vogue* magazine. Dr. Friedman completed a three-year fellowship in neuroendocrinology at Beth Israel Deaconess Medical Center in Boston and was granted a research fellowship award by the Epilepsy Foundation of America.

BraVada Garrett-Akinsanya, Ph.D., is a licensed psychologist and the president of Brakins Consulting & Psychological Services. Dr. Garrett-Akinsanya has written a number of scholarly articles and monologues on topics of wellness and mental health across the life span. Currently, she writes a biweekly column entitled "The Wellness Wheel" for the Insight Health Section of *Insight Newspaper* in Minneapolis.

Patricia A. Geller, Ed.D., is a licensed psychologist with a degree from the Harvard Graduate School of Education. She has a private practice in psychotherapy in Lexington, Massachusetts, and is an EMDRIA-approved consultant in EMDR.

Beverly Greene, Ph.D., ABPP, is a diplomate in clinical psychology and a professor of psychology at St. John's University. A practicing psychologist, she has written numerous publications on the psychologies of women of color.

Janet Shibley Hyde, Ph.D., is a Helen Thompson Woolley Professor of Psychology and Women's Studies at the University of Wisconsin–Madison. She has published several academic books, including *Half the Human Experience: The Psychology of Women.*

Dana Crowley Jack, Ed.D., holds a degree in human development and psychology. She is a professor at Fairhaven College/Western Washington University and the author of *Silencing the Self: Women and Depression, Behind the Mask: Destruction and Creativity in Women's Aggression,* and *Moral Vision and Professional Decisions,* as well as other articles and chapters on women's psychology.

Judith V. Jordan, Ph.D., is the co-director of the Jean Baker Miller Training Institute at Wellesley College and an assistant professor of psychology at Harvard Medical School. She is the co-author of *Women's Growth in Connection* and editor of *Women's Growth in Diversity.*

Lori Kaplowitz, M.D., is an instructor in adult psychiatry at Harvard Medical School. She has a private practice in psychotherapy and psychopharmacology in Cambridge, Massachusetts, and specializes in issues related to women's reproductive health.

Laura Kramer, M.D., is a psychiatrist in private practice in the Boston area.

Jane MacDonald, Ph.D., a psychologist who practices in Newton, Massachusetts, is on the faculty of the Jean Baker Miller Training Institute at Wellesley College.

Susan Mahler, M.D., is a writer and a psychiatrist practicing in the Boston area. Her essays have appeared in *The American Scholar, The Threepenny Review, Pandora,* and other publications.

Martha Brown Martin, M.D., is a psychiatrist and psychoanalyst in private practice in Bethesda, Maryland. She recently completed an M.F.A. in creative nonfiction at Goucher College, receiving the Christine White Memorial Award at graduation for her memoir, *Sister Sally.*

Susan J. Miller, Psy.D., is a psychologist in private practice in Belmont, Massachusetts. She is also a clinical supervisor at McLean Hospital in Belmont.

Cynthia W. Moore, Ph.D., is a clinical instructor in psychiatry at Harvard Medical School. She is also the project director for the Close Relationships Project at the Judge Baker Children's Center.

Bonnie Ohye, Ph.D., is an assistant clinical professor at Harvard Medical School and a clinical associate in psychiatry in the Massachusetts General Hospital Department of Psychiatry. She is also the author of *Mothering From the Heart: Lessons on Listening to Our Children and Ourselves.*

Lucia F. O'Sullivan, Ph.D., is an assistant professor of clinical psychology at Columbia University. She is also a co-editor of *Sexual Coercion in Dating Relationships.*

Karen Propp, Ph.D., is the author of two memoirs, *In Sickness & In Health: A Love Story* and *The Pregnancy Project: Encounters with Reproductive Therapy.* She has written for *Lilith, The Sun, Women's Review of Books,* and many other publications.

Susan Kushner Resnick is the author of *Sleepless Days: One Woman's Journey Through Postpartum Depression.* She is also a health reporter for *The Providence Journal.* She lives in Massachusetts with her husband and two children.

Joy K. Rice, Ph.D., is a clinical professor of psychiatry, emerita professor of Educational Policy Studies and Women's Studies at the University of Wisconsin–Madison, and a clinical psychologist in private practice. She is the co-author of *Living through Divorce: A Developmental Approach to Divorce Therapy.*

Laurie Rosenblatt, M.D., is a psychiatrist in the Dana Farber Cancer Institute's Department of Psychosocial Oncology. She is also an instructor at Harvard Medical School.

Janis V. Sanchez-Hucles, Ph.D., is a professor of psychology at Old Dominion University and does part-time clinical and consulting work in her private practice. She writes and consults on issues focusing on women, work and relationships, diversity, and cultural competence. Dr. Sanchez-Hucles is the author of *The First Session with African Americans: A Step-by-Step Guide.*

Audrey Schulman is the author of three novels, *The Cage, Swimming with Jonah,* and *A House Named Brazil.* She has written for *Ms., Hope,* and *E,* among other publications.

Angel Seibring, Ph.D., is an instructor in psychiatry at Harvard Medical School, a psychologist at Brigham and Women's Hospital, and a consultant at Boston IVF, an outpatient fertility and in-vitro fertilization center. She also has a private practice in Arlington, Massachusetts.

Elizabeth B. Simpson, M.D., is a clinical instructor in psychiatry at the Harvard Medical School and the director of the Dialectical Behavior Therapy program at Massachusetts Mental Health Center (MMHC) in Boston. She is a senior trainer in dialectical behavior therapy.

Lauren Slater, Ed.D., is a psychologist and Knight-Ridder Science Journalist Fellow at the Massachusetts Institute of Technology. Her writing has appeared in the *Best American Science Writing 2002,* and she is the author of *Love Works Like This, Lying: A Metaphorical Memoir, Prozac Diary,* and *Welcome to My Country.*

Carole Sousa is a nationally recognized leader in the movement to end domestic violence. She has led intervention groups for abusive men, developed curriculum for abusive men on the effects of domestic violence on their children, and co-developed and taught the Massachusetts Department of Public Health certification course for professionals and others who plan to work with abusive men. Ms. Sousa has received numerous awards and has been an appointee to the Massachusetts Governor's Commission on Domestic Violence since 1994.

Meg I. Striepe, Ph.D., is a research scientist at the Center for Research on Women, Wellesley College. She also works as a staff psychologist at the Trauma Center and has a psychotherapy practice, specializing in sexual health, in Concord, Massachusetts.

Lisa A. Tieszen, M.A., LICSW, is the co-director for the Center for Violence Prevention and Recovery at Beth Israel Deaconess Medical Center. She is a co-founder of the Advocacy for Women and Kids in Emergencies (AWAKE) Project at Children's Hospital, Boston, and has been working with victims/survivors of domestic violence and their children for over twenty years.

Deborah L. Tolman, Ed.D., is a professor of Human Sexuality Studies at San Francisco State University. She is the author of several books, including *Dilemmas of Desire: Teenage Girls Talk about Sexuality.*

Pratyusha Tummala-Narra, Ph.D., is an assistant professor at Georgetown University School of Medicine and a lecturer in psychology at Harvard Medical School. She works in the Department of Psychiatry at Georgetown University Hospital.

Melba J. T. Vasquez, Ph.D., ABPP, is in independent practice in Austin, Texas. She is co-author, with Ken Pope, of *Ethics in Psychotherapy and Counseling: A Practical Guide.* She has also published in the areas of psychology of women, ethnic minority psychology, and training and supervision.

Maureen Walker, Ph.D., is a psychologist with an independent practice in Cambridge, Massachusetts. She is on the faculty and coordinating committee of the Jean Baker Miller Training Institute, Stone Center, Wellesley College. She is also the associate director of MBA Support Services at Harvard Business School.

Karen Fraser Wyche, Ph.D., is an associate professor of psychology at the University of Miami. She is also the editor of *Women's Ethnicities: Journeys Through Psychology.*

Janet Yassen, LICSW, is the coordinator of Crisis Services for the Victims of Violence Program at Cambridge Health Alliance. She is also the co-founder of the Boston Area Rape Crisis Center. Her private practice focuses on individual and group psychotherapy, supervision, training, and consultation.

Dale Young, Psy.D., M.P.H., is a clinical psychologist in private practice in Boston and an instructor at Harvard Medical School. In addition, she is director of training for a local health center and is a clinical associate in the Department of Psychiatry at Brigham and Women's Hospital.

Celexa, 203, 205, 278, 282, 292

cervix, 87

change: of addictive behaviors, 245–246; five stages of, 245

change process in therapy, 347–348

Changing Woman (Navajo archetype), 53

cheese effect, 279

Chernin, Kim, 223, 377

child abuse, 164–172; abuse history as a factor in, 168–169; of adolescents, 169–170; causes of, 166–168; commonly used terms in, 171b; common reactions to, 169–170; definition of, 165; and economic stress, 166; effects of, 164–165; identifying, 169–170; and inadequate parenting models, 168; and lack of social support, 166–167; of preschool children, 169; psychological difficulties as a contributing factor to, 167; reporting, 170–172; and safety planning, 172; of school age children, 169; and special needs children, 167–168; statistics of, 165; and substance abuse, 167

Child Abuse Prevention and Treatment Act, 165

child care and relationship conflicts, 117

childlessness, 40–47; of lesbians, 46; and shame, 47

child maltreatment. See child abuse

child protection agency, 171b

child-related stress, 27

children: and common reactions to abuse, 169–170; effect of domestic violence on, 151–152; and reactions to trauma, 138–139; as witnesses of domestic violence, 170

child survivors of sexual assault, 157

chlorpromazine, 287, 288

Chodorow, Nancy, 116

Chrisler, Joan, 364

chromium for depression, 301

chronic-fatigue lifestyle, 257

chronic fatigue syndrome, 178, 181, 184

chronic illness, 177–184; alternative treatments for, 184; combination of symptoms in, 178; and definition of chronic, 177; diagnosis and acceptance of, 178–179; and education, 183; and fertility, 180; and miscarriage, 180; myths and stigmas regarding, 181–182; and Post-Traumatic Stress Disorder, 184; and poverty, 187; recommendations for those suffering from, 183–184; relational implications of adjusting to, 179–181; side effects of medications for, 182–183; stages of coping with, 179–180; and stress, 183; and support, 184; treatment approaches for, 182–183

chronic pelvic pain, 178

Cisler, Lucinda, 7

Clemente, C., 245

climacteric, 51, 266

clitoral therapy device, 83

clitoris, 85–87

Clorazil, 252, 288

cocaine, 243b

cognitive behavioral therapy, 307–313; and anger, 132–133; for anxiety disorders, 202, 310b, 311; assessment of, 308; and automatic responses, 307; as behavioral medicine, 310b, 311; and body dysmorphic disorder, 227; core beliefs of, 307, 308; and depression, 208, 307–309; and eating disorders, 236–237, 310b, 311, 312–313; and group psychotherapy, 335; and habit control, 310b, 311; and infertility, 14–16; and mood disorders, 310b, 311; for phobias, 311; and Post-Traumatic Stress Disorder, 220; and sexual assault, 156–157

cognitive difficulties and child abuse, 165

cognitive restructuring in infertility, 15

Cognitive Therapy and the Emotional Disorders, 307

Collins, Patricia Hill, 92, 97

Coltart, Nina, 327

committed relationships, 113–115; friendship as, 107–108; and gender differences, 115; types of, 113–115

companionship model (of committed relationships), 113

complementary treatment for depression and anxiety, 300–306

Complex Post-Traumatic Stress Disorder, 140, 141–142

compulsions, 202

concentration and depression, 206

confidentiality, 152, 351–352

"confinement" in pregnancy, 6

conflict, 117; and gender differences in handling, 115; and growth, 95

connection, 92–99; feelings in, 96–99; in psychotherapy, 103; and recovery, 103

connective tissue disorders, 178

contraception and the history of feminism, 7

co-parenting, 30

cortisol, 205, 217, 217

cortisol-releasing factor (CRF), 217, 217

cosmetic surgery, 225

Cotton, N. S., 240

Coumadin, 304

couple's therapy for domestic violence, 152

Cowan, Carolyn, 29, 30

Cowan, Philip, 29, 30

Cox, Deborah, 133

crisis intervention therapy, 156

Crittendon, Ann, 258

Crohn's disease, 178, 181

cultural expectations and girls' sexual health, 78–80

culture and spirituality, 382

culture camps, 37

Cumming, Elaine, 60

Cutrona, Carolyn, 27, 28

cyclothymia, 209

Cziksszentmihaly, Mihaly, 375

dance and movement as sexual assault therapy, 158

dating, 111, 112

death and dying, 62–64, 65–73

Deaux, Kay, 112

debilitating illness. See chronic illness

defenses in psychotherapy, 330

dehydroepiandrosterone (DHEA), 306

delirium tremens, 242

delivery and psychological preparation for, 22–23

delusions and antipsychotic medications, 287–290

demand–withdraw pattern, 115

Denning, Patt, 245, 246

Depakote, 285

dependency, drug. See addiction; substance abuse

depression, 102; and acupuncture and bodywork, 305; and adaptation to motherhood, 27; and anger, 129, 130, 132; and antidepressants, 72–73, 280; and artists, 204; atypical, 207, 278; and Bipolar Disorder, 211; and body image, 224; and cognitive behavioral therapy, 307–309; compared to grief, 71b; complementary treatments for, 300–306; and domestic violence, 147; and empty nest syndrome, 48; and ethnic minorities, 207; and eye movement desensitization and reprocessing, 325–326; gender differences in, 207, 208; and genetics, 208; herbal therapy for, 303–305; hormone treatment for, 305–306; and hormones, 208; and infertility, 12–13; light therapy for, 306; and marital status, 207; and marriage, 253; and mood stabilizers, 283; neurobiology of, 205; and nutrition, 300–303; and perimenopause, 271; and poverty, 187, 188; during pregnancy, 296, 297b, 298; and psychotherapy, 208; and selective serotonin-reuptake inhibitors, 278; and sexual assault, 155; and suicide, 209–210; and transition from adolescence to young adulthood, 5; and trauma, 138; treatment for, 208–209, 280; and tricyclic antidepressants, 277; typical, 207. See also antidepressants; depressive disorders; grief; Major Depression

depressive disorders, 204–210; clinical features of, 206–207; epidemiology of, 207–209; etiology of, 205–206; historical overview of, 204; and related disorders, 209. See also antidepressants; depression; Major Depression

disorders, 198, 305–306; and breast-feeding, 24; and depression, 208, 305–306; and love, 91; and menopause, 49, 266; and mood and cognition, 267–268; and postpartum depression, 262; reproductive, 83–84; and trauma, 140

Hoschild, Arlie, 257

hospitalization and domestic abuse therapy, 151

hot flashes, 52

household chores and relationship conflicts, 117

hyperforin, 303

hypericin, 303

hypersomnia, 206

hypertension, 129

hypertensive crisis, 279

hypnotics and withdrawal, 243*b*

hypomania, 211

hypothalamic function, in menopause, 266

hypothalamic-pituitary-adrenal (HPA) axis, 205, 217, 217

hypothalamus, 83, 84, 87, 271

hysteria, 182, 197

identity and spirituality, 381–382

identity development and adoptees, 34–35

illness, chronic. *See* chronic illness

illness, debilitating. *See* chronic illness

immigrants: and domestic violence, 152; and sexual assault, 161

immune-suppressant drugs, 183

independent model (of committed relationships), 113

individualism versus interdependence, 100–101

inequality and anger, 131

infertility, 10–17; and adoption, 36–37; and anger, 16; and anxiety, 12–13; causes of, 11; and cognitive therapy, 14–16; and depression, 12–13; emotional impact of, 10–11, 12–13; ending treatment for, 16–17; evaluation and treatment of, 11–12; and grief, 17; and lesbians, 13; organizations and resources for, 15*b*; pregnancy after, 8; relaxation training for, 13–14; and shame, 10; and stress, 11; support groups for, 15, 16; and survival skills, 13–16; and women of color, 13

infertility industry, 7

informed consent, 352

"In Search of How People Change: Applications to Addictive Behaviors," 245

insidious traumatization, 137

insight-oriented psychotherapy, 327–332; description and origins of, 327–329; and feminist thinking, 329; and how it creates change, 329–331; problems addressed by, 331–332; value of, 332

insomnia, 206

Institute for Mind and Biology, 90

integration and domestic violence, 148

integrity versus despair, 57

interdependence versus individualism, 100–101

interdependent model (of committed relationships), 114

international adoption, 32

interpersonal effectiveness, 315, 316

interpersonal group psychotherapy, 336

interpretation (in psychotherapy), 329–330

interracial relationships, 112–113

intimacy, 116–117; development of, 2

intimate relationships, 104–120; female, 119–120; gendered nature of, 104–105

intimate strangers, 113

intimidation, 173

intracytoplasmic sperm injection (ICSI), 8

Inuit, 160

in vitro fertilization (IVF), 11

irritable bowel syndrome, 129, 178

isolation, 94–95, 102; and child abuse, 165; and domestic abuse, 145; feelings in, 96–99

Jack, Dana C., 130

Jagger, Allison, 129

James, William, 206

Jamison, Kay Redfield, 284

Janoff-Bulman, Ronnie, 136, 137

Jarvis, Cheryl, 254

jealousy and gender, 118

Jellinek, E. M., 247

Jordan, Judith, 92

Josselson, Ruthellen, 18

Journal of the American Medical Association (JAMA), 89

Journet, Leslie, 44

justice (moral principle of therapy), 346

juvenile and family courts, 171*b*

Kasl, Charlotte, 239, 248

Kaslo, Nadine, 189

Kaufman, Edward, 240

kava (*piper methysticum*), 304–305

Keys, Ancel, 232

Kitchener, Karen, 345, 346

Klein, Laura Cousin, 105

Kleinman, Arthur, 181

Klonopin, 203, 281

Koenig, Harold G., 380

Koko, 90

Krasnow, Iris, 256

Kuba, Sue A., 235

Kubler-Ross, Elizabeth, 68

labeling (cognitive distortion), 309, 309*b*

Lamictal, 285

Lamott, Anne, 25

Lang, Karen, 97

Langley, Jackie, 61

Latinas: and body image, 222, 223; and

interracial relationships, 113; and sexual assault, 160. *See also* ethnicity; ethnic minorities; Hispanics; racism; women of color

Lazell, Edward, 333

Lederman, R. P., 21, 23

left-handedness and hormonal sensitivity, 271

Leifer, Myra, 20, 23, 25

lesbians: and abusive relationships, 152; and adoption, 32; and anger, 131; and body image, 222; and childlessness, 46; of color, 100, 102; and domestic violence, 144; and eating disorders, 235; and egalitarian relationships, 114; and friendship, 119; and gender roles, 112; health of, in older adulthood, 62; and infertility, 13; and insidious traumatization, 137; and interracial relationships, 112–113; and older adulthood, 56, 61; and sexual assault, 161–162

Lewis, C. S., 65, 66, 67, 68

libido loss, 303

Librium, 281

life stages: adoption, 31–39; childlessness, 40–47; grief and bereavement, 65–73; infertility, 10–17; menopause, 51–55; middle age, 48–50; motherhood, 18–30; older adulthood, 56–64; pregnancy, 6–8; spirituality, 380–381; transition from adolescence to adulthood, 1–5

light therapy, 306

Lindemann, Eric, 68, 70, 71

Linehan, Marsha, 314, 318, 320

liposuction, 225

lithium, 209, 212, 213, 283–284; side effects of, 284; toxicity of, 284–285

longevity, 63

Lorde, Audrey, 131

loss: and adoptees, 34–35; and adoption, 33, 39; and adoptive parents, 36–37; and birth parents, 39

love, 116–117; romantic, 255; and sex, 90–91

Love and Addiction, 247

Lowell, Robert, 204

lupus, 178. *See also* autoimmune disorders

Luvox, 203, 278

Maccoby, Eleanor, 106

Mackey, Mary, 44–46

Major Depression, 69, 204–210; and antidepressants, 72; compared to Disthymic Disorder, 209; and complicated bereavement, 71–72; and polypharmacy, 292. *See also* antidepressants; depression; depressive disorders

male–female friendships, 110–111

maltreatment of children. *See* child abuse

mandated reporter, 171*b*

mania, 209, 211, 283

manic depression. *See* Bipolar Disorder

Mansfield, Jayne, 223

sexual health, 74–81; definition of, 74–75; and feminine ideals, 78–80; of girls, 78–80; positive model of, 81; and sex education, 80

sexuality, 82–91; and anatomy, 85–97; claiming, 81; and cultural scripts for women, 78–80; and menopause, 54, 85; of men versus women, 82–83; normal female, 82–83; and pregnancy, 85; and social context, 76–78

sexual orientation: and health in older adulthood, 62; and sexual assault, 161–162. *See also* lesbians

sexual problems, 88–90; economic factors in, 76*b*; medical factors in, 77*b*; new classification of, 76–77*b*, 77; and partner, 76*b*, 77*b*; political factors in, 76*b*; psychological factors in, 77*b*; and relationship, 76*b*, 77*b*; sociocultural factors in, 76*b*

sexual stereotypes, 78–80

shamanism, 382

shame, 96–97; and childlessness, 47; and gender stereotyping, 98; and infertility, 10

Shapiro, Francine, 322, 323, 324

shared abundance, 98

Shelley, Mary, 6

shell shock, 214

Shereshefsky, Pauline, 20, 24–25

Sherman, Jeffrey J., 184

short-term treatment (cognitive behavioral therapy), 311

Shou, Mogens, 283

should statements (cognitive distortion), 309, 309*b*

Shulgold, Barbara, 8

Sichel, Deborah, 269

side effects: of antipsychotic medications, 288–289, 288*b*; of medications for chronic illness, 182–183; and polypharmacy, 291–292

single-hood: societal disapproval of, 119; versus marriage, 118–119

single parent adoption, 32

Sisterhood Is Powerful, 7

skeletal asymmetry and hormonal sensitivity, 271

Sleepless Days, 256

slender ideal, 221–223

SMART (Self Management and Recovery Training), 248, 248*b*

Smith, Joseph Carmen, 182

Smith, M. L., 333

Social Phobia, 198, 201; alternative medications for, 282; and antianxiety medications, 281; and antidepressants, 282

social roles model of dating preferences, 112

social support: and child abuse, 166–167; and mothers' emotional well-being, 27–28; and sexual assault therapy, 159

Society for Psychiatry and Neurology, 182

special needs children and child abuse, 167–168

Spelman, Elizabeth, 129

spiritual alienation in bereavement, 67

spirituality, 379–382; in adolescence to elder years, 371–380; compared to religion, 379; and culture, 382; and friendship, 98–99; and gender identity, 382; and identity, 381–382; and menopause, 54; New Age, 380; and sexual assault therapy, 158–159; and surviving child abuse, 170; and trauma, 139

SSRIs. *See* selective serotonin-reuptake inhibitors

Stabb, Sally, 133

stereotyped threat, 372

stereotypes: and gender, 98, 101, 112, 372; and older adults, 57–58; and poverty, 185; and relationships, 111–112; sexual, 78–80; and spirituality, 380

Stern, Daniel, 21

Sternberg, Robert, 104

Stevens-Johnson Syndrome, 285

stigmas and "women's diseases," 181–182

stimulants and withdrawal, 243*b*

Stiver, Irene, 92, 180, 184, 233

stomach-stapling, 225

Stone Center for Developmental Services and Studies, 92, 93, 94, 132

stress: and adaptation to motherhood, 27; of caregiver, 188; child-related, 27; and chronic illness, 183; cognitive and perceptual signs of, 371b, 372; coping with, 373–374; definition of, 369–370; emotional signs and symptoms of, 370*b*, 371–372; and ethnic minorities, 372–373; factors unique to women, 372–373; and infertility, 11; physiological signs and symptoms of, 370–371; and poverty, 188; and racism, 191; relaxation techniques for, 374; and signs and symptoms of overload, 370–372; and terrorism, 175; and women's response to, 183

stress management, 369–374

stress response, 217

Stuart, Eileen M., 15

Styron, William, 204

substance abuse: adaptive model of, 247; and child abuse, 165, 167; definition of, 246–247; disease model of, 247; and domestic violence, 147, 152; and Post-Traumatic Stress Disorder, 215; and poverty, 187; and self-help groups, 248, 248*b*; and trauma, 239; and treatment, 244–245. *See also* addiction

Substance Abuse and Mental Health Services Administration Clearinghouse for Alcohol and Drug Information, 240

suicidal thoughts, 207

suicide, 209–210; and anger, 129; assisted, 64; and Bipolar Disorder, 213; and eth-

nicity, 63; and grief, 65; and older adulthood, 63; and poverty, 189

support and chronic illness, 184

support groups for infertility, 15, 16

Surrendering to Motherhood: Losing Your Mind, Finding Your Soul, 256

Surrey, Janet, 92, 132

Surviving Infertility, 17

synapse, 218, *218*

Tannen, Deborah, 115

tardive dyskinesia, 289

Taylor, Shelley, 105, 183

Tegretol, 285

Teifer, Leonore, 75

temporolimbic system, 271

tend-and-befriend response, 105, 183

terrorism, 173–176; and abusive relationships, 174; aftermath of, 175–176; and anger, 175; definition of, 173; and emotional recovery, 175–176; and fear, 175; and stress, 175; symptoms after experiencing, 175; and trauma, 174; and vicarious traumatic experience, 175. *See also* trauma

testosterone, 83, 84, 90, 267, 269, 270

testosterone therapy, 273

thalidomide, 295

Theory and Practice of Group Psychotherapy, The, 333

therapeutic alliance: barriers to, 345–346; and ethics of care, 345

therapeutic relationship: asking questions in, 349–350; bartering in, 351; basic risks of, 348; boundary issues in, 348; and confidentiality, 351–352; and gifts, 350; and informed consent, 352; and insurance problems, 353–354; nonsexual touch in, 350; and oppressive exploitation of women, 348; and overlapping relationships, 350–351; and record-keeping guidelines, 353; and self-disclosure by therapist, 348–349; and sexual violations, 348, 349; and terminating therapy, 354

therapeutic touch, 305

therapists: choosing, for victims of domestic abuse, 150; education of, 343–344; finding and choosing, 340–343; work of, 344–345

therapy: and anger, 132–133; change process in, 347–348; and choosing a therapist, 340–343; cognitive behavioral therapy, 307–313; and depression, 208; dialectical behavior therapy, 314–321; and domestic violence, 150–153; eye movement desensitization and reprocessing, 322–326; feminist, 132; goals for, 344–345; group psychotherapy, 333–339; insight-oriented psychotherapy, 327–332; moral principles of, 346–347; and postpartum depression, 263–265; and